Design and Analysis of Bridging Studies

Chapman & Hall/CRC Biostatistics Series

Chapman & Hall/CRC Biostatistics Series

Adaptive Design Methods in Clinical Trials, Second Edition
Shein-Chung Chow and Mark Chang

Adaptive Design Theory and Implementation Using SAS and R
Mark Chang

Advanced Bayesian Methods for Medical Test Accuracy
Lyle D. Broemeling

Advances in Clinical Trial Biostatistics
Nancy L. Geller

Basic Statistics and Pharmaceutical Statistical Applications, Second Edition
James E. De Muth

Bayesian Adaptive Methods for Clinical Trials
Scott M. Berry, Bradley P. Carlin, J. Jack Lee, and Peter Muller

Bayesian Analysis Made Simple: An Excel GUI for WinBUGS
Phil Woodward

Bayesian Methods for Measures of Agreement
Lyle D. Broemeling

Bayesian Missing Data Problems: EM, Data Augmentation and Noniterative Computation
Ming T. Tan, Guo-Liang Tian, and Kai Wang Ng

Bayesian Modeling in Bioinformatics
Dipak K. Dey, Samiran Ghosh, and Bani K. Mallick

Biostatistics: A Computing Approach
Stewart J. Anderson

Causal Analysis in Biomedicine and Epidemiology: Based on Minimal Sufficient Causation
Mikel Aickin

Clinical Trial Data Analysis using R
Ding-Geng (Din) Chen and Karl E. Peace

Clinical Trial Methodology
Karl E. Peace and Ding-Geng (Din) Chen

Computational Methods in Biomedical Research
Ravindra Khattree and Dayanand N. Naik

Computational Pharmacokinetics
Anders Källén

Controversial Statistical Issues in Clinical Trials
Shein-Chung Chow

Data and Safety Monitoring Committees in Clinical Trials
Jay Herson

Design and Analysis of Animal Studies in Pharmaceutical Development
Shein-Chung Chow and Jen-pei Liu

Design and Analysis of Bioavailability and Bioequivalence Studies, Third Edition
Shein-Chung Chow and Jen-pei Liu

Design and Analysis of Bridging Studies
Jen-pei Liu, Shein-Chung Chow, and Chin-Fu Hsiao

Design and Analysis of Clinical Trials with Time-to-Event Endpoints
Karl E. Peace

Design and Analysis of Non-Inferiority Trials
Mark D. Rothmann, Brian L. Wiens, and Ivan S. F. Chan

Difference Equations with Public Health Applications
Lemuel A. Moyé and Asha Seth Kapadia

DNA Methylation Microarrays: Experimental Design and Statistical Analysis
Sun-Chong Wang and Arturas Petronis

DNA Microarrays and Related Genomics Techniques: Design, Analysis, and Interpretation of Experiments
David B. Allison, Grier P. Page, T. Mark Beasley, and Jode W. Edwards

Dose Finding by the Continual Reassessment Method
Ying Kuen Cheung

Elementary Bayesian Biostatistics
Lemuel A. Moyé

Frailty Models in Survival Analysis
Andreas Wienke

Generalized Linear Models: A Bayesian Perspective
Dipak K. Dey, Sujit K. Ghosh, and Bani K. Mallick

Handbook of Regression and Modeling: Applications for the Clinical and Pharmaceutical Industries
Daryl S. Paulson

Measures of Interobserver Agreement and Reliability, Second Edition
Mohamed M. Shoukri

Medical Biostatistics, Third Edition
A. Indrayan

Meta-Analysis in Medicine and Health Policy
Dalene Stangl and Donald A. Berry

Monte Carlo Simulation for the Pharmaceutical Industry: Concepts, Algorithms, and Case Studies
Mark Chang

Multiple Testing Problems in Pharmaceutical Statistics
Alex Dmitrienko, Ajit C. Tamhane, and Frank Bretz

Randomized Clinical Trials of Nonpharmacological Treatments
Isabelle Boutron, Philippe Ravaud, and David Moher

Sample Size Calculations in Clinical Research, Second Edition
Shein-Chung Chow, Jun Shao and Hansheng Wang

Statistical Design and Analysis of Stability Studies
Shein-Chung Chow

Statistical Evaluation of Diagnostic Performance: Topics in ROC Analysis
Kelly H. Zou, Aiyi Liu, Andriy Bandos, Lucila Ohno-Machado, and Howard Rockette

Statistical Methods for Clinical Trials
Mark X. Norleans

Statistics in Drug Research: Methodologies and Recent Developments
Shein-Chung Chow and Jun Shao

Statistics in the Pharmaceutical Industry, Third Edition
Ralph Buncher and Jia-Yeong Tsay

Translational Medicine: Strategies and Statistical Methods
Dennis Cosmatos and Shein-Chung Chow

Chapman & Hall/CRC Biostatistics Series

Design and Analysis of Bridging Studies

Edited by

Jen-pei Liu

Shein-Chung Chow

Chin-Fu Hsiao

CRC Press
Taylor & Francis Group
Boca Raton London New York

CRC Press is an imprint of the
Taylor & Francis Group, an **informa** business
A CHAPMAN & HALL BOOK

CRC Press
Taylor & Francis Group
6000 Broken Sound Parkway NW, Suite 300
Boca Raton, FL 33487-2742

Printed in the United States of America on acid-free paper
Version Date: 20120525

International Standard Book Number: 978-1-4398-4634-6 (Hardback)

Library of Congress Cataloging-in-Publication Data

Design and analysis of bridging studies / editors, Chin-Fu Hsiao, Jen-Pei Liu, Shein-Chung Chow.
p. ; cm. -- (Chapman & Hall/CRC biostatistics series)
Includes bibliographical references and index.
ISBN 978-1-4398-4634-6 (hardcover : alk. paper)
I. Hsiao, Chin-Fu, 1964- II. Liu, Jen-pei, 1952- III. Chow, Shein-Chung, 1955- IV. Series: Chapman & Hall/CRC biostatistics series (Unnumbered)
[DNLM: 1. Clinical Trials as Topic--standards. 2. Drug Evaluation, Preclinical--standards. 3. Biostatistics--methods. 4. Guidelines as Topic. 5. Internationality. 6. Research Design. QV 771.4]

615.1072'4--dc23 2012015476

Visit the Taylor & Francis Web site at
http://www.taylorandfrancis.com

and the CRC Press Web site at
http://www.crcpress.com

Contents

Preface

In recent years, the variations of pharmaceutical products in efficacy and safety among different geographic regions due to ethic factors have become a matter of great concern for sponsors as well as for regulatory authorities. However, the key issues lie on when and how to address the geographic variations of efficacy and safety for product development. To address this issue, a general framework has been provided by the International Conference Harmonisation (ICH) E5 in a document titled "Ethnic Factors in the Acceptability of Foreign Clinical Data" for evaluation of the impact of ethnic factors on the efficacy, safety, dosage, and dose regimen. The ICH E5 guideline provides regulatory strategies for minimizing duplication of clinical data and requirements for bridging evidence to extrapolate foreign clinical data to a new region. More specifically, the ICH E5 guideline suggests that a bridging study should be conducted in the new region to provide pharmacodynamic or clinical data on efficacy, safety, dosage, and dose regimen to allow extrapolation of the foreign clinical data to the population of the new region.

However, a bridging study may require significant development resources and also delay availability of the tested medical product to the needing patients in the new region. To accelerate the development process and shorten approval time, the design of multiregional trials incorporates subjects from many countries around the world under the same protocol. After showing the overall efficacy of a drug in all global regions, one can also simultaneously evaluate the possibility of applying the overall trial results to all regions and subsequently support drug registration in each of them. Recently, the trend for clinical development in Asian countries being undertaken simultaneously with clinical trials conducted in Europe and the United States has been rapidly rising.

With increasing globalization of the development of medicines, creating strategies on when and how to address the geographic variations of efficacy and safety for the product development is now inevitable. This book explicitly addresses the issues arising from bridging studies and multiregional clinical trials. For bridging studies, we will explore issues including ethnic sensitivity, necessity of bridging studies, types of bridging studies, and assessment of similarity between regions based on bridging evidence. For multiregional clinical trials, we dig into issues such as consideration of regional difference, assessment of the consistency of treatment effect across regions, and sample size determination for each region. Although several statistical procedures have been proposed for designing bridging studies and multiregional clinical trials, the statistical work is still in the preliminary stages. This book provides a comprehensive and unified summary of the growing literature and research activities on regulatory requirements, scientific and practical issues, and statistical methodology on designing and evaluating bridging studies and multiregional clinical trials. Most importantly, we sincerely hope that this book can inspire in academia new research activities in the design and analysis of bridging studies and multiregional clinical trials.

Contributors

Herng-Der Chern
Center for Drug Evaluation
Taipei, Taiwan

Shein-Chung Chow
Duke University School of Medicine
Duke University
Durham, North Carolina

Christy Chuang-Stein
Statistical Research and Consulting Center
Pfizer, Inc.
Kalamazoo, Michigan

Chin-Fu Hsiao
Institute of Population Health Sciences
National Health Research Institutes
Miaoli County, Taiwan

Eric Tsung-Cheng Hsieh
Buddhist Tzu-Chi University and Hospital
Hualien, Taiwan

Hsien-Ming James Hung
Center for Drug Evaluation and Research
U.S. Food and Drug Administration
Silver Spring, Maryland

Yoichi Ii
Clinical Statistics
Pfizer Japan Inc.
Tokyo, Japan

Mari Ikuta
GlaxoSmithKline
Tokyo, Japan

Norisuke Kawai
Clinical Statistics
Pfizer Japan Inc.
Tokyo, Japan

Osamu Komiyama
Clinical Statistics
Pfizer Japan Inc.
Tokyo, Japan

Kazuhiko Kuribayashi
Clinical Statistics
Pfizer Japan Inc.
Tokyo, Japan

Kuang-Kuo Gordon Lan
Janssen Pharmaceutical Companies of Johnson & Johnson
Raritan, New Jersey

Yeong-Liang Lin
Center for Drug Evaluation
Taipei, Taiwan

Jen-pei Liu
Department of Agronomy
National Taiwan University
Taipei, Taiwan

Ying Lu
Beijing University of Technology
Beijing, China

Hiromu Nakajima
GlaxoSmithKline
Tokyo, Japan

Robert O'Neill
Center for Drug Evaluation and Research
U.S. Food and Drug Administration
Silver Spring, Maryland

José Pinheiro
Janssen Pharmaceutical Companies of Johnson & Johnson
Raritan, New Jersey

Hui Quan
Department of Biostatistics and Programming
Sanofi
Bridgewater, New Jersey

Weichung J. Shih
Department of Biostatistics
University of Medicine and Dentistry of New Jersey–School of Public Health
Piscataway, New Jersey

Kihito Takahashi
GlaxoSmithKline
and
Japanese Association of Pharmaceutical Medicine
and
Japanese Center of Pharmaceutical Medicine
Tokyo, Japan

Yi Tsong
Center for Drug Evaluation and Research
U.S. Food and Drug Administration
Silver Spring, Maryland

Hsiao-Hui Tsou
National Health Research Institutes
Miaoli County, Taiwan

Mey Wang
Center for Drug Evaluation
Taipei, Taiwan

Sue-Jane Wang
Center for Drug Evaluation and Research
U.S. Food and Drug Administration
Silver Spring, Maryland

Yuh-Jenn Wu
Chung Yuan Christian University
Chung Li City, Taiwan

Lan-Yan Yang
National Cheng Kung University
Taiwan City, Taiwan

1

Bridging Diversity: Extrapolating Foreign Data to a New Region

Shein-Chung Chow
Duke University

Chin-Fu Hsiao
National Health Research Institutes

1.1 Introduction

In recent years, the possible influence of ethnic factors on clinical outcomes for evaluating the efficacy and safety of study medications under investigation has attracted much attention from both the pharmaceutical/biotechnology industry and regulatory agencies such as the U.S. Food and Drug Administration (FDA), especially when the sponsor is interested in bringing an approved drug product from the original region, such as the United States or the European Union, to a new region such as the Asia-Pacific region. As indicated in Caraco (2004), genetic determinants may mediate variability among persons in the response to a drug, which implies that patient response to therapeutics may vary from one racial/ethnic group to another. Some ethnic groups may exhibit clinically significant side effects, whereas others may have no therapeutic responses. Other ethnic factors that can distinguish new and original regions may include the social and cultural aspects of a region such as medical practice (e.g., diagnostic criteria), epidemiological difference (e.g., diet, tobacco or alcohol use, exposure to pollution and sunshine), and compliance with prescribed medications. As a result, the dose and dose regimen approved in the original region may not be appropriate (for achieving the desired therapeutic effect) for patients in a new region. Thus, it is important to demonstrate that the approved treatment at the original region will achieve *similar* or *equivalent* therapeutic effects (in terms of efficacy and safety) when applied to patients in the new region before it can be approved and used there. However, it should be noted that if there is evidence of therapeutic differences due to race or ethnicity, the dose and dose regimen of the test treatment is necessarily modified to achieve similar therapeutic effect as observed in the original region.

In practice, the sponsor can conduct studies in a new region with similar dose and dose regimens and sample sizes to confirm clinical efficacy and safety observed in the original region for regulatory approval at the new region. However, duplicating clinical evaluation in the new region will not only require (and waste) already limited resources but also delay the availability of the approved treatment at the original region to patients in the new region. To overcome this dilemma, in 1998, the International Conference on Harmonization (ICH) issued a guideline titled "Ethnic Factors in the Acceptability of Foreign Clinical Data" (known as ICH E5) to determine if clinical data generated from the original region are acceptable in a new region. The purpose of this guideline is not only to permit adequate evaluation of the influence of ethnic factors but also to minimize duplication of clinical studies and consequently not to delay the availability of the approved test treatment to patients in the new region. This guideline is usually referred to as the ICH E5 guideline.

Following the 1998 ICH E5 guideline, regulatory authorities in different regions (e.g., Japan, South Korea, and Taiwan in the Asia-Pacific region) have developed similar but different regulatory requirements for bridging studies, which have led to different bridging strategies in different regions. These bridging strategies also raise some practical issues such as criteria for assessment of similarity in therapeutic effect between regions, sample size calculation and allocation, and statistical methods for data analysis and interpretation in bridging or multiregion studies.

In the next section, the possible influence of racial and ethnic differences on clinical outcomes is discussed. This justifies the need to conduct bridging studies when a sponsor is seeking regulatory approval in a new region. Section 1.3 provides a brief summary of ICH guideline and regulatory guidelines from the Asia-Pacific region (e.g., South Korea and Japan). Some current issues and bridging strategies are discussed in Section 1.4. Two successful examples for bridging evaluations are given in Section 1.5. Some concluding remarks are given in Section 1.6, followed in Section 1.7 by the aim and scope of the book.

1.2 Impact of Ethnic Differences

Since the completion of the Human Genome Project, there has been increasing evidence that genetic determinants may mediate variability among persons in the response to a drug, which implies that patient response to therapeutics may vary from one racial or ethnic group to another. As an example, Caraco (2004) pointed out that some diversity in the rate of responses can be ascribed to differences in the rate of drug metabolism, particularly by the cytochrome P-450 superfamily of enzymes. While 10 isoforms of cytochrome P-450 are responsible for the oxidative metabolism of most drugs, the effect of genetic polymorphisms on catalytic activity is most prominent for three isoforms—CYP2C9, CYP2C19, and CYP2D6. Among these three, CYP2D6 has been most extensively studied and is involved in the metabolism of about 100 drugs including beta-blockers and anti-arrhythmic, antidepressant, neuroleptic, and opioid agents. Several studies revealed that some patients are classified as having "poor metabolism" of certain drugs due to lack of CYP2D6 activity. On the other hand, patients having some enzyme activity are classified into three subgroups: (1) those with *normal* activity (or extensive metabolism), (2) those with reduced activity (intermediate metabolism), and (3) those with markedly enhanced activity (ultrarapid metabolism). Dosages for most drugs are commonly determined by their pharmacokinetic behavior in a group of healthy patients, most of whom have extensive metabolism of CYP2D6 substrates. It is clear that for the CYP2D6-inactivated drugs, the "average doses" are too much for people with poor metabolism and too little for those with ultrarapid metabolism. It should be noted that the distribution of CYP2D6 phenotypes varies with race. For instance, the frequency of the phenotype associated with poor metabolism is 5% to 10% in the Caucasian population but only 1% in the Chinese and Japanese populations (Caraco, 2004). In other words, Caucasians are more likely than Asians to have abnormally low levels of CYP2D6, which metabolizes drugs such as antidepressants, antipsychotics, and beta-blockers.

Another example regarding the impact of ethnic factors on the responses to therapeutics is the epidermal growth factor receptor (EGFR) tyrosine kinase inhibitor gefitinib (Iressa). Recently, Iressa was approved in Japan and the United States for the treatment of non-small cell lung cancer (NSCLC). The EGFR is a promising target anticancer therapy because it is more abundantly expressed in lung carcinoma tissue than in adjacent normal lung tissue. However, clinical trials have revealed significant variability in the response to gefitinib with higher responses observed in Japanese patients than in a predominantly European-derived population (27.5% vs. 10.4%, in a multi-institutional phase II trial; Fukuoka et al., 2003). Paez et al. (2004) also show that somatic mutations of the EGFR were found in 15 of 58 unselected tumors from Japan and 1 of 61 from the United States. Treatment with Iressa causes tumor regression in some patients with NSCLC, more frequently in Japan. Finally, the striking differences in the frequency of EGFR mutation and response to Iressa between Japanese and American patients raise general questions regarding variations in the molecular pathogenesis of cancer in different ethnic, cultural, and geographic groups.

Recently, geotherapeutics has attracted much attention from sponsors as well as regulatory authorities. However, the key issues lie in when and how to address the geographic variations of efficacy and safety for the product development. It will strongly depend on the size of the market, development cost, and the factors influencing the clinical outcomes for evaluation of efficacy and safety. If the size of the market for some new geographic region is sufficiently large, then it is understandable that the sponsor may be willing to repeat the whole clinical development program after the test product has completed its development plan and maybe obtain the market approval in the original region.

1.3 Regulatory Guidelines

1.3.1 ICH E5 Guideline on Bridging Studies

The ICH E5 guideline suggests that the new region's regulatory authority assess the ability to extrapolate foreign data based on the bridging data package by gathering information including pharmacokinetic (PK) data and any preliminary pharmacodynamic (PD) and dose-response data from the complete clinical data package (CCDP) that is relevant to the population of the new region and by conducting a bridging study to extrapolate the foreign efficacy data or safety data to the new region. In addition, the ICH E5 guideline also points out that evaluation of the ability of extrapolation of the foreign clinical data relies on the similarity of dose response, efficacy, and safety between the new and original regions either with or without dose adjustment.

By the ICH E5 guideline, the ethnic factors are classified into two categories. *Intrinsic ethnic factors* define and identify the population in the new region and may influence the ability to extrapolate clinical data between regions. They are more genetic and physiologic in nature (e.g., genetic polymorphism, age, gender). *Extrinsic ethnic factors* are associated with the environment and culture and are more social and cultural in nature (e.g., medical practice, diet, practices in clinical trials, conduct).

The ICH E5 guideline indicates that bridging studies may not be necessary if the study medicines are insensitive to ethnic factors. For medicines characterized as insensitive to ethnic factors, the type of bridging studies (if needed) will depend on experience with the drug class and on the likelihood that extrinsic ethnic factors could affect the medicine's safety, efficacy, and dose response. On the other hand, for medicines that are ethnically sensitive, a bridging study is usually needed since the populations in the two regions are different. The ICH E5 guideline has also listed critical properties of a compound that make it more likely to be sensitive to ethnic factors. These critical properties include nonlinear PK, a steep PD curve for both efficacy and safety, a narrow therapeutic dose range, high metabolizing rate, extent of bioavailability, potential for protein binding, potential for interactions, genetic polymorphism, intersubject variability, systemic mode of action, and potential for inappropriate use. However, the ICH E5 guideline also points out that no one property of the medicine is predictive of the compound's relative sensitivity to ethnic factors.

The ICH E5 guideline also provides a summary of the types of bridging studies required in the new region. A bridging study could be a PK–PD study or a controlled clinical trial depending on the ethnic sensitivity of the study medicine, clinical experience of the drug class, extrinsic ethnic factors, and ethnic differences between the new and original regions. For example, if the regions are ethnically dissimilar and the medicine is ethnically sensitive but extrinsic factors such as medical practice, design, and conduct of clinical trials are generally similar and the drug class is a familiar one in the new region, a PK–PD study in the new region could provide assurance that the efficacy, safety, dose, and dose regimen data derived from the original region are applicable to the new region. On the other hand, if there are doubts about the choice of dose, there is little or no experience with acceptance of controlled clinical trials carried out in the foreign region, medical practices (e.g., use of concomitant medications and design or conduct of clinical trials) are different, or the drug class is not a familiar one in the new region, a controlled clinical trial will usually need to be carried out in the new region.

Although the ICH E5 guideline has provided a general framework for evaluation of the impact of ethnic factors, many questions still remain. First, the ICH E5 guideline did not provide precise and definitive criteria for assessment of the sensitivity to ethnic factors for determining whether a bridging study is needed. Consequently, both regulatory authority in the new region and the sponsor will not have criteria and a method for an objective and impartial evaluation of ethnic sensitivity and necessity of a bridging study. Under the circumstances, any proposed approach for the assessment of the necessity of bridging studies could be subjective and controversial and may not be accepted by the regulatory authority and sponsors in the new region. Second, when a bridging study is conducted, the ICH E5 guideline indicates that the study is readily interpreted as capable of bridging the foreign data if it shows that dose response, safety, and efficacy in the new region are similar to those in the original region. However, the ICH E5 guideline does not clearly define the similarity. For assessment of similarity, a number of different statistical procedures have been proposed based on different definitions or concepts of similarity—for example, batch similarity in stability analysis for shelf-life estimation, similarity in drug release for comparison of dissolution profiles between drug products, similarity in drug absorption for assessment of bioequivalence between drug products, and the concept of consistency between clinical results. While those statistical procedures may be useful, well-defined, and scientifically justifiable, criteria for assessment of similarity based on bridging evidence need to be addressed in the future.

Note that following the ICH E5 guideline, many countries in the Asia-Pacific region including Japan, South Korea, and Taiwan not only have developed similar but slightly different guidelines for bridging studies but also have formally announced the implementation of regulatory requirements for bridging studies. For example, in Japan, more than 40 medicines have been approved based on a bridging strategy articulated in the ICH E5 guideline (Uyama et al., 2005).

1.3.2 Regulatory Guidelines in Asia-Pacific Region

Currently, Japan, South Korea, and Taiwan are the three regions that are more frequently demanding data on ethnical differences than others. The regulatory requirements for bridging studies adopted by the health authority of Taiwan will be described in Chapter 13. In what follows, for illustration purposes, we will focus on the regulatory guidelines for Japan and South Korea.

The Japanese government has made efforts to promote Japan's participation in global development and international clinical study. On September 28, 2007, the Japanese Ministry of Health, Labour and Welfare (MHLW) published the *Basic Principles on Global Clinical Trials* guidance related to the planning and implementation of global clinical studies. It outlines, in a question-and-answer format, the basic concepts for planning and implementing multiregional trials. By the guidelines, global clinical studies refers to studies planned with the objective of world-scale development and approval of new drugs in which study sites of a multiple number of countries and regions participate in a single study based on a common protocol and conducted at the same time in parallel. Special consideration was placed on establishing consistency of treatment effects between the Japanese group and the entire group. The Japanese MHLW provides two methods as examples for deciding on the number of Japanese subjects in a multiregional trial for establishing the consistency of treatment effects between the Japanese group and the entire group.

In 1999, the South Korean government announced the elimination of compulsory conduction of local clinical trials in South Korea as a condition of registration for products with fewer than 3 years' market experience or for products marketed only in the original developing country and simultaneously introduced in bridging studies. In June 2001, the South Korea Food and Drug Administration (FDA) adopted the bridging concept. The need for a bridging study would always have to be assessed, since applying foreign clinical data directly to the Korean population might raise problems due to ethnical differences. Studies on Koreans living in South Korea are required. Data generated on Asians of other nationalities may not be accepted. However, there may be instances where bridging study requirements could be exempted. In Korea, there are seven bridging waiver categories: (1) orphan (or former orphan) drugs, (2) drugs for life-threatening disease or AIDS, (3) anticancer therapy for no standard therapy or therapy after failure of a standard therapy, (4) new drugs for which clinical trials have been conducted on Koreans, (5) diagnostic or radioactive drugs, (6) topical drugs with no systemic effect, and (7) drugs that have no ethnic differences.

1.4 Current Issues

1.4.1 Criteria for Similarity

Although the ICH E5 guideline establishes the framework for the acceptability of foreign clinical data, it does not clearly define the similarity in terms of dose response, safety, and efficacy between the original region and a new region. In practice, similarity is often interpreted as *equivalence* or *comparability* between the original region and the new region. However, there is no universal agreement regarding similarity. In addition, it is not clear how similar is considered similar and what degree of similarity is considered acceptable for regulatory approval.

Shih (2001) interpreted similarity as *consistency* among study centers by treating the new region as a new center of multicenter clinical trials. Under this definition, Shih proposed a method for assessment of consistency to determine whether the study is capable of bridging the foreign data to the new region. Alternatively, Shao and Chow (2002) proposed the concepts of *reproducibility* and *generalizability* probabilities for assessing bridging studies. If the influence of the ethnic factors is negligible, then we may consider the reproducibility probability to determine whether the clinical results observed in the original region are reproducible in the new region. If there is a notable ethnic difference, the concept of generalizability probability can be used to determine whether the clinical results in the original region can be generalized in a similar but slightly different patient population due to the difference in ethnic factors. In addition, Chow, Shao, and Hu (2002) proposed to assess similarity by analysis using a *sensitivity index,* which is a measure of population shift between the original region and the new region. Along these lines, Hung (2003) and Hung, Wang, Tsong, Lawrence, and O'Neil (2003) considered the assessment of similarity based on testing for *noninferiority* based on bridging studies conducted in the new region compared with those previously conducted in the original region. This method, however, leads to the argument regarding the selection of a noninferiority margin (Chow and Shao, 2006).

Under different interpretations of similarity, several methods have been proposed in the literature. For example, Liu, Hsueh, and Chen (2002) used a hierarchical model approach to incorporating the foreign bridging information into the data generated by the bridging study in the new region. Lan, Soo, Siu, and Wang (2005) introduced weighted Z-tests, in which the weights may depend on the prior observed data for the design of bridging studies.

Alternatively, Liu, Hsiao, and Hsueh (2002) proposed a Bayesian approach to synthesize the data generated by the bridging study and foreign clinical data generated in the original region for assessment of similarity based on superior efficacy of the test product over a placebo control. Even if both regions have positive treatment effect, their effect sizes might in fact be different. Liu, Hsueh, and Hsiao (2004) therefore proposed a Bayesian noninferiority approach to evaluating bridging studies. However, the results of the bridging studies using these Bayesian approaches will be overwhelmingly dominated by the results of the original region due to an imbalance of sample sizes between the regions. Hsiao, Hsu, Tsou, and Liu (2007) therefore proposed a Bayesian approach with the use of mixed prior information for assessing the similarity between the new and original region based on the concept of positive treatment effect. For Bayesian methods, the foreign clinical data provided in the CCDP from the original region and those from the bridging study in the new region were not generated in the same study and are not internally valid. Therefore, a group sequential method (Hsiao, Xu, and Liu, 2003) and a two-stage design (Hsiao, Xu, and Liu, 2005) were proposed to overcome the issue of internal validity.

1.4.2 Sample Size Estimation and Allocation

Recently, the trends of clinical development in Asian countries and clinical trials conducted in Europe and the United States have simultaneously been speedily on the rise. In particular, Taiwan, South Korea, Hong Kong, and Singapore have already had much experience in planning and conducting multiregional trials.

The Japanese government has also made efforts to promote Japan's participation in global development and international clinical study. As mentioned, the Japanese MHLW has published guidelines related to planning and implementing global clinical studies. In the ICH E5 "Guidance for Industry Questions and Answers" (ICH, 2006), Q11 discusses the concept of a multiregional trial and states, "It may be desirable in certain situations to achieve the goal of bridging by conducting a multi-regional trial under a common protocol that includes sufficient numbers of patients from each of multiple regions to reach a conclusion about the effect of the drug in all regions" (p. 6). Both guidelines have established a framework on how to demonstrate the efficacy of a drug in all participating regions while also evaluating the possibility of applying the overall trial results to each region by conducting a multiregional bridging trial. Recent approaches for sample size determination in multiregional trials developed by Kawai, Stein, Komiyama, and Li (2008); Quan, Zhao, Zhang, Roessner, and Aizawa (2010); and Ko, Tsou, Liu, and Hsiao (2010) are all based on the assumption that the effect size is uniform across regions. For example, assume that we focus on the multiregional trial for comparing a test product and a placebo control based on a continuous efficacy endpoint. Let X and Y be some efficacy responses for patients receiving the test product or the placebo control, respectively. For convention, both X and Y are normally distributed with variance σ^2. We assume that is known, although it can generally be estimated. Let μ_T and μ_P be the population means of the test and placebo, respectively, and let $\Delta = \mu_T - \mu_P$. Assume that effect size (Δ/σ) is uniform across regions. The hypothesis of testing for the overall treatment effect is given as

$$H_0{:}\Delta \le 0 \text{ versus } H_a{:}\Delta > 0$$

Let N denote the total sample size for each group planned for detecting an expected treatment difference $\Delta = \delta$ at the desired significance level α and with power of $1 - \beta$. Thus,

$$N = 2\sigma^2 \left\{ \left(z_{1-\alpha} + z_{1-\beta} \right) / \delta \right\}^2$$

where $z_{1-\alpha}$ is the $(1-\alpha)$th percentile of the standard normal distribution. Once N is determined, special consideration should be placed on the determination of the number of subjects from the Asian region in the multiregional trial. The selected sample size should be able to establish the consistency of treatment effects between the Asian region and the regions overall. Let D_{Asia} be the observed treatment effect for the Asian region and D_{All} the observed treatment effect for all regions. Given that the overall result is significant at α level, we will judge whether the treatment is effective in the Asian region by the following criterion:

$$D_{Asia} \ge \rho\, D_{All} \text{ for some } 0 < \rho < 1 \tag{1.1}$$

Other consistency criteria can be found in Uesaka (2009) and Ko et al. (2010). Selection of the magnitude, ρ, of consistency trend may be critical. All differences in ethnic factors between the Asian region and other regions should be taken into account. The Japanese MHLW suggests that ρ be 0.5 or greater. However, the determination of ρ will be and should be different from product to product and from therapeutic area to therapeutic area. For example, in a multiregional liver cancer trial, the Asian region can definitely require a larger value of ρ, since it will contribute more subjects than other regions. To establish the consistency of treatment effects between the Asian region and the entire group, it is suggested that the selected sample size should satisfy that the assurance probability of the consistency criterion in Equation 1.1, given that $\Delta = \delta$ and the overall result is significant at α level, is maintained at a desired level, say, 80%. That is,

$$P_\delta(D_{Asia} \ge \rho\, D_{All} \mid Z > z_{1-\alpha}) > 1 - \gamma \tag{1.2}$$

for some prespecified $0 < \gamma \le 0.2$. Here Z represents the overall test statistic.

Ko et al. (2010) calculated the sample size required for the Asian region based on Equation 1.2. For $\beta = 0.1$, $\alpha = 0.025$, and $\rho = 0.5$, the sample size for the Asian region has to be around 20% of the overall sample size to maintain the assurance probability at 80% level. On the other hand, by considering a two-sided test, Quan et al. (2010) derived closed-form formulas for the sample size calculation for normal, binary, and survival endpoints based on the consistency criterion. For examples, if we choose $\rho = 0.5$, $\gamma = 0.2$, $\alpha = 0.05$, and $\beta = 0.9$, then the Asian sample size has to be at least 22.4% of the overall sample size for the multiregional trial.

It should be noted that the sample size determinations given in Kawai et al. (2008), Quan et al. (2010), and Ko et al. (2010) are all derived under the assumption that the effect size is uniform across regions. In practice, a difference in treatment effect due to ethnic difference might be expected. Thus, the sample size calculation derived by Kawai et al. and Ko et al. may not be of practical use. More specifically, some other assumptions addressing the ethnic difference should be explored. For example, we may consider the following assumptions:

1. Δ is the same but σ^2 is different across regions.
2. Δ is different but σ^2 is the same across regions.
3. Δ and σ^2 are both different across regions.

Statistical methods for the sample size determination in multiregional trials should be developed based on these assumptions.

1.5 Examples

Here we have two successful stories to tell. In the European Stroke Prevention Study 2 (ESPS 2) conducted among Caucasians (Diener et al., 1996), a drug with a fixed combination of 200 mg dipyridamole and 25 mg 1 bid aspirin, both given twice daily, has been shown to be more effective than either agent prescribed singly in the secondary prevention of ischaemic strokes. Data from the 6,602 patients in ESPS 2 revealed that stroke risk when compared with placebo was reduced by 18% with acetylsalicylic acid alone, 16% with dipyridamole alone, and 37% with the combination therapy. In the ESPS 2 study, headache was the most common adverse event occurring approximately 15% higher with the dipyridamole-treated patients compared with those given the placebo. Due to the headaches experienced by some of their patients, Filipino neurologists are strongly concerned with prescribing high doses of dipyridamole. Subsequently, an open noncomparative study was conducted to document the frequency, severity, and pattern of occurrence of the headaches among Filipinos taking acetylsalicylic acid plus dipyridamole. Subjects in the Filipino study received 25 mg of acetylsalicylic acid and 200 mg of dipyridamole twice a day for 2 weeks. Number of dropouts due to headache was used as the primary endpoint.

A total of 105 patients was recruited in the Filipino study (Chua et al., 2003). The results showed that a total of 70 patients (67%) experienced headaches during the 2-week study period, and a total of 22 patients dropped out during the study with 17 patients (16%) dropping out due to headache. However, in ESPS 2, headache only developed in 38% of patients taking acetylsalicylic acid and dipyridamole, and only around 8% of those taking the drugs had to discontinue therapy primarily because of headaches. As a result, ethnic differences may exist in the headache-associated dropout rate between Filipino and Caucasian patients given the same combination of acetylsalicylic acid and dipyridamole.

After the standard bridging study evaluation process, Taiwan's regulatory agency decided to request a bridging study due to an ethnic difference in medical practice (much lower dose for one of the components in Taiwan) and higher headache-associated dropout rate in the Filipino study. Therefore, a study was conducted to evaluate the tolerance of headache and safety in Taiwanese patients who are receiving two different dosing regimens of acetylsalicylic acid plus dipyridamole. In the first 4 weeks, the local bridging study results showed that the headache dropout rate of patients with reduced-dose for 2 weeks and full-dose for 2 weeks was 6.7%, which was not different from the dropout rate of placebo (8.7%) but was statistically different from the dropout rate of patients with full-dose 4 weeks (16.3%). Consequently, Taiwan decided to change the label instructions for use.

Note that the rationale for dose reduction is understandable in some situations. But why such a reduction can still maintain the efficacy of the combination of dipyridamole and aspirin may be a generic problem with bridging studies or multiregional clinical trials where different doses are used for different regions. Unless some kind of consistency is articulated, we shall never know whether dose reduction is ever good from the standpoint of both efficacy and safety.

Another drug studied is a new potent lipid-lowering agent, Crestor. The PK study in the Japanese showed that the C_{max} of the Japanese is 1.9 to 2.5 times of that for Caucasian, whereas area under the curve (AUC) is 2 to 2.5 times. Although the mean interracial difference is not substantial, Taiwan approved the drug with reduced maximal dosage due to the dose-dependent, drug-related rare serious adverse effect (SAE) of rhabdomyolysis. Since clinical trials revealed that patients in Asian countries reacted differently to Crestor than patients in U.S. trials, most of whom were white, the medical community was uncertain if these differences also applied to Asians in the United States. Subsequently, the FDA requested more studies by the manufacturer. A study by the drug's manufacturer, AstraZeneca, indicated that Asians appear to process the drug differently; half the standard dose can have the same cholesterol-lowering benefit in those patients, but a full dose could increase the risk of side effects. Consequently, the FDA urged physicians to use caution in prescribing Crestor to patients of Asian heritage. In March 2005, the FDA issued a public health advisory, made changes to prescribing information for doctors, and said that Asian patients should be started at the lowest approved dose, 5 milligrams a day.

1.6 Concluding Remarks

In recent years, global collaboration has led to a new strategy for drug development. However, the possible geographic variations of efficacy and safety may have influence on the global drug development. In this chapter, two examples are provided to see the impact of ethnic differences. One example shows that significant ethnic differences seem to exist in the enzymatic activity of several drug metabolizing enzymes. The other shows that patient response to therapeutics may vary from one racial or ethnic group to another.

In 1998, the ICH issued a guideline on *Ethnic Factors in the Acceptability of Foreign Clinical Data* to determine if clinical data generated from the original region are acceptable in a new region. The purpose of this guideline is to permit adequate evaluation of the influence of ethnic factors on clinical efficacy and safety of the approved test treatment (at the original region) for regulatory review and approval in the new region. However, it also minimizes duplication of clinical studies and consequently does not to delay the availability of the approved test treatment in the new region. In particular, the ICH E5 guideline suggests that a bridging study be conducted in the new region to generate additional information to bridge the foreign clinical data when the foreign clinical data contained in the CCDP cannot provide sufficient bridging evidence. In this chapter, the main points of the ICH E5 are described and followed with a critique. Following the 1998 ICH E5 guideline, Japan, South Korea, and Taiwan have developed similar but slightly different bridging strategies to extrapolating foreign (e.g., the United States and European Union) data to their respective countries. In this chapter, the regulatory guidances for Japan and South Korea are also described briefly. In addition, some practical issues that are commonly encountered when conducting bridging studies are discussed. These practical issues include criteria for assessment of similarity between regions and sample size calculation and allocation for bridging and multiregional studies. Finally, two successful examples of drugs approved based on a bridging strategy articulated in the ICH E5 guideline are given.

Although a bridging review and evaluation or study might be required before submitting an application for *new* drug application in the Asia-Pacific region, for example, Japan, South Korea, and Taiwan, replicated clinical trials may be waived if no evidence of possible ethnic difference is found. As an example, in Taiwan, after regulatory requirement for bridging study evaluation (BSE) was announced at the beginning of 2004, 132 applications were received by the regulatory agency of Taiwan by the end of that year. Among these, 121 (completed cases) have been reviewed, in which 82 (68%) cases were waived, 38 (31%) cases were not waived, and 1 (1%) was judged not related to BSE. Also, among the 121 completed cases, 51 (42%) did not provide Asian clinical and pharmacokinetic information. For those 51 cases, while bridging studies were not waived in 19 cases, they were waived in the other 32 cases despite lack of Asian clinical and pharmacokinetic data. From the 38 cases that were not waived for bridging study, the most common reasons were lack of pharmacokinetic information (71.1%), efficacy (55.3%), and safety concerns (47.4%). On the other hand, in South Korea, based on the new chemical entity approved by the South Korea FDA, from 2002 to September 2007, 72% of applications were waived for bridging studies (Kim, 2008). The waiver rates are quite similar between Taiwan and South Korea.

The purpose of ICH E5 is to facilitate the registration of medicines among ICH regions (United States, European Union, and Japan). This chapter expands this guidance for approval of new drugs in other countries and areas. Since pharmaceuticals are of large trade value for the United States and the European Union–based international manufacturers, this chapter focuses on the issue of "one-way bridging," or bridging from the United States and the European Union to the Asia-Pacific region. Many Asian countries and areas including Japan, South Korea, and Taiwan have already had much experience in the implementation of bridging studies. However, O'Neill (2002) indicated, "Few examples of formal bridging studies done in the US that were performed subsequent to development of a complete clinical data package, and that were carried out in response to an FDA request. Generally, when FDA asks for more data/studies, it is because the clinical trial evidence in the NDA is not convincing and other formal phase III studies conducted in the US are needed." "Despite the inclusion of foreign clinical data in an NDA, sponsors have anticipated an FDA request by carrying out US trials without being asked. Sometime these trials are ongoing at the time of NDA submission" (p. 12). Currently, the FDA may not have much experience in implementing bridging studies. As we know, the biopharmaceutical industry may be the most vital and important industry in the 21st century. Although Asian regional native-owned drug companies are relatively small in capital capabilities compared with U.S.- and EU-based international manufacturers, the biopharmaceutical industry is indeed blooming in the Asian region. It might be possible in the future that the U.S. FDA may have to consider the bridging strategy for approval of new drugs, especially for the drugs targeted to the diseases that have higher prevalence rates in the Asia-Pacific region compared with the United States and the European Union.

1.7 Aim and Structure of the Book

This book is intended to be the first entirely devoted to designing and analyzing bridging studies in clinical research and development. It covers issues that are commonly encountered during bridging studies. It is our goal to provide a useful desk reference and state-of-the-art examination of issues in design and analysis of bridging studies to clinical scientists who are engaged in pharmaceutical and clinical research and development, those in government regulatory agencies who have to make decisions on bridging review and evaluation of test treatments under investigation, and biostatisticians who provide the statistical support for design and analysis to bridging studies or related projects. We hope that this book can serve as a *bridge* among pharmaceutical industry scientists, governmental regulatory agency medical/statistical reviewers, and academic researchers.

This chapter provides the background for bridging diversity by extrapolating foreign data to a new region in pharmaceutical and clinical research and development. In the next chapter, a group sequential method and a two-stage design are introduced to incorporate foreign clinical data information into evaluating bridging data observed in the new region within the same study based on Hsiao, Xu, and Liu (2003, 2005). In Chapter 3, methods of consistency assessment and associated issues are reviewed. Chapter 4 discusses the possibility for assessing similarity based on the reproducibility and generalizability and sensitivity index proposed by Shao and Chow (2002) and Chow et al. (2002), respectively. Chapter 5 focuses on a combination of information of the type used in bridging studies, in which information is leveraged from previous foreign clinical studies to reduce the resource requirements (e.g., number of patients) for domestic registration of a new compound. A Bayesian approach for assessment of bridging studies is discussed in Chapter 6. Chapters 7 and 8 give a comprehensive overview of statistical methods for bridging studies and multiregional clinical trials conducted in global development. Chapter 9 illustrates the application of genomic technologies in bridging studies. Chapter 10 provides a thorough discussion regarding interaction and confounding effects that are commonly encountered in bridging studies. Chapter 11 discusses the issues, details, and impacts of designing a multiregional clinical trial to assess the overall effect of a test treatment when there are differences in authority requirements between the regions. Feasibility and implementation of bridging studies in the Asia-Pacific region countries of Japan and Taiwan are discussed in Chapter 12 and Chapter 13, respectively.

In each chapter, examples and possible recommendations or resolutions of issues that are commonly encountered during the conduct of bridging studies in pharmaceutical or clinical development are provided whenever possible.

References

Caraco, Y. (2004). Genes and the response to drugs. *New England Journal of Medicine*, 351(27): 2867–2869.

Chow, S. C., and Shao, J. (2006). On non-inferiority margin and statistical tests in active control trials. *Statistics in Medicine*, 25: 1101–1113.

Chow, S. C., Shao, J., and Hu, O. Y. P. (2002). Assessing sensitivity and similarity in bridging studies. *Journal of Biopharmaceutical Statistics*, 12: 385-400.

Chua, C., Navarro, J., Luis, A. S., Espiritu, A. G., Esagunde, R., Lao, R. et al. (2003). Tolerance study among Filipinos on acetylsalicylic acid and dipyridamole. *Neurological Journal of Southeast Asia*, 8: 9–13.

Diener, H. C., Cunha, L., Forbes, C., Sivenius, J., Smets, P., and Lowenthal, A. (1996). European dipyridamole and acetylsalicylic acid in the secondary prevention of stroke. *Journal of Neurological Sciences*, 143: 1–13.

Fukuoka, M., Yano, S., Giaccone, G., Tamura, T., Nakagawa, K., Douillard, J. Y. et al. (2003). Multi-institutional randomized phase II trial of gefitinib for previously treated patients with advanced non-small-cell lung cancer. *Journal of Clinical Oncology*, 21(12): 2237–2246.

Hsiao, C. F., Hsu, Y. Y., Tsou, H. H., and Liu, J. P. (2007). Use of prior information for Bayesian evaluation of bridging studies. *Journal of Biopharmaceutical Statistics*, 17(1): 109–121.

Hsiao, C. F., Xu, J. Z., and Liu, J. P. (2003). A group sequential approach to evaluation of bridging studies. *Journal of Biopharmaceutical Statistics*, 13: 793–801.

Hsiao, C. F., Xu, J. Z., and Liu, J. P. (2005). A two-stage design for bridging studies. *Journal of Biopharmaceutical Statistics*, 15: 75–83.

Hung, H. M. J. (2003). Statistical issues with design and analysis of bridging clinical trial. Paper presented at the Symposium on Statistical Methodology for Evaluation of Bridging Evidence, Taipei, Taiwan.

Hung, H. M. J., Wang, S. J., Tsong, Y., Lawrence, J., and O'Neil, R. T. (2003). Some fundamental issues with non-inferiority testing in active controlled trials. *Statistics in Medicine*, 22: 213–225.

International Conference on Harmonization. (ICH). (1998). Tripartite guidance E5 ethnic factors in the acceptability of foreign data. *U.S. Federal Register*, 83: 31790–31796.

International Conference on Harmonization. (ICH). (2006). Technical requirements for registration of pharmaceuticals for human use. *Q&A for the ICH E5 Guideline on Ethnic Factors in the Acceptability of Foreign Data*. Available at: http://www.ich.org/fileadmin/Public_Web_Site/ICH_Products/Guidelines/Efficacy/E5_R1/Q_As/E5_Q_As_R5_.pdf.

Kawai, N., Stein, C., Komiyama O., and Li, Y. (2008). An approach to rationalize partitioning sample size into individual regions in a multiregional trial. *Drug Information Journal*, 42: 139–147.

Kim, I. B. (2008). Review policies for global drug development: Korea's perspective. Paper presented at the East Asian Pharmaceutical Regulatory Symposium, Tokyo, Japan, April 14–15.

Ko, F. S., Tsou, H. H., Liu, J. P., and Hsiao, C. F. (2010). Sample size determination for a specific region in a multi-regional trial. *Journal of Biopharmaceutical Statistics*, 20(4): 870–885.

Lan, K. K., Soo, Y., Siu, C., and Wang, M. (2005). The use of weighted Z-tests in medical research. *Journal of Biopharmaceutical Statistics*, 15(4): 625–639.

Liu, J. P., Hsiao, C. F., and Hsueh, H. M. (2002). Bayesian approach to evaluation of bridging studies. *Journal of Biopharmaceutical Statistics*, 12: 401–408.

Liu, J. P., Hsueh, H. M., and Chen, J. J. (2002). Sample size requirement for evaluation of bridging evidence. *Biometrical Journal*, 44: 969–981.

Liu, J. P., Hsueh, H. M, and Hsiao, C. F. (2004). Bayesian non-inferior approach to evaluation of bridging studies. *Journal of Biopharmaceutical Statistics*, 14: 291–300.

Ministry of Health, Labour and Welfare of Japan. (2007). Basic principles on global clinical trials. Notification No. 0928010, September 28. Available at: http://www.pmda.go.jp/english/service/pdf/notifications/0928010-e.pdf.

O'Neill, R. (2002). The ICH E5 guidance: An update on experiences with its implementation. Paper presented at the 3rd Kitasato University-Harvard School of Public Health Symposium, Tokyo, Japan.

Paez, J. G., Janne, P. A., Lee, J. C., Tracy, S., Greulich, H., Gabriel, S. et al. (2004). EGFR mutations in lung cancer: Correlation with clinical response to gefitinib therapy. *Science*, 304(5676): 1497–1500.

Quan, H., Zhao, P. L., Zhang, J., Roessner, M., and Aizawa, K. (2010). Sample size considerations for Japanese patients based on MHLW guidance. *Pharmaceutical Statistics*, 9: 100–112.

Shao, J., and Chow, S. C. (2002). Reproducibility probability in clinical trials. *Statistics in Medicine*, 21: 1727–1742.

Shih, W. J. (2001). Clinical trials for drug registration in Asian-Pacific countries: Proposal for a new paradigm from a statistical perspective. *Controlled Clinical Trials*, 22: 357–366.

Uesaka, H. (2009). Sample size allocation to regions in multiregional trial. *Journal of Biopharmaceutical Statistics*, 19: 580–595.

Uyama, Y., Shibata, T., Nagai, N., Hanaoka, H., Toyoshima, S., and Mori, K. (2005). Successful bridging strategy based on ICH E5 guideline for drugs approved in Japan. *Clinical Pharmacological Therapy*, 78(2): 102–113.

2

Two-Stage Designs of Bridging Studies

Chin-Fu Hsiao and Hsiao-Hui Tsou
National Health Research Institutes

Jen-pei Liu
National Taiwan University

Yuh-Jenn Wu
Chung Yuan Christian University

2.1 Introduction

In recent years, global collaboration has led to a new strategy for drug development. After a pharmaceutical product has been approved for commercial marketing in one region (e.g., the United States or European Union) based on its proven efficacy and safety, the pharmaceutical sponsor might seek registration of the product in a new region, such as an Asian country. However, to extrapolate the original clinical data to new populations, the differences in race, diet, environment, culture, and medical practice among regions might cause impact upon a medicine's effect. In 1998, the International Conference on Harmonisation (ICH) published a guideline titled "Ethnic Factors in the Acceptability of Foreign Clinical Data" known as ICH E5 to provide a general framework for evaluating the impact of ethnic factors on a medicine's effect such as its efficacy and safety at a particular dosage or dose regimen. More specifically, the ICH E5 guideline suggests that a bridging study be conducted in the new region to extrapolate the inference based on the foreign efficacy data or safety data to a new region.

Several statistical procedures have been proposed to assess the similarity based on the additional information from the bridging study and the foreign clinical data in the complete clinical data package (CCDP). Shih (2001) used the method of Bayesian to find the most plausible prediction for drug approval for countries in the Asia-Pacific region. Since substantial information from multicenter studies has already shown efficacy in the original regions (e.g., the United States or the European Union), when a drug manufacturer seeks marketing approval in another new region (e.g., an Asian country), the result from the new region is consistent with the previous results if it falls within the previous experience. Chow, Shao, and Hu (2002) proposed the use of reproducibility, probability, and generalizability to assess the necessity of bridging studies in the new region. Liu, Hsueh, and Chen (2002) used a hierarchical model approach to incorporating the foreign bridging information into the data generated by the bridging study in the new region. They proposed an empirical Bayesian approach to synthesize the data generated by the bridging study and foreign clinical data generated in the original region to assess the similarity based on superior efficacy of the test product over a placebo control. Liu, Hsueh, and Hsiao (2006) proposed a Bayesian approach to assess the similarity between the new and original region based on the concept of noninferiority. Lan, Soo, Siu, and Wang (2005) introduced weighted Z-tests in which the weights may depend on the prior observed data for the design of bridging studies. Hsiao, Hsu, Tsou, and Liu (2007) then proposed a Bayesian approach using a mixture prior, which is a weighted average of two points, for assessment of similarity between the new and original region based on the concept of positive treatment effect.

For the aforementioned approaches, the foreign clinical data provided in the CCDP from the original region and those from the bridging study in the new region were not generated in the same study. One of the current issues for evaluating bridging studies is a cross-study comparison. Bias occurs when the study is not internally valid. Hsiao, Xu, and Liu (2003, 2005) therefore proposed a group sequential method and a two-stage design to overcome the issue of internal validity. Within this framework, regions are treated as group sequence or stages. In particular, we use the regions as group sequence or stages to enroll the patients from the original region first and then to enroll patients from the new region. This chapter introduces a group sequential method and a two-stage design to incorporate the information of the foreign clinical data into evaluation of the positive treatment effect observed in the new region within the same study based on Hsiao et al. (2003, 2005). Section 2.2 introduces a two-stage design structure to synthesize the data from both the bridging study and the original region for assessment of bridging evidence. In Section 2.3, a group sequential approach to evaluation of bridging studies will be described. Some concluding remarks are given in Section 2.4.

2.2 Two-Stage Design for Bridging Studies

For simplicity, we focus only on the trials for comparing a test product and a placebo control. We consider the problem for assessment of similarity between the new and original region based on the structure of two-stage design. Let X_i and Y_j be some efficacy responses for patients i and j receiving the test product and the placebo control, respectively. For simplicity, assume that both X_i's and Y_j's are normally distributed with a known variance σ^2. Let μ_1 and μ_2 be the population means of the test product and the placebo, respectively, and let $\Delta = \mu_1 - \mu_2$. The hypothesis of testing for the overall treatment is given as

$$H_0 : \Delta = 0 \text{ vs. } H_A : \Delta > 0 \tag{2.1}$$

Although the hypothesis is one-sided, the method proposed next can be straightforwardly extended to the two-sided hypothesis.

2.2.1 Two-Stage Design

The idea of the two-stage approach to evaluating bridging is presented as follows. When we design adequate and well-controlled studies for submission to the original region, we include the patients in the new region as part of recruitment for the whole study. In other words, the bridging study is a substudy. More specifically, we use the two-stage design to enroll the patients from the original region in the first stage and then to enroll patients from the new region in the second stage. Without loss of generality, an equal number of patients should be enrolled into test and placebo groups at both regions. Let n_O and n_N denote the number of patients studied for each treatment group in the original region and the new region, respectively. Let T_O and C_O be the test statistic and the critical values in the first stage, and T_N and C_N the test statistic and the critical value in the second stage. The subscript O in T_O and C_O represents the original region, while the subscript N in T_N and C_N indicates the new region.

When the study is completed in the original region, we perform the statistical analysis with the data from the original region. If the observed value of test statistic T_O does not exceed C_O, then a bridging substudy is not needed. On the other hand, if the results from the first stage based on the data of the original region demonstrate a statistically significantly positive treatment effect, then data are ready to support registration in the original region and we also proceed to enroll the patients in the new region. After recruitment of patients in the new region is complete, we then perform the final analysis with additional data from the new region. If the accumulated results in the second stage are similar to those in the first stage, then the results of the new region can be declared similar to the original region. Here, the similarity is defined as the similar treatment effect to meet requirement of exceeding the critical value C_N at the second stage.

2.2.2 Determining Sample Size and Critical Values

As stated in the previous section, n_O and n_N represent the numbers of patients studied per treatment in the original and new region, respectively.

The decision of whether to conduct the bridging study in the new region will be based on the results observed in the original region. Let T_O and T_N represent the test statistics obtained from the first stage in the original region and the second stage in the new region, respectively, which can be expressed by

$$T_O = \frac{\sum_{i=1}^{n_O}(X_i - Y_i)}{\sigma\sqrt{2n_O}}$$

and

$$T_N = T_O\{n_O/(n_O + n_N)\}^{1/2} + W_N\{n_N/(n_O + n_N)\}^{1/2}$$

where

$$W_N = \frac{\sum_{i=n_O+1}^{n_O+n_N}(X_i - Y_i)}{\sigma\sqrt{2n_N}}$$

In addition, let C_O and C_N denote the critical values for rejecting the null hypothesis in the original and new regions. Therefore, the probability of failing to reject H_0 with true treatment difference Δ is a function of Δ, n_O, n_N, C_O, and C_N and is given by

$$\begin{aligned}
&\phi(\Delta, n_O, n_N, C_O, C_N) \\
&= P_\Delta(T_O < C_O) + \int_{C_O}^{\infty} f_\Delta(t) P_\Delta(T_N < C_N)dt \\
&= P_\Delta(T_O < C_O) + \int_{C_O}^{\infty} f_\Delta(t) P_\Delta\{W_N < C_N((n_O + n_N)/n_N)^{1/2} - t(n_O/n_N)^{1/2}\}dt
\end{aligned}$$

where P_Δ denotes the probability measure with respect to Δ and $f_\Delta(t)$ represents the probability density function of T_O with respect to Δ.

Let α denote the overall type I error rate. Consequently, α can be expressed as

$$\begin{aligned}
\alpha &= 1 - \phi(0, n_O, n_N, C_O, C_N) \\
&= 1 - P_0(T_O < C_O) - \int_{C_O}^{\infty} f_0(t) P_0(T_N < C_N)dt
\end{aligned}$$

which can be rewritten as

$$P_0(T_O < C_O) + \int_{C_O}^{\infty} f_0(t) P_0(T_N < C_N) dt = 1 - \alpha \tag{2.2}$$

The first and the second term on the left-hand side of Equation 2.2 can be thought of as the "power" (the probability of "accepting" H_0 giving that H_0 is true) for null hypothesis H_0 at the first and the second stage, respectively. As seen in Equation 2.2, the critical value C_O could be smaller than the critical value of 1.96 used in a single test of hypothesis with $\alpha = 0.025$. However, many data-monitoring committees might wish to be somewhat conservative. With that in mind, we introduce a type I error adjustment factor (TIEAF) τ, where $0 < \tau < 1$, so that Equation 2.2 is rewritten as

$$P_0(T_O < C_O) + \int_{C_O}^{\infty} f_0(t) P_0(T_N < C_N) dt = 1 - \tau\alpha \tag{2.3}$$

One attractive feature of TIEAF is that the critical value used at the first stage can be adjusted to be close to that of a single test and at the same time the type I error rate is preserved at the desired level. The smaller the τ is, the more likely C_O will be increased. We suggest that τ be between 0.8 and 1.0. Based on Equation 2.3, the regulatory agencies in both original and new regions and the sponsor have to determine how they want to spend the "power" under H_O, $1 - \tau\alpha$, at each stage. Therefore, we use a weighting factor γ_1 such that

$$P_0(T_O < C_O) = \gamma_1(1 - \tau\alpha) \tag{2.4}$$

and

$$\int_{C_O}^{\infty} f_0(t) P_0(T_N < C_N) dt = (1 - \gamma_1)(1 - \tau\alpha) \tag{2.5}$$

where $0 < \gamma_1 < 1$. It should be noted that the larger the γ_1 is, the larger the C_O is.

Next let β be the type II error with a specified alternative hypothesis Δ. We can derive that

$$\begin{aligned}\beta &= \phi(\Delta, n_O, n_N, C_O, C_N) \\ &= P_\Delta(T_O < C_O) + \int_{C_O}^{\infty} f_\Delta(t) P_\Delta(T_N < C_N) dt\end{aligned}$$

Again the regulatory agencies in both original and new regions and the sponsor need to determine how they want to spend the type II error probability at each stage. Consequently, we introduce another weighting factor γ_2 such that

$$P_\Delta(T_O < C_O) = \gamma_2\beta \tag{2.6}$$

and

$$\int_{C_O}^{\infty} f_\Delta(t) P_\Delta(T_N < C_N) dt = (1-\gamma_2)\beta \tag{2.7}$$

where $0 < \gamma_2 < 1$. As seen, the larger the γ_2 is, the smaller the n_O is. The two-stage design considered here is to specify design parameters Δ, α, β, τ, γ_1, and γ_2 to determine n_O, n_N, C_O, and C_N based on Equations 2.4, 2.5, 2.6, and 2.7.

Tables 2.1, 2.2, and 2.3 illustrate the two-stage designs for different combinations of design parameters. Table 2.1 applies to trials with $\Delta = 0.2$, Table 2.2

TABLE 2.1

Designs for $\Delta = 0.2$

γ_1	γ_2	n_O	n_N	C_O	C_N
0.8	0.8	239	458	0.786	1.934
	0.7	255	393	0.786	1.960
	0.6	273	342	0.786	1.985
	0.5	295	297	0.786	2.004
	0.4	321	254	0.786	2.020
	0.3	355	209	0.786	2.036
	0.2	403	154	0.786	2.051
	0.2	484	72	0.786	2.053
0.9	0.9	318	396	1.185	1.850
	0.8	335	312	1.185	1.903
	0.7	354	252	1.185	1.931
	0.6	375	206	1.185	1.971
	0.5	400	164	1.185	2.001
	0.4	430	125	1.185	2.016
	0.3	469	81	1.185	2.029
	0.2	524	26	1.185	2.034
0.95	0.9	398	283	1.483	1.853
	0.8	417	201	1.483	1.928
	0.7	437	148	1.483	1.970
	0.6	461	107	1.483	2.011
	0.5	489	71	1.483	2.039
	0.4	522	34	1.483	2.053

Source: *Journal of Biopharmaceutical Statistics,* 15, 75–83.

TABLE 2.2

Designs for $\Delta = 0.3$

γ_1	γ_2	n_O	n_N	C_O	C_N
0.8	0.8	106	204	0.786	1.936
	0.7	113	175	0.786	1.963
	0.6	121	152	0.786	1.983
	0.5	131	132	0.786	2.004
	0.4	142	113	0.786	2.018
	0.3	158	93	0.786	2.037
	0.2	179	69	0.786	2.049
	0.1	215	32	0.786	2.053
0.9	0.9	141	176	1.185	1.850
	0.8	149	140	1.185	1.900
	0.7	157	113	1.185	1.944
	0.6	166	92	1.185	1.971
	0.5	177	74	1.185	1.997
	0.4	191	56	1.185	2.019
	0.3	208	37	1.185	2.034
	0.2	233	12	1.185	2.039
0.95	0.9	177	126	1.483	1.850
	0.8	185	89	1.483	1.925
	0.7	194	66	1.483	1.974
	0.6	205	48	1.483	2.013
	0.4	232	15	1.483	2.052

Source: *Journal of Biopharmaceutical Statistics*, 15, 75–83.

is for trials with $\Delta = 0.3$, and Table 2.3 is for trials with $\Delta = 0.4$. For each Δ, we consider $\alpha = 0.025$, $\beta = 0.1$, $\tau = 0.8$, $\sigma = 1$, and various values of γ_1 and γ_2. The tabulated results include the sample size per treatment group for the original region (n_O), the sample size per treatment group for the new region (n_N), the critical value at the end of the first stage (C_O), and the critical value at the end of the second stage (C_N). For instances, the first line in Table 2.1 corresponds to a design with $\Delta = 0.2$, $\gamma_1 = 0.8$, and $\gamma_2 = 0.8$. The original region needs to recruit 239 patients per treatment group. When the study is completed in the original region and if the observed value of the test statistic T_O does not exceed 0.786, then the trial is terminated and a bridging substudy is not needed. Otherwise, data are ready to support the registration in the original region, and the new region is required to enroll 458 patients per treatment group. After the recruitment of the patients in the new region is completed and if the observed statistic at the end of the trial is larger than 1.934, the results of the new region can be declared similar to the original region.

As shown in the tables, the required total sample size for the bridging study in the new region is smaller than those required by the original

TABLE 2.3

Designs for $\Delta = 0.4$

γ_1	γ_2	n_O	n_N	C_O	C_N
0.8	0.8	59	115	0.786	1.934
	0.7	63	98	0.786	1.955
	0.6	68	85	0.786	1.978
	0.5	73	74	0.786	1.996
	0.4	80	64	0.786	2.024
	0.3	88	52	0.786	2.027
	0.2	100	39	0.786	2.045
	0.1	121	18	0.786	2.050
0.9	0.9	79	99	1.185	1.850
	0.8	83	78	1.185	1.901
	0.7	88	64	1.185	1.946
	0.6	93	52	1.185	1.971
	0.5	100	41	1.185	2.001
	0.4	107	32	1.185	2.021
	0.3	117	21	1.185	2.036
	0.2	131	7	1.185	2.042
0.95	0.9	99	71	1.483	1.852
	0.8	104	50	1.483	1.924
	0.7	109	37	1.483	1.972
	0.6	115	27	1.483	2.012
	0.5	122	18	1.483	2.040
	0.4	130	9	1.483	2.055

region when the weighting factor, γ_2, is sufficiently small. As γ_2 decreases, the required sample size per treatment group in the new region decreases, but the required sample size per treatment group in the original region increases. This makes sense, since the original region will spend more power than the new region as γ_2 decreases. In addition, the critical value at the final analysis also increases as γ_2 decreases. This phenomenon can be observed from Equation 2.7. On the other hand, it is notable that the sample size in the original region increases as γ_1 increases. This fact is because that the larger the γ_1, the more power under H_O will be spent by the original region. In other words, the regulatory agencies in both original and new regions and the sponsor should make considerable decision on how they want to spend the type I and type II error probabilities at each stage.

There are several points we wish to make. First, if $T_O > 1.96$ and $T_N < C_N$, then the drug product shows its efficacy in the original region and can thus be supported by the data to register in the original region, but the results from the new region fail to show similarity. As a result, the data from the original region cannot be extrapolated (or bridged) to the new region. Second, the occurrence for the situation where T_O is much greater than C_O, $T_N > C_N$, but W_N is zero or even negative is possible. However, this phenomenon can occur only when W_N shows extreme negative result, since C_N is much larger than C_O in our design. In this case, the contribution of the patients from the new region strongly decreases indicating the test product should not be supported to register in the new region.

2.3 Group Sequential Approach to Evaluating Bridging Studies

In the preceding two-stage design, the overall type I error and power spent at each stage are controlled by the weighting factors γ_1 and γ_2, respectively. At the design stage, once γ_1 and γ_2 are specified, the corresponding stopping boundary and sample size required for each stage can be derived. Although the two-stage design can allow flexibility on how we want to spend the type I error rate and power at each stage, it cannot avoid the calculation of numerical integration. An alternative way to resolve the difficulties arising from complex calculation is to consider adopting a group sequential approach for designing and evaluating bridging studies.

2.3.1 Group Sequential Approach

Again, we focus only on the trials for comparing a test product and a placebo control. We consider the problem for assessment of similarity between the new and original region based on the structure of group sequential design. We shall continue to use much of the notation developed in Equation 2.2. Let X_i and Y_j be some efficacy responses for patients i and j receiving the test product and the placebo control, respectively. For simplicity, assume that both X_i's and Y_j's are normally distributed with a known variance σ^2, say, $\sigma^2 = 1$. In actual practice, σ^2 is unknown and must be estimated from some data. Let μ_1 and μ_2 be the respective means, and let $\Delta = \mu_1 - \mu_2$. The hypothesis of testing for the overall treatment is given in Equation 2.1.

Similar to the two-stage design, we use the region as group sequence to enroll the patients from the original region first and then to enroll patients from the new region. Let N denote the total sample size for each treatment group planned in the protocol for detecting an expected treatment difference $\Delta = \delta$ at the desired significance level α and with power $1 - \beta$, that is,

$$N = 2\{(z_\alpha + z_\beta)/\delta\}^2$$

where z_α is the $(1 - \alpha)$th percentile of the standard normal distribution. Let N_O represent the planned sample size recruited per treatment group in the original region. Then $t_O = N_O/N$ is the total information observed at the time when accrual is completed in the original region. Since the sample size for the new region depends on the specification of t_O, t_O can be determined jointly by the regulatory authorities in the original and new regions and of the sponsor. After t_O is specified, we then prespecify an α-spending function $\alpha(t)$ in the protocol, where t indexes the information time with $\alpha(0) = 0$ and $\alpha(1) = \alpha$. Let C_O and C_N be the respective boundary values at time t_O and at the final analysis. C_O and C_N can be derived by Lan and DeMets (1983).

The idea of our group sequential approach proceeds as follows. When the study is completed in the original region, we then perform an interim analysis with the data from the original region. If the resulting test statistic does not cross the boundary C_O, then a bridging substudy is not needed. On the other hand, if the results from the interim analysis based on the data of the original region show significant test product effect, then we proceed to enroll the patients in the new region. After the recruitment of the patients in the new region is complete, we then perform the final analysis with additional data from the new region. If the results obtained for the final analysis are similar to those from the interim analysis, then the results of the new region can be declared similar to the original region. Here, the similarity is defined as the similar treatment effect to meet requirement of crossing the boundary C_N at the final analysis.

2.3.2 Sample Size Determination

As stated in previous section, N represents the total sample size per population planned for detecting an expected treatment difference $\Delta = \delta$ with power $1 - \beta$ at the significance level α. When N_O, the planned sample size recruited per treatment group in the original region, is determined, the planned sample size per treatment group for the new region is $N - N_O$. After the study is completed in the original region, the estimated treatment difference $\hat{\Delta}_O$ obtained from the interim analysis with N_O patients in the original region is smaller than the expected difference. The sample size required for the new region needs to be revised to preserve the overall power. The sample size can be adjusted based on the conditional power given the interim results of the original region and required boundary for the final analysis (Lan, Simon, and Halperin, 1982). Let T_O and T_N be the respective test statistics for Equation 2.1 at time t_O and at the final analysis. When the study is completed in the original region, the conditional power can be evaluated by

$$CP_O(\Delta) = \Pr(T_N > C_N \mid T_O, \Delta)$$

$$= \Phi(-\{C_N - T_O t_O^{1/2} - (1 - t_O)(N/2)^{1/2}\Delta\}/(1 - t_O)^{1/2})$$

Following the approach suggested by Cui, Hung, and Wang (1999) and conditional power, we may adjust the sample size according to the following plan. If $CP_O(\hat{\Delta}_O) < \gamma_N CP_O(\delta)$ for some conditional power adjustment factor

(CPAF) γ_N, where, $0 < \gamma_N \leq 1$, then we can increase the total sample size per treatment group by

$$M = N(\delta/\hat{\Delta}_O)^2 \tag{2.8}$$

That is, the sample size per treatment group in the new region becomes $M - N_O$. As noted, the need for an increase of sample size in the new region is strongly influenced by γ_N. Therefore, the specification of γ_N is critical and may be determined by the regulatory authority in the new region and the sponsor. However, the larger the γ_N, the more likely the sample size will be increased in the new region. We suggest that γ_N be between 0.8 and 1.0. Cui, Hung, and Wang (1999) showed that increasing sample size based on the observed treatment difference can preserve the unconditional power at $1 - \beta$ when $\Delta = \hat{\Delta}_O$ but can substantially inflate the type I error rate. Lan and Trost (1997) pointed out that, with the increase of sample size, the alpha spending function needs to be adjusted and so do critical values. To preserve the type I error probability at the desired level, Cui et al. also developed a new test procedure in which they used the same critical values as those for the original test procedure but different test statistic from the original procedure for interim analyses. When an increase of sample size is not needed, the test statistic at the final analysis is given by

$$T_N = T_O(N_O/N)^{1/2}\, W_N\{(N - N_O)/N\}^{1/2} \tag{2.9}$$

where

$$W_N = \frac{\sum_{i=N_O+1}^{N} (X_i - Y_i)}{\sqrt{2(N - N_O)}}$$

When sample size per treatment group in the new region is needed to increase from $N - N_O$ to $M - N_O$, the test statistic in Equation 2.9 at the final analysis may be replaced by

$$T_N^* = T_O(N_O/M)^{1/2} + W_N^*\{(M - N_O)/M\}^{1/2}$$

where

$$W_N^* = \frac{\sum_{i=N_O+1}^{M} (X_i - Y_i)}{\sqrt{2(M - N_O)}}$$

Using the same critical values C_N, Cui et al. (1999) showed that the total type I error probability of the new test procedure allowing increasing sample size is equal to that of the original test procedure without increase. That is,

$$\Pr((T_O > C_O) \cup (T_N^* > C_N)|H_0) = \Pr((T_O > C_O) \cup (T_N > C_N)|H_0) = \alpha$$

Also the power of the new test procedure is greater than that of the original test procedure.

The following example illustrates the situation regarding the sample size increase in the new region. We set the total sample size per treatment group to $N = 250$ for detecting $\delta = 0.30$ at $\alpha = 0.025$ and with power 0.90. We further restrict ourselves to three designs of interim analysis times (t_O,1.0): (0.5, 1.0), (0.8, 1.0), and (0.9, 1.0). The O'Brien-Fleming alpha spending function is used. The program of DeMets, Kim, Lan, and Reboussin (available at http://www.medsch.wisc.edu/landemets/) yields respective boundary values of (2.9626, 1.9686), (2.2504, 2.0249), and (2.0937, 2.0531) for those three designs (1992). When the observed difference $\hat{\Delta}_O = 0.20$, the results from the original region are not significant for $t_O = 0.5$ and $t_O = 0.8$, and thus there is no necessity of a bridging study. However, for $t_O = 0.9$, the observed test statistic from the original region does cross $C_O = 2.0937$ implying the necessity of a bridging study. Note that the results from the original region are significant even if the observed $\hat{\Delta}_O = 0.20$ deviates to a large extent from the expected difference $\delta = 0.30$, since we test for the hypothesis $H_0{:}\Delta = 0$. With $t_O = 0.9$, the sample size per treatment group for the original region is 225, and thus the sample size planned per treatment group for the new region is 250 – 225 = 25. After observing = 0.20 and let $\gamma_N = 1$, it follows that $CP_O(\hat{\Delta}_O) = 0.7186 < CP_O(\delta) = 0.8244$. This implies that we may increase the total sample size per treatment group based on Equation 2.8 by

$$M = N(\delta/\hat{\Delta}_O)^2 = 250(0.3/0.2)^2 = 563$$

In other words, the sample size required per treatment group in the new region becomes 563 – 225 = 338 with $\gamma_N = 1.0$. This example illustrates that although a significant result is obtained from the interim analysis, since the estimated treatment effect is 67% of the expected, the required sample size for the new region is even larger than that planned for the original region. We have applied the group sequential approach to other choices of $\hat{\Delta}_O$. Table 2.4 gives the estimation of sample size per treatment group in the original and new region for various observed $\hat{\Delta}_O$ with $\gamma_N = 0.85$ and $\gamma_N = 1.0$ based on Equation 2.8 for the O'Brien-Fleming boundary. Sample sizes based on the Pocock α-spending function are given in Table 2.5.

Tables 2.4 and 2.5 show that increase in sample size is needed when the estimated treatment difference is smaller than the expected treatment difference $\delta = 0.30$. In other words, it could give a large increase for the sample

TABLE 2.4

The Sample Size Estimation in the Original and New Region for the O'Brien-Fleming Boundary

	$t_O = 0.5$		$t_O = 0.8$		$t_O = 0.9$	
$\hat{\Delta}_O$	**Original**	**New**	**Original**	**New**	**Original**	**New**
0.20	No efficacy		No efficacy		225	338(25)
0.25	No efficacy		200	160(50)	225	135(25)
0.30	No efficacy		200	50(50)	225	25(25)
0.35	No efficacy		200	50(50)	225	25(25)
0.40	125	125(125)*	200	50(50)	225	25(25)

Note: $\delta = 0.30$, $\gamma_N = 0.85$, and $\gamma_N = 1.0$.

* Number in the parentheses is the sample size required per treatment for the new region with $\gamma_N = 0.85$.

Source: *Journal of Biopharmaceutical Statistics*, 13, 793–801.

TABLE 2.5

The Sample Size Estimation in the Original and New Region for the Pocock Boundary

	$t_O = 0.5$		$t_O = 0.8$		$t_O = 0.9$	
$\hat{\Delta}_O$	**Original**	**New**	**Original**	**New**	**Original**	**New**
0.20	No efficacy		No efficacy		225	338(338)
0.25	No efficacy		200	160(50)	225	135(25)
0.30	125	125(125)*	200	50(50)	225	25(25)
0.35	125	125(125)	200	50(50)	225	25(25)
0.40	125	125(125)	200	50(50)	225	25(25)

Note: $\delta = 0.30$, $\gamma_N = 0.85$, and $\gamma_N = 1.0$

* Number in the parentheses is the sample size required per treatment for the new region with $\gamma_N = 0.85$.

Source: *Journal of Biopharmaceutical Statistics*, 13, 793–801.

size in the new region only when the observed treatment difference, $\hat{\Delta}_O$, is smaller than the expected difference, δ. Another point we wish to make is that the specification of γ_N and alpha spending function can strongly influence the determination of sample size increase. For instance, suppose that $\gamma_N = 0.85$ is selected and consider $t_O = 0.9$. With $\hat{\Delta}_O = 0.20$, we can derive that, for the type of O'Brien-Fleming boundary,

$$CP_O(\hat{\Delta}_O) = 0.7186 > \gamma_N \, CP_O(\delta) = 0.85 \times 0.8244 = 0.7007$$

and thus the sample size increase in the new region is not needed based on Equation 2.8. In other words, the sample size required per treatment group in the new region remains 25. However, with the same $\hat{\Delta}_O$, if the Pocock boundary is used, then we can obtain

$$CP_O(\hat{\Delta}_O) = 0.4931 < \gamma_N\, CP_O(\delta) = 0.85 \times 0.6317 = 0.5369$$

which yields that the sample size required per treatment group in the new region needs to increase to 338. Therefore, the general specification of γ_N and the alpha spending function may be rather critical.

2.4 Concluding Remarks

In this chapter, we propose a group sequential structure and a two-stage design to synthesize the data from both the bridging study and the original region for assessing bridging evidence. Under this group sequential or two-stage structure, a bridging study is a substudy prespecified in the same protocol with the same inclusion–exclusion criteria, the same study design, the same control, the same dose, the same methods for evaluation, and the same efficacy and safety endpoints. Except for the region and order of enrollment, the bridging study in the new region is conducted in the same way as the study in the original region with respect to the same protocol. In addition, the data from the new and original regions are managed and analyzed according to the plans prespecified in the protocol. In other words, the data from both the new and original regions are generated within the same study. Therefore, they are internally valid. In addition, the study protocol can specify that the data obtained from the original region are for registration for the original region and that the additional data from the new region will be for the registration for the new region and will be acquired only if a statistically significant result is obtained in the original region. With this approach, the registration in the original region will not be delayed.

The proposed group sequential structure for the bridging study is very easy to implement. Most importantly, the total information of the original region, t_O, and conditional power adjustment factor, γ_N, can be used by the regulatory agencies in both original and new regions and by the sponsor as tools to formulate a regulatory and development strategy for minimizing duplication of data and facilitating acceptance of foreign clinical data in the new region. Under our group sequential approach, a bridging substudy is conducted only after the interim results based on the data from the original region provide strong evidence that the test drug is superior. In addition, when the estimated treatment effect of the interim analysis is greater than or equal to the expected treatment effect, no increase in sample size is required for the new region. As a result, the proposed group sequential approach for evaluating bridging evidence not only can minimize unnecessary duplication of clinical data but also can save considerable valuable resource and development time and cost.

On the other hand, the proposed two-stage design structure for the bridging study is also very easy to implement. Tables 2.1, 2.2, and 2.3 show that to achieve the goal of minimizing unnecessary duplication of clinical data in the new region it is possible to reduce the total sample size for the bridging study in some cases. Most importantly the type I error adjustment factor, τ, and the weighting factors, γ_1 and γ_2, can be used by regulatory agencies in both original and new regions and by the sponsor as tools to formulate a regulatory and development strategy for minimizing duplication of data and facilitating acceptance of foreign clinical data in the new region. Similar to determining equivalence margins for the noninferiority trials, TIEAF τ, γ_1, and γ_2 will be and should different from product to product, from therapeutic area to therapeutic area, and from region to region.

References

Chow, S. C., Shao, J., and Hu, O. Y. P. (2002). Assessing sensitivity and similarity in bridging studies. *Journal of Biopharmaceutical Statistics,* 12: 385–400.

Cui, L., Hung, H. M. J., and Wang, S.-J. (1999). Modification of sample size in group sequential clinical trials. *Biometrics,* 55: 853–857.

Hsiao, C. F., Hsu, Y. Y., Tsou, H. H., and Liu, J. P. (2007). Use of prior information for Bayesian evaluation of bridging studies. *Journal of Biopharmaceutical Statistics,* 17(1): 109–121.

Hsiao, C. F., Xu, J. Z., and Liu, J. P. (2003). A group sequential approach to evaluation of bridging studies. *Journal of Biopharmaceutical Statistics,* 13: 793–801.

Hsiao, C. F., Xu, J. Z., and Liu, J. P. (2005). A two-stage design for bridging studies. *Journal of Biopharmaceutical Statistics,* 15: 75–83.

International Conference on Harmonisation. (ICH). (1998). Tripartite guidance E5 ethnic factors in the acceptability of foreign data. *U.S. Federal Register,* 83: 31790–31796.

Lan, K. K. G., Soo, Y., Siu, C., and Wang, M. (2005). The use of weighted Z-tests in medical research. *Journal of Biopharmaceutical Statistics,* 15(4): 625–639.

Lan, K. K. G., and DeMets, D. L. (1983). Discrete sequential boundaries for clinical trials. *Biometrika,* 70: 659–663.

Lan, K. K. G., Simon, R., and Halperin, M. (1982). Stochastically curtailed tests in long-term clinical trials. *Communications in Statistics,* C1: 207–219.

Lan, K. K. G., and Trost, D. C. (1997). Estimation of parameters and sample size reestimation. American Statistical Association Proceedings (Biopharmaceutical Section), 48–51.

Liu, J. P., Hsiao, C. F., and Hsueh, H.-M. (2002). Bayesian approach to evaluation of bridging studies. *Journal of Biopharmaceutical Statistics,* 12: 401–408.

Liu, J. P., Hsueh, H. M., and Chen, J. J. (2002). Sample size requirement for evaluation of bridging evidence. *Biometrical Journal,* 44: 969–981.

Liu, J. P., Hsueh, H. M., and Hsiao, C. F. (2004). A Bayesian noninferiority approach to evaluation of bridging studies. *Journal of Biopharmaceutical Statistics,* 14(2): 291–300.

Reboussin, D. M., DeMets, D. L., Kim, K., and Lan, K. K. G. (1992). Programs for computing group sequential boundaries using the Lan–DeMets method. Technical Report 60, Department of Biostatistics, University of Wisconsin–Madison.

Shih, W. J. (2001). Clinical trials for drug registration in Asian-Pacific countries: Proposal for a new paradigm from a statistical perspective. *Controlled Clinical Trials*, 22: 357–366.

3

Consistency of Treatment Effects in Bridging Studies and Global Multiregional Trials

Weichung J. Shih
University of Medicine and Dentistry of New Jersey–School of Public Health

Hui Quan
Sanofi

3.1 Introduction

The idea and function of conducting *bridging studies* after a medical product has been approved in one or more of the three major International Conference on Harmonisation (ICH) regions— the United States, the European Union, and Japan—as described in ICH (1998a) E5 guidance are discussed in other chapters of this book. Moving forward toward a simultaneous drug development, the pharmaceutical industry has globalized its research and development (R&D) to provide quality medical products around the world to meet patients' needs in various regions and countries. One of the key R&D globalization components is to conduct *global clinical trials*—also called multiregional clinical trials (MRCTs)—in which patients from multiple regions, countries, and medical institutions around the world are accrued and studied simultaneously in accordance with a common clinical trial protocol.

Conducting global clinical trials helps increase the developmental efficiency while promoting local regional clinical research. These trials also provide a way for local regulatory authorities to evaluate the medical product using a large body of data including the local countries' own patients studied with the same standard and hence the possibility of making the drug available to their patients around the same times as other regions. Because of these advantages, participating in a global clinical trial is a recent trend for many nations as a popular alternative to conducting a *bridging study.*

There are two main aims in a global clinical trial. The primary one is to show the overall treatment effect of a medical product. The other is, when the overall effect has been shown, to assess region/nation-specific effects to satisfy individual nations' requirements. (The definition of the overall treatment is model dependent; see later discussion.) The associated issues include how to design a suitable global clinical trial, how many patients and their distribution for the regions or nations to accrue, how to analyze the data to show the overall effect, and how to use the whole data to assess individual region effect. In a bridging study, the premise is that the overall treatment effect has already been shown to be positive in the original complete clinical data package (CCDP); hence, only the second aim is of interest here: to assess the region/nation-specific effect for the *region of interest* (*ROI*) with its requested bridging study and the CCDP. Linking all these issues is a very pertinent concept, the so-called *consistency* in treatment effects.

No matter whether a multiregional trial or a bridging trial strategy is used for global or regional drug development, we have to separate issues for trial design and data analysis. For trial design, regions have to be predefined, the consistency criterion has to be prespecified, and overall sample size and sample size distribution for individual regions have to be determined in the study protocol to ensure power for the overall treatment effect assessment and power for consistency assessment. A principle for the specification of consistency criterion for a global trial design is to treat all regions equally regardless of the market volumes of individual regions and countries. Otherwise, it may be difficult for the protocol to pass the review of the health authorities of individual regions and countries. For data analysis, customized analyses can be performed to meet the specific needs of health authorities in individual regions and countries. Results from these exploratory analyses should be interpreted with great caution. For bridging studies, the focus is on a specific region or country after the CCDP has been completed. Therefore, the objective for the trial can be easily specified.

There are two categories of consistency assessment. One is based on formal hypothesis testing on the true treatment effects, and the other is based on criteria or rules on the observed treatment effects. For the one based on hypothesis testing, consistency of treatment effects can be specified as the null hypothesis or as the alternative hypothesis. Sample size requirements for these two hypothesis testing approaches can be substantially different. In this chapter we delineate the different concepts and give an overview of some methods of consistency assessment and associated issues.

3.2 Global Clinical Trial

Since a global clinical trial is "a trial designed for a new drug aiming for worldwide development and approval ..." (Ministry of Health, Labour and Welfare of Japan, 2007), there are some basic requirements for its conduct. For instance, the participating countries and clinical trial sites must be ICH-GCP (Good Clinical Practice) compliant, and prior considerations need to be given regarding ethnic factors specific to individual regions for the efficacy and safety of the investigational drug. The primary endpoints and dose regimens should be acceptable to all individual regions. Also, when the entire study population across regions is defined as a primary analysis population for its sample size calculation, justification should be given for using the entire population as one population. This translates to the overall treatment effect denoted here as θ for the primary efficacy endpoint. However, the statistical expression of the overall treatment effect θ is model dependent. For a fixed-effect model, it is a weighted average of the (fixed) individual treatment effects of the participating regions. Weights are proportions of the sample sizes. Hence, the overall treatment effect is trial specific. For a random-effect model, the individual treatment effects are random, with θ as their parent mean.

It is fundamental for a rational global trial design to hold a plausible belief that participating regions have reasonable similarity of treatment effects. If there is a strong a priori reason to suspect that the effect within a region is likely to differ substantially from the other regions—perhaps based on genetics, pharmacokinetics, disease biology, local culture, or medical practice—then that region may warrant a separate evaluation. Such a separate evaluation could be performed within the multiregional trial. Another design to incorporate this a priori belief may be considered, such as a stratified trial with the designated strata having sufficient sample size. Notice, however, that including a region with a much smaller treatment effect in the primary population for the primary analysis will dilute the power for the overall analysis, underestimate the treatment effects for other regions, and result in potentially uninterpretable treatment evaluation.

The individual regional treatment effect can be denoted as $\{\theta_i, i = 1, \ldots, K\}$ for K prospectively defined regions or countries. As stated earlier, the two related key research aims in a global trial are to make inferences regarding the overall and the individual regional treatment effects. In performing both research aims, the literature often refers to *consistency* as a key concept or strategy in the assessment. However, it is important to point out that there is a difference in the concept of *consistency* for these two research aims.

3.3 Consistency in Making Inference Regarding the Overall Treatment Effect θ

In making inference regarding the overall treatment effect θ, *consistency* refers to the similarity of treatment effects across regions represented by $\{\theta_i, i = 1, \ldots, K\}$. We call this *consistency across regions (CAR)*. From the basic requirement of conducting a global clinical trial as discussed in Section 3.2, it is clear that the premise of a global clinical trial is assuming *consistency* across regions. However, when a global clinical trial is also serving as an alternative bridging study, this assumption is subject to verification for possible influence with ethnic factors, as explained in ICH E5. In this regard, the assessment of consistency, or lack of it, among regions is essentially under the same spirit as that for assessing homogeneity among centers by testing center-by-treatment interaction in the usual multicenter clinical trial setting. Most discussions of *treatment-by-region interaction* including quantitative or qualitative interactions are parallel to that for the treatment-by-center interaction as discussed in depth in the document ICH (1998b) E9. When an interaction test is used for this type of consistency assessment, consistency is claimed when the null hypothesis of homogeneity fails to be rejected. Under the null hypothesis, the probability for showing consistency is 1 minus the significance level of the interaction test, which is independent of the sample size. Therefore, sample size planning in this setting should be based on the probability for detecting potential heterogeneity to control the type II error rate. With such an approach, it can be shown that, given the total sample size, the larger the number of regions and the smaller the sample sizes for individual regions, the higher the chance for claiming consistency. Chen et al. (2010) reviewed three categories of statistical methods for assessing this type of consistency across all regions when making inference regarding the overall treatment effect.

Another CAR category of criteria and rules is based on *observed* treatment effects. The Japanese Pharmaceutical Medical Device Agency (JPMDA) Method 2 (Ministry of Health, Labour and Welfare of Japan, 2007) is one of them, corresponding to assessing no *observed* qualitative treatment-by-region interaction:

$$\hat{\theta}_1 > 0,\ \hat{\theta}_2 > 0,\ \ldots,\ \hat{\theta}_K > 0 \tag{3.1}$$

where $\hat{\theta}_i$ is the estimated (observed) treatment effect for country/region *i*. (JPMDA Method 1 is described in Section 3.4.) With this method, the number of regions should not be large so that there are enough patients from individual regions to ensure the probability for consistency assessment. Kawai, Chuang-Stein, Komiyama, and Li (2007) discussed sample sizes to ensure probability for showing consistency based on this method when the true treatment effects for all regions are identical. For example, if there are three regions in a study that is designed with a 90% power for claiming a significant overall treatment effect and we desire an 80% chance of satisfying this consistency criterion, the smallest region must contribute at least 15% of all patients in the study. If the study is designed for 80% overall power, the smallest region must contain at least 21% of all patients.

Quan, Li, Chen et al. (2010) also provided a review but extended definitions and assessments of consistency in this setting—simultaneous consistency assessment of treatment effects across all regions. They further demonstrated the relationships between the power for consistency assessment and the configurations of sample sizes across the regions for these definitions. For example, they combined Method 1 and Method 2 in the Japanese guidance to form their Definition 1 for simultaneous consistency assessment as

$$\hat{\theta}_1 > \lambda\hat{\theta},\ \hat{\theta}_2 > \lambda\hat{\theta},\ \ldots,\ \hat{\theta}_K > \lambda\hat{\theta} \tag{3.2}$$

where $\hat{\theta}$ is the estimated (observed) overall treatment effect, $\hat{\theta}_i$ is the estimated treatment effect for country/region *i*, and λ (≥0) is a prespecified quantity. This definition also relies on only the observed treatment effects and is not in any formal hypothesis testing framework. Obviously, this definition includes Method 2 of the Japanese guidance (see Equation 3.1) as a special case with $\lambda = 0$ and is more stringent than Method 2.

Let *S* be a consistency statement. *P*(*S*) is called the assurance probability (Uesaka, 2009). The total sample size is determined by the desirable power of the overall effect. Given this total sample size, the sample size distribution across the regions also impacts the assurance probability for consistency assessment. In addition, consistency assessment is meaningful only when the overall treatment effect is significant. Therefore, for trial design, we may also be interested in the relationship between sample size distribution across the regions and the conditional probability of showing treatment effect consistency given a significant overall treatment effect.

Let

$$N_i/N = f_i \quad \text{and} \quad \theta_i/\theta = u_i \cdot \sum_{i=1}^{K} f_i = 1$$

Under the fixed-effect model,

$$\theta = \sum_{i=1}^{K} f_i\theta_i$$

Then

$$\sum_{i=1}^{K} u_i f_i = 1$$

When $u_i = 1$, the treatment effect in the *i*-th region is the same as the overall effect; if all u_i's are 1, the effects in all regions are identical. Quan, Li, Chen et al. (2010) provided the joint distribution for calculating the probability of Equation 3.2 and the corresponding conditional probability given the significant overall treatment effect. Results are summarized in Table 3.1, where the overall sample size is to detect the standardized overall treatment effect

TABLE 3.1

Unconditional and Conditional Probabilities (%) for Claiming Consistency Based on Equation 3.2

$(f_1, f_2, \ldots, f_K)$	$(u_1, u_2, \ldots, u_K)$	Uncond.	Cond.
	$K = 3, \lambda = 1/K = 1/3$		
(1/3,1/3,1/3)	(1,1,1)	76	81
(0.2,0.2,0.6)	(1,1,1)	69	73
(1/3,1/3,1/3)	(0.9,1,1.1)	75	80
(1/3,1/3,1/3)	(0.6,1.2,1.2)	65	69
(0.2,0.2,0.6)	(0.7, 0.7, 1.2)	49	53
(0.2,0.2,0.6)	(1.2, 1.1, 0.9)	76	80
(0.2,0.4,0.4)	(0.8,1.1,1)	68	72
(0.1,0.45,0.45)	(1.9,0.9,0.9)	80	85
	$K = 4, \lambda = 1/K = 1/4$		
(1/4,1/4,1/4,1/4)	(1,1,1,1)	64	69
(0.1,0.3,0.3,0.3)	(1,1,1,1)	60	65
(1/4,1/4,1/4,1/4)	(0.7,0.8,0.8,1.7)	51	55
(1/4,1/4,1/4,1/4)	(0.7,1.1,1.1,1.1)	61	66
(0.1,0.3,0.3,0.3)	(1.3,1,0.9,1)	64	69
(0.1,0.3,0.3,0.3)	(1.9,0.9,0.9,0.9)	67	72
(0.15,0.15,0.35,0.35)	(0.65,0.65,1.1,1.2)	44	48
(0.15,0.15,0.15,0.55)	(1.3,1.4,1.4,0.7)	70	75

Notes: One-sided $\alpha = 0.025$, $\beta = 0.90$, $\theta = 0.25$, $\sigma = 1$.

of $\theta = 0.25$ with a 90% power based on a one-sided test at a significance level of 0.025.

To ensure probability for consistency assessment based on Equation 3.2, λ should be a decreasing function of the number of regions due to the reduced sample sizes for individual regions and the multiplicity issue. For Table 3.1, $\lambda = 1/K$ is used. Even so, the assurance probability for $K = 4$ is still much smaller than that of $K = 3$. When true treatment effects for all regions are identical ($u_i = 1$), evenly distributing sample sizes among the regions will have the highest assurance probability. If one region has larger treatment effect, distributing fewer patients to that region so that more patients can be reserved for the other regions can actually increase the assurance probability.

A key characteristic for all the methods in this CAR setting is that each and every region is considered. The assessment of CAR is for making an appropriate inference and interpretation regarding the *overall treatment effect*. As long as consistency is demonstrated based on the prespecified criterion regardless of the type I or type II error rate, the overall treatment effect is usually applied to all regions even in some cases where a region yields a barely positive observed effect that is visually very different from the other regions with stronger results.

However, in discussing global trials, sometimes it is easy to mix CAR with the other type of consistency for ROI (see the next section for clarification) when considering an individual region's interest, thus causing confusion between the two distinct concepts of consistency. An example is the following statement: "By ensuring consistency of each region, it could be possible to appropriately extrapolate the result of full population to each region" (Ministry of Health, Labour and Welfare of Japan, 2007, p. 7). When only a specific ROI is the concern (such as Japan; Ministry of Health, Labour and Welfare of Japan, 2007), it is not necessary to consider each region unless assessment of the overall treatment is the objective in the discussion or when a random-effect model is used as a method in the discussion. But the previous example statement obviously was referring to neither scenario. Most authors would agree that treatment-by-region interaction is not the pivotal method of assessing consistency when using a global trial for making a specific ROI market application.

3.4 Consistency as a Method for Region-Specific Registration

After the overall treatment effect is demonstrated in a confirmatory global trial, a certain region or country may be of special interest (ROI) for marketing approval of the new drug. This is a common research aim shared by both bridging studies and global trials. The only difference is that for bridging studies, the CCDP already exists prior to the local bridging study, while for the global trial, all the data are collected concurrently under the same study protocol. In this scenario, showing consistency for ROI (i.e., CROI) between a specifically targeted country/region treatment effect, say, θ_T (i.e., a particular θ_i), and the overall treatment effect θ, is relevant as a method to demonstrate the treatment effect in the specific ROI directly or as a way of "bridging" (Shih, 2001, 2006). The assessment of CROI is not necessarily a universal document to be submitted to each and every regulatory agency around the world; rather, it is country/region-specific. The criterion for the CROI (see following for examples) is subject to negotiation and may vary from one ROI to another. Therefore, methods of assessing CROI should emphasize the consistency between a particular θ_T and θ, not among all $\{\theta_i, i = 1, \ldots, K\}$. For example, JPMDA Method 1 (Ministry of Health, Labour and Welfare of Japan, 2007) is for this type of consistency between the Japanese population (say, θ_J) and the entire population in the global trial (see the following sequel for its definition).

However, this is not to say that data from other participating countries or regions cannot contribute to the assessment. On the contrary, Bayesian or random-effect model approaches, which render shrinkage estimates by borrowing information from other participating countries or regions, have been advocated in the literature for this purpose (Ko, Tsou, Liu, and Hsiao, 2010; Liu, Hsiao, and Hsueh, 2002; Quan, Li, Shih et al., 2010).

Criteria that emphasize consistency between a country/region-specific treatment effect and the overall treatment effect have been proposed. Some examples suggested in Uesaka (2009), Shih (2001), and Ko et al. (2010) are given here and can be seen as quite different from the treatment-by-region interaction setting in Equation 3.1 or the simultaneous consistency assessment in Equation 3.2 as discussed in the previous section. Recall that $\hat{\theta}$ is the estimated (observed) overall treatment effect and $\hat{\theta}_i$ is the estimated treatment effect for country/region i (for which $i = T$ is for the particular ROI). Let $\bar{\theta}_T$ be the treatment effect excluding the specific country/region T and $\hat{\bar{\theta}}_T$ be its estimate. Positive sign implies favoring the investigational treatment. The following are six possible criteria of region/country T-specific consistency. For some threshold value $0 < \lambda < 1$:

$$\hat{\theta}_T \geq \lambda\hat{\theta}\ (> 0) \tag{i}$$

$$\hat{\theta}_T \geq \lambda\hat{\bar{\theta}}_T\ (>0) \tag{ii}$$

$$\lambda \leq \hat{\theta}_T / \hat{\theta} \leq 1/\lambda \tag{iii}$$

$$\lambda \leq \hat{\theta}_T / \hat{\bar{\theta}}_T \leq 1/\lambda \tag{iv}$$

$$\hat{\theta}_T \geq (1/\lambda)\min(\hat{\theta}_i;\ i = 1,\ldots,K, i \neq T) \tag{v}$$

$$g(\hat{\theta}_T \mid [\hat{\theta}_i;\ i = 1,\ldots,K, i \neq T]) \geq \text{a percentile of the distribution of} \tag{vi}$$

$$\{g(\hat{\theta}_j \mid [\hat{\theta}_i;\ i = 1,\ldots,K, i \neq j]);\ j = 1,\ldots,K, j \neq T\}$$

where $g(y|A)$ is the predictive probability of y given A.

Criteria (i)–(v) are discussed in Uesaka (2009) and Ko et al. (2010) for global trials. Usually, $\hat{\theta}$ is a weighted combination of $\hat{\theta}_T$ and $\hat{\bar{\theta}}_T$. Therefore, (ii) may be obtained from (i) through a new λ. An obvious deficiency for these (and Equation 3.1 and Equation 3.2) criteria/rules is that they are based on point estimates, not on confidence intervals. In contrast, criterion (vi) is predictive-distribution based and is a slight variant of the consistency criterion originally suggested by Shih (2001) in the bridging study framework, where the minimum instead of a percentile was specified on the right-hand side of the inequality. There is no universal regulation around the world for assessing CROI. Hence, the strategy of which criterion to use and what threshold value λ [for (i)–(v)] or percentile [for (vi)] to select is subject to negotiation between the specific ROI and the sponsor. For example, Japan in its JPMDA Method 1 recommends criterion (i) with $\lambda = 0.5$ or more.

Let S be a consistency statement chosen from (i)–(vi) above. $P(S)$ is the assurance probability (Uesaka, 2009). The proportion of sample size for the specific region of interest can be determined by requiring $P(S)$ to be at least x%. This minimum level of assurance probability is also subject to negotiation between the specific ROI and the sponsor. For example, the Japanese guidance requires enough patients from Japan to have at least 80% power for demonstrating treatment effect consistency for Japanese patients based on (i) when $\lambda = 0.5$.

Quan, Zhao, Zhang et al. (2010) derived a formula for sample size from Region T based on (i) under a general setting with a fixed-effect model without assuming the same treatment effects for all regions. When the true treatment effect for Region T equals the overall treatment effect, the proportion of patients from Region T has the following simple closed-form solution:

$$f_T = \frac{z_{\beta'}^2}{(z_\alpha + z_\beta)^2(1-\lambda)^2 + z_{\beta'}^2(2\lambda - \lambda^2)} \tag{3.3}$$

where z_a is the $(1-a) \times 100$ percentile of the standard normal distribution, the overall sample size is for $1-\beta$ overall power via a one-sided test at significance level α, and $1-\beta'$ is the desired assurance probability for (i). Clearly, f_T is an increasing function of λ but a decreasing function of β, α, and β'. Note that this fraction f_T remains the same no matter whether the trial has a balanced or imbalanced design.

Table 3.2 presents the required f_T for various parameter configurations. $P(S$ and significant positive overall treatment effect) = Ψ for criterion (i) is also provided in the table. For example, if $\lambda = 0.5$, $1-\beta = 0.9$, $\alpha = 0.025$, and $1-\beta' = 0.8$, then $f_T = 22.4\%$. Thus, in such a case, if there are five or more regions/countries, it will be impossible to satisfy simultaneously all their demands. If $\lambda = 0.7$, $1-\beta = 0.9$, and $1-\beta' = 0.8$, f_T is as high as 44.5%. Therefore, the increase in λ has a big impact on f_T. Also shown in Table 3.2, for criterion (i), $\Psi = P(S$ and significant positive overall treatment effect) is generally very close to $P(S|\theta_T = \theta) \times P(\text{significant positive overall treatment effect}|\theta) = (1-\beta')(1-\beta)$. Hence, the conditional probability $P(S|\text{significant positive overall treatment effect})$ is also close to $P(S)$. Results of required proportions of patients for Region T to reach the desired $P(S)$ when θ_T is slightly different from θ can be found in Quan, Zhao, Zhang et al. (2010).

As we can see, criteria (i)–(vi) focus on consistency assessment for a specific Region T and ignore the assessments for the other regions. This posts no difficulty for a bridging study with a ROI, which is conducted after the CCDP is completed. But with a global trial, if any of the criteria is specified in the study protocol for a specific ROI, the protocol may encounter objections by the health authorities of other regions that may prefer other criteria.

TABLE 3.2

Values of f_T and Ψ when $\theta_T = \theta$

λ	$1-\beta$	$1-\beta'$	f_T	$(1-\beta)(1-\beta')$	Ψ
0.5	0.90	0.80	0.224	0.720	0.735
0.5	0.95	0.80	0.187	0.760	0.768
0.5	0.90	0.85	0.313	0.765	0.781
0.5	0.95	0.85	0.265	0.808	0.816
0.5	0.90	0.90	0.426	0.810	0.826
0.5	0.95	0.90	0.367	0.855	0.864
0.6	0.90	0.80	0.311	0.720	0.735
0.6	0.95	0.80	0.265	0.760	0.768
0.6	0.90	0.85	0.416	0.765	0.781
0.6	0.95	0.85	0.360	0.808	0.816
0.6	0.90	0.90	0.537	0.810	0.826
0.6	0.95	0.90	0.475	0.855	0.864
0.7	0.90	0.80	0.445	0.720	0.735
0.7	0.95	0.80	0.390	0.760	0.768
0.7	0.90	0.85	0.559	0.765	0.781
0.7	0.95	0.85	0.500	0.808	0.816
0.7	0.90	0.90	0.673	0.810	0.826
0.7	0.95	0.90	0.616	0.855	0.864

Note: One-sided $\alpha = 0.025$.

Therefore, the adoption of any of these criteria for a global trial needs to be considered through negotiation with individual regions at the design stage to enroll appropriate numbers of patients from the regions. On the other hand, these criteria can be used for post hoc exploratory analyses of consistency. Recently, two-stage designs for specific region of interest have also been proposed (Luo, Shih, Ouyang, and DeLap, 2010; Wang, 2009). When the observed treatment effect of a specific region from the original global trial fails to meet the prespecified consistency criteria, additional data may be obtained from the region through a follow-up trial. The sample size for this follow-up trial can be determined based on the conditional power given the observed results from the earlier global trial. Data from the original global trial and the follow-up trial can be combined for consistency assessment based on perhaps a new criterion via the negotiation with the health authority.

The estimate of treatment effects in the aforementioned consistency criteria depends on the statistical model and methods used in the analysis of the primary endpoint. The drawback of a fixed-effect model is that, as mentioned previously, the overall treatment effect depends on proportions of sample sizes, which are trial specific. For a bridging study with CCPD or a global study, it is necessary to consider possible but unrecognized heterogeneity among regions caused by ethnic or environmental factors. Therefore, a random effect or frailty model or Bayesian approach in general, which express this variation among regions, is preferred. Under a random-effect model (Quan, Li, Shih et al., 2010) or a Bayesian approach, the overall treatment effect is the mean of the random individual treatment effects of the regions, and hence, not sample-size dependent. The derived shrinkage estimate of θ_T borrows information from all other regions and is a weighted average of the estimate of the regional treatment effect using its own data alone and the overall treatment effect using all the data. It is closer to the estimate of the overall treatment effect and has smaller variability. Therefore, the use of such an estimate makes it much easier to demonstrate consistency.

3.5 Other Considerations

Issues with bridging studies are discussed in other chapters. For consistency assessment in a global trial, besides what has been discussed, other issues should be kept in mind when we design and conduct a global trial. We discuss these in this section.

3.5.1 Time-to-Event and Binary Endpoints

Bridging studies are mostly short-term and, relatively speaking, small sample size. Global trials, however, are often long-term and require a large number of patients (as one of the reasons to conduct it globally). Hence, using time to event as the primary endpoint would not be an unusual scenario for a global trial. For a time-to-event endpoint, the number of events (not directly the sample size) is the index of the quantity of information. It is anticipated for a global trial that the trial initiations for all regions are at about the same time. However, if certain regions have delayed enrollment of patients until much later than other regions, to reach the desired numbers of events for these regions to ensure power for consistency assessment, relatively larger sample sizes should be assigned to these regions. Otherwise, the completion of the trial will be delayed if we wait until all regions reach their targeted numbers of events. A formula for the relationships between sample size, enrollment curve, study duration, and the number of events for individual regions should be used for more precise study planning (Quan, Li, Shih et al., 2010; Quan, Zhao et al., 2010).

For a binary endpoint, even when the treatment effects (measured either through the difference of rates, ratio of rates, or odds ratio) are similar across regions, the event rates for individual treatment groups can still be very different across regions due to the differences in intrinsic and extrinsic factors. Since the variances of the estimates of the treatment effects of individual regions depend on these event rates, the calculation of power for consistency assessment for trial design will be much more complicated.

Care should be exercised when we plan a global trial with a binary endpoint as the primary endpoint.

3.5.2 Noninferiority Trial

For a noninferiority trial, the true treatment effect or the estimate of the treatment effect of the experimental drug compared with the control can be very close to zero. Thus, many definitions for consistency assessment for superiority trials relying on preserving certain proportion of the overall treatment effect for individual regions may not be applicable to noninferiority trials. The quantitative or qualitative interaction test for a noninferiority trial is also different from that for a superiority trial. Thus, we have to use another interaction test that is suitable for noninferiority trials if we want to apply an interaction test for CAR assessment. After certain modifications, some other definitions for consistency assessment for superiority trials can be applied to noninferiority trials. For example, Method 2 in the Japanese guidance can be applied to noninferiority trials after replacing the zero lower bound by the noninferiority margin (Quan, Li, Chen et al., 2010). In addition, we can replace the observed overall treatment effect by zero or even the noninferiority margin in the funnel plot discussed in Hung, Wang, and O'Neill (2010) and Chen et al. (2010).

3.5.3 MRCT Monitoring

Ongoing blinded trial monitoring during a study is an essential component of trial conduct to ensure the high quality of the trial and data integrity. Special attention should be paid when monitoring an MRCT to anticipate potential sources of inconsistency of treatment effects across regions when the unblinded analysis is performed. During monitoring, we have to ensure investigators from all regions uniformly follow the protocol including the inclusion and exclusion criteria. Any systematic deviation from the protocol or inclusion–exclusion criteria made by some of the regions should be corrected promptly. Missing data rates and patterns should also be evaluated to ensure consistent data quality across regions. If certain patient characteristics are very different across regions and these characteristics have known impact on treatment effect (e.g., imbalance in use of concomitant medication), the overall sample size or distribution of sample sizes across regions may need adjustment to have enough information to address potential questions from regulatory agencies. Any trial adjustments or modifications based on blinded data review during the trial will not create bias for treatment effect assessment and, therefore, are likely to be acceptable by regulatory agencies (FDA guidance on adaptive designs). For sequential MRCTs, robustness of trial results and consistency of treatment effects should be verified before trial early stopping.

3.6 Example

A multiregional trial was designed to evaluate the effect of an investigational drug on change from baseline in HbA_{1c}. To have more safety data for the investigational drug, the trial used an unbalanced design, allocating patients in a 2-to-1 ratio to receiving either the active treatment or the matched placebo. Also, the study was overpowered with regard to efficacy to obtain an amount of safety data required for regulatory purposes. With 558 patients, 186 receiving placebo and 372 in the active treatment group, there was > 99% power to detect a between-treatment difference of $\delta = 0.005$ with $\sigma = 0.013$ for a significance level $\alpha = 0.025$ one-sided test.

At the design stage, we would like to determine the minimum required proportion of sample size for a particular region (e.g., Region 1) so that there will be an 80% probability of demonstrating CAR based on Equation 3.2. Table 3.3 shows such proportion f_1 when there are four regions in total and the region effect sizes are assumed equal. For example, if the sample sizes of the other three regions are the same ($f_1 < f_2 = f_3 = f_4$) and if the conditional probability is the concern, then using Equation 3.2 with $\lambda = 1/K = ¼$, f_1 should be 13%, that is, 13% of all patients should be in the minimum region, Region 1; and around 29% of all patients should be in each of the other three regions. Values of f_1 for other scenarios could also be easily derived.

If one specific region, say, Region T, is the focus and CROI criterion (i) is used for consistency assessment, assuming equal treatment effects for the regions, we first calculate f_T using the formula of Equation 3.3 and results are provided in Table 3.4. As mentioned earlier, f_T remains the same for both balanced and imbalanced designs. Because of the high power for the overall treatment effect assessment, the proportions provided in Table 3.4 are smaller than those presented in Table 3.2. We then multiply the overall sample sizes for the two treatment groups by f_T to get the sample sizes for Region T. For $\lambda = 0.5$ and $1 - \beta' = 0.8$, the sample sizes for Region T are 26 and 51 (or 52 to satisfy the 2:1 ratio) for the placebo and active treatment groups, respectively. If $1 - \beta'$ is increased from 0.8 to 0.9, the sample sizes for Region T need to be approximately doubled.

TABLE 3.3

The Minimum f_1 to Have an 80% Probability of Showing Consistency Based on Equation 3.2

	Uncond.	Cond.
$f_1 < f_2 = f_3 = f_4$	0.14	0.13
$f_1 = f_2 < f_3 = f_4$	0.18	0.17
$f_1 = f_2 = f_3 < f_4$	0.20	0.20

Note: $K = 4$.

TABLE 3.4
Sample Size for Region T in a HbA_{1c} Trial

			N_T Based on f_T	
λ	$1-\beta'$	f_T	Placebo	Treatment
0.5	0.80	0.138	26	51
0.5	0.85	0.199	37	74
0.5	0.90	0.282	52	105
0.6	0.80	0.200	37	75
0.6	0.85	0.280	52	104
0.6	0.90	0.380	71	141
0.7	0.80	0.308	57	115
0.7	0.85	0.408	76	152
0.7	0.90	0.522	97	194

3.7 Discussion

This chapter discusses assessment of consistency in bridging studies and global multiregional trials. A bridging study is conducted in a specific country/region of interest (ROI) after the medicine is already approved for marketing in other ICH regions and the large complete clinical data package is readily available. A bridging study may be a small-scale pharmacokinetic (PK)/pharmacodynamic (PD) study or, when deemed necessary by the specific ROI (often the case), a study with the same primary clinical endpoint as in the phase III study contained in the CCDP. A global multiregional study trial, on the other hand, includes many countries/regions in the same megastudy under the same study protocol simultaneously. The goal of a bridging study is to show that the treatment effect in the ROI is consistent with that shown in the CCDP. This is clear. However, in a global multiregional study, consistency of treatment effects is of two different kinds since there are many regions involved, and any can be the ROI at the design stage. One kind is consistency across/among all regions (CAR), and the other is consistency for the specific region of interest (CROI). CAR is essential for the overall effect to be meaningful. CROI is the basis for thing as the marketing application for the specific country/region. It would be logical that CAR is more stringent and implies CROI. However, this may not be so if the specific ROI poses a different criterion of consistency. After all, there is no such thing as a global submission for approval and every marketing authorization is handled by each country/region individually. This is a fundamental challenge for the global multiregional trial. At the design stage with only one global trial protocol, all regions are treated equally, and the premise is that there is no substantial difference in treatment effect among countries/regions to plan for the regional sample size distribution and the total sample size to show the meaningful overall treatment effect.

Therefore, it is difficult to have different criteria for consistency for any specific region in one protocol. However, for some criteria, it is impossible to accommodate all regions the same if the number of regions becomes large. When data are analyzed and results are submitted to each country/region, the ROI may have the right to require its own consistency criterion to be satisfied, however ad hoc it may be.

Because the assessments of consistency all involve some sort of comparison of data between the ROI and other regions, there is an underlying assumption of exchangeability under the null hypothesis of consistency. The global trial setting, although it poses more challenges with the study design and conduct, has better assurance of exchangeability than the bridging study strategy, since it is conducted under the same protocol simultaneously. Also, the within-country variances are likely to be different from region to region. To further improve the exchangeability, multilevel hierarchical Bayesian or stratified random effects modeling can be used, especially when more countries in regions are included in the trial. This is a topic for future research. Methods for this topic are still evolving, and it is our hope that the discussions in this chapter provide some assistance to the manufacturers and the regulatory authorizes in clarifying the concept and issues with current methods of assessment for consistency in the treatment effect for bridging studies and global multiregional trials.

References

Chen, J., Quan, H., Binkowitz, B., Ouyang, S. P., Tanaka, Y., Li, G. et al. (2010). Assessing consistent treatment effect in a multi-regional clinical trial: A systematic review. *Pharmaceutical Statistics*, 9: 242–253.

Hung, H. M. J., Wang, S. J., and O'Neill, R. T. (2010). Consideration of regional difference in design and analysis of multi-regional trials. *Pharmaceutical Statistics*, 9: 173–178.

International Conference on Harmonisation (ICH). (1998a). Tripartite guidance E5 ethnic factor in the acceptability of foreign data. *US Federal Register*, 83, 31790–31796.

International Conference on Harmonisation. (ICH). (1998b). Tripartite guidance E9 statistical principles for clinical trials. *US Federal Register*, Section V.G. 33–34.

Kawai, N., Chuang-Stein, C., Komiyama, O., and Li, Y. (2007). An approach to rationalize partitioning sample size into individual regions in a multiregional trial. *Drug Information Journal*, 42: 139–147.

Ko, F. S., Tsou, H. H., Liu, J. P., and Hsiao, C. F. (2010). Sample size determination for a specific region in a multiregional trial. *Journal of Biopharmaceutical Statistics*, 20(4): 870–885.

Liu, J. P., Hsiao, C. F., and Hsueh, H. M. (2002). Bayesian approach to evaluation of bridging studies. *Journal of Biopharmaceutical Statistics*, 44: 969–981.

Luo, X., Shih, W. J., Ouyang, S. P., and DeLap, R. J. (2010). An optimal adaptive design to address local regulations in global clinical trials. *Pharmaceutical Statistics*, 9: 179–189.

Ministry of Health, Labour and Welfare of Japan. (2007). Basic principles on global clinical trials. Notification No. 0928010, September 28.

Quan, H., Li, M., Chen, J., Gallo, P., Binkowitz, B., Ibia, E. et al. (2010). Assessment of consistency of treatment effects in multiregional clinical trials. *Drug Information Journal*, 44: 617–632.

Quan, H., Li, M., Shih, W. J., Ouyang, S. P., Chen, S., Zhang, J. et al. (2010). Empirical shrinkage estimator for consistency assessment of treatment effects in multiregional clinical trials. Sanofi-Aventis Technical Report #48.

Quan, H., Zhao, P. L., Zhang, J., Roessner, M., and Aizawa, K. (2010). Sample size considerations for Japanese patients in a multi-regional trial based on MHLW guidance. *Pharmaceutical Statistics*, 9: 100–112.

Shih, W. J. (2001). Clinical trials for drug registrations in Asian-Pacific countries: Proposal for a new paradigm from a statistical perspective. *Controlled Clinical Trials*, 22: 357–366.

Shih, W. J. (2006). From bridging studies to global trial development. Paper presented at the FDA/Pharmaceutical Industry Annual Conference, Washington DC, September 29.

Uesaka, H. (2009). Sample size allocation to regions in a multiregional trial. *Journal of Biopharmaceutical Statistics*, 19: 580–594.

Wang, S. J. (2009). Bridging study versus prespecified regions nested in global trials. *Drug Information Journal*, 43: 27–34.

4

Assessing Similarity Using the Reproducibility and Generalizability Probabilities and the Sensitivity Index

Shein-Chung Chow
Duke University

Ying Lu
Beijing University of Technology

Lan-Yan Yang
National Cheng Kung University

4.1 Introduction

In clinical research and development, it is well recognized that ethnic factors may have significant influence on clinical outcomes for evaluation of efficacy and safety of study medications under investigation, especially when the sponsor is interested in bringing an approved drug product from the original region (e.g., the United States or the European Union) to a new region (e.g., Asia-Pacific region). To determine if clinical data generated from the original region are acceptable in the new region, the International Conference on Harmonisation (ICH) issued a guideline titled "Ethnic Factors in the Acceptability of Foreign Clinical Data" in 1998. The purpose of this guideline is not only to permit adequate evaluation of the influence of ethnic factors but also to minimize duplication of clinical studies in the new region.

As indicated in the previous chapter, the ICH guideline suggests the regulatory authority of the new region to assess the ability to extrapolate foreign data based on the bridging data package. The bridging package typically includes (1) information including pharmacokinetic (PK) data and any preliminary pharmacodynamic (PD) and dose-response data from the complete clinical data package (CCDP) that is relevant to the population of the new region and (2) if needed, a bridging study to extrapolate the foreign efficacy data or safety data to the new region. Bridging studies are necessary if the study medicines are ethnically sensitive since the populations in two regions are different. In the ICH guideline, however, no criteria are provided for assessing the sensitivity to ethnic factors for determining whether a bridging study is needed. Moreover, when a bridging study is conducted, the ICH guideline indicates that the study is readily interpreted as capable of bridging the foreign data if it shows that dose response, safety, and efficacy in the new region are similar to those in the original region. However, the ICH guideline does not clearly define the similarity in terms of dose response, safety, and efficacy between the original region and a new region.

In practice, similarity is often interpreted as *equivalence* or *comparability* between the original region and the new region. However, there exists no universal agreement regarding similarity. In the past decade, several criteria for assessing similarity have been proposed in the literature (see, e.g., Chow, Shao, and Hu, 2002; Hsiao, Xu, and Liu, 2003, 2005; Hung, 2003; Hung, Wang, Tsong, Lawrence, and O'Neil, 2003; Liu and Chow, 2002; Shih, 2001). During this time, several statistical methods have also been proposed. This chapter focuses on assessing similarity by testing the reproducibility and generalizability probability proposed by Shao and Chow (2002). In addition, similarity between regions will be assessed based on the sensitivity index suggested by Chow et al. (2002).

In the next section, several criteria for assessing similarity are briefly reviewed. Statistical methods for assessing similarity by testing using the reproducibility and generalizability probability are introduced in Section 4.3. Section 4.4 discusses statistical methods for assessing similarity using the sensitivity index to determine possible population shifts between the original region and a new region. Some concluding remarks are given in the final section.

4.2 Criteria for Assessing Similarity

Shih (2001) interpreted similarity as *consistency* among study centers by treating the new region as a new center of multicenter clinical trials. Under this definition, the assessment of consistency can be used to determine whether the study is capable of bridging the foreign data to the new region. In other words, if there is statistical evidence of consistency (e.g., in terms of effect size) among the centers, we conclude that the foreign data can be bridged to the new region.

Shao and Chow (2002) proposed the concepts of *reproducibility* and *generalizability* probabilities for assessing similarity in bridging studies. If the influence of the ethnic factors is negligible, then we may consider the reproducibility probability to determine whether the clinical results observed in the original region are reproducible in the new region. If there is a notable ethnic difference, the generalizability probability can be assessed to determine whether the clinical results in the original region can be generalized in a similar but slightly different patient population due to the difference in ethnic factors.

In addition, Chow et al. (2002) proposed to assess similarity using a *sensitivity index*, which is a measure of possible shift from one patient population (the original region) to another (a new region), assuming that the shift (location, scale, or both) in population is due to ethnic differences. If the sensitivity index falls within a prespecified range, we conclude that the foreign (the original region) data can be bridged to the new region.

On the other hand, Hung (2003) and Hung et al. (2003) suggested assessing similarity by testing for *noninferiority* based on bridging studies conducted in the new region compared with those previously conducted in the original region. This method, however, raises the question of how to select the noninferiority margin (Chow and Shao, 2006).

Under different interpretations of similarity, several methods have been proposed in the literature. For example, Shih (2001) derived a way to test for consistency among study centers under a statistical model by treating the new region as a new center of a multicenter trial. Liu, Hsueh, Hsieh, and Chen (2002) used a hierarchical model approach to incorporating the foreign bridging information into the data generated by the bridging study in the new region. Lan, Soo, Siu, and Wang (2005) introduced the weighted Z-tests in which the weights may depend on the prior observed data for the design of bridging studies. Hsiao, Hsu, Tsou, and Liu (2007) then proposed a Bayesian approach with the use of a mixture prior for assessment of similarity between the new and original regions based on the concept of positive treatment effect.

4.3 Reproducibility and Generalizability

As indicated in the previous section, Shao and Chow (2002) proposed considering the reproducibility to determine whether the clinical results observed in the original region are reproducible in the new region if there is no evidence of ethnic influence on clinical outcomes. When there is a notable ethnic difference, the authors suggested assessing the generalizability probability to determine whether the clinical results in the original region can be generalized in a similar but slightly different patient population due to the difference in ethnic factors. In what follows, Shao and Chow's statistical tests for the reproducibility and generalizability probabilities are briefly introduced.

4.3.1 Test for Reproducibility

Under the assumption that the ethnic difference is negligible, as suggested by Shao and Chow (2002), we may test for reproducibility probability to assess similarity between clinical results from a bridging study and studies conducted in the CCPD. Shao and Chow proposed three methods: the estimated power approach, the confidence bound approach, and the Bayesian approach for assessing the reproducibility probability. They are briefly described in the following sections. Note that these methods can be directly applied to assess similarity of clinical data between the original region and a new region.

4.3.1.1 Estimated Power Approach

To study the reproducibility probability, we need to specify the test procedure, that is, the form of the test statistic, T. We will first consider the case of two samples with equal variances. Suppose that a total of $n = n_1 + n_2$ patients are randomly assigned to two groups, a treatment group and a control group. In the treatment group, n_1 patients receive the treatment (or a test drug) and produce responses $x_{11}, \ldots, x_{1n_1}$. In the control group, n_2 patients receive the placebo (or a reference drug) and produce responses $x_{21}, \ldots, x_{2n_2}$. This design is a typical two-group parallel design in clinical trials. We assume that x_{ij}'s are independent and normally distributed with means μ_i, $i = 1,2$, and a common variance σ^2. Suppose that the hypotheses of interest are

$$H_0 : \mu_1 - \mu_2 = 0 \quad versus \quad H_a : \mu_1 - \mu_2 \neq 0 \tag{4.1}$$

The discussion for a one-sided is similar. Consider the commonly used two-sample t-test, which rejects H_0 if and only if $|T| > t_{0.975,n-2}$, where $t_{0.975,n-2}$ is the 97.5th percentile of the t-distribution with $n - 2$ degrees of freedom

$$T = \frac{\bar{x}_1 - \bar{x}_2}{\sqrt{\dfrac{(n_1 - 1)s_1^2 + (n_2 - 1)s_2^2}{n-2}}\sqrt{\left(\dfrac{1}{n_1} + \dfrac{1}{n_2}\right)}} \tag{4.2}$$

and are, respectively, the sample mean and variance based on the data from the i-th treatment group. The power of T for the second trial is

$$\begin{aligned} p(\theta) &= P(|T(y)| > t_{0.975,n-2}) \\ &= 1 - \Im_{n-2}(t_{0.975,n-2} \mid \theta) + \Im_{n-2}(-t_{0.975,n-2} \mid \theta) \end{aligned} \tag{4.3}$$

where

$$\theta = \frac{\mu_1 - \mu_2}{\sigma\sqrt{\left(\frac{1}{n_1} + \frac{1}{n_2}\right)}} \tag{4.4}$$

and $\Im_{n-2}(\bullet \mid \theta)$ denotes the distribution function of the noncentral t-distribution with $n - 2$ degrees of freedom and the noncentrality parameter θ. Note that $p(\theta) = p(|\theta|)$.

Values of $p(\theta)$ as a function of $|\theta|$ are provided in Table 4.1. Using the idea of replacing θ by its estimate $T(x)$, which is defined by Equation 4.2, we obtain the following reproducibility probability:

$$\hat{P} = 1 - \Im_{n-2}(t_{0.975,n-2} \mid T(x)) + \Im_{n-2}(-t_{0.975,n-2} \mid T(x)) \tag{4.5}$$

which is a function of $|T(x)|$. When $|T(x)| > t_{0.975,n-2}$

$$\hat{P} \approx \begin{cases} 1 - \Im_{n-2}(t_{0.975,n-2} \mid T(x)) & \textit{if } T(x) > 0 \\ \Im_{n-2}(-t_{0.975,n-2} \mid T(x)) & \textit{if } T(x) < 0 \end{cases} \tag{4.6}$$

If $\Im_{n-2}$ is replaced by the normal distribution and $t_{0.975,n-2}$ is replaced by the normal percentile, then Equation 4.6 is the same as that in Goodman (1992), who studied the case where the variance σ^2 is known. Table 4.1 can be used to find the reproducibility probability $\hat{P}$ in Equation 4.6 with a fixed sample size n. For example, if $T(x) = 2.9$ was observed in a clinical trial with $n = n_1 + n_2 = 40$, then the reproducibility probability is 0.807. If was observed in a clinical trial with $n = 36$, then an extrapolation of the results in Table 4.1 (for $n = 30$ and 40) leads to a reproducibility probability of 0.803.

Now, consider the case of two samples with unequal variances. Consider the problem of testing the hypotheses in Equation 4.1 under the two-group parallel design without the assumption of equal variances. That is, x_{ij}'s are independently distributed as $N(\mu_i, \sigma_i^2), i = 1, 2$. When $\sigma_1^2 \neq \sigma_2^2$, there exists no exact testing procedure for the hypotheses in Equation 4.1. When both n_1 and n_2 are large, an approximate 5% level test rejects H_0 when $|T| > z_{0.975}$ where

$$T = \frac{\bar{x}_1 - \bar{x}_2}{\sqrt{\left(\frac{s_1^2}{n_1} + \frac{s_2^2}{n_2}\right)}} \tag{4.7}$$

Since T is approximately distributed as $N(\theta,1)$ with

TABLE 4.1

Values of the Power Function in Equation 4.3

	Total Sample Size							
θ	10	20	30	40	50	60	100	∞
1.96	0.407	0.458	0.473	0.480	0.484	0.487	0.492	0.500
2.02	0.429	0.481	0.496	0.504	0.508	0.511	0.516	0.524
2.08	0.448	0.503	0.519	0.527	0.531	0.534	0.540	0.548
2.14	0.469	0.526	0.542	0.550	0.555	0.557	0.563	0.571
2.20	0.490	0.549	0.565	0.573	0.578	0.581	0.586	0.594
2.26	0.511	0.571	0.588	0.596	0.601	0.604	0.609	0.618
2.32	0.532	0.593	0.610	0.618	0.623	0.626	0.632	0.640
2.38	0.552	0.615	0.632	0.640	0.645	0.648	0.654	0.662
2.44	0.573	0.636	0.654	0.662	0.667	0.670	0.676	0.684
2.50	0.593	0.657	0.675	0.683	0.688	0.691	0.697	0.705
2.56	0.613	0.678	0.695	0.704	0.708	0.711	0.717	0.725
2.62	0.632	0.698	0.715	0.724	0.728	0.731	0.737	0.745
2.68	0.652	0.717	0.735	0.743	0.747	0.750	0.756	0.764
2.74	0.671	0.736	0.753	0.761	0.766	0.769	0.774	0.782
2.80	0.690	0.754	0.771	0.779	0.783	0.786	0.792	0.799
2.86	0.708	0.772	0.788	0.796	0.800	0.803	0.808	0.815
2.92	0.725	0.789	0.805	0.812	0.816	0.819	0.824	0.830
2.98	0.742	0.805	0.820	0.827	0.831	0.834	0.839	0.845
3.04	0.759	0.820	0.835	0.842	0.846	0.848	0.853	0.860
3.10	0.775	0.834	0.849	0.856	0.859	0.862	0.866	0.872
3.16	0.790	0.848	0.862	0.868	0.872	0.874	0.879	0.884
3.22	0.805	0.861	0.874	0.881	0.884	0.886	0.890	0.895
3.28	0.819	0.873	0.886	0.892	0.895	0.897	0.901	0.906
3.34	0.832	0.884	0.897	0.902	0.905	0.907	0.911	0.916
3.40	0.844	0.895	0.907	0.912	0.915	0.917	0.920	0.925
3.46	0.856	0.905	0.916	0.921	0.924	0.925	0.929	0.932
3.52	0.868	0.914	0.925	0.929	0.932	0.933	0.936	0.940
3.58	0.879	0.923	0.933	0.937	0.939	0.941	0.943	0.947
3.64	0.889	0.931	0.940	0.944	0.946	0.947	0.950	0.953
3.70	0.898	0.938	0.946	0.950	0.952	0.953	0.956	0.959
3.76	0.907	0.944	0.952	0.956	0.958	0.959	0.961	0.965
3.82	0.915	0.950	0.958	0.961	0.963	0.964	0.966	0.969
3.88	0.923	0.956	0.963	0.966	0.967	0.968	0.970	0.973
3.94	0.930	0.961	0.967	0.970	0.971	0.972	0.974	0.977

Source: Chow, S. C., J. Shao, and O. Y. P. Hu, *Journal of Biopharmaceutical Statistics*, 12, 385–400, 2002. With permission.

$$\theta = \frac{\mu_1 - \mu_2}{\sqrt{\left(\frac{\sigma_1^2}{n_1} + \frac{\sigma_2^2}{n_2}\right)}} \tag{4.8}$$

the reproducibility probability obtained by using the estimated power approach is given by

$$\hat{P} = \Phi(T(x) - z_{0.975}) + \Phi(-T(x) - z_{0.975}) \tag{4.9}$$

When the variances under different treatments are different and the sample sizes are not large, a different study design such as a matched-pair parallel design or a 2 × 2 crossover design is recommended. A matched-pair parallel design involves pairs of matched patients. One patient in each pair is assigned to the treatment group, and the other is assigned to the control group. Let x_{ij} be the observation from the j-th pair and the i-th group. It is assumed that the differences $x_{1j} - x_{2j}$, $j = 1,\ldots,m$, are independent and identically distributed as $N(\mu_1 - \mu_2, \sigma_D^2)$. Then, the null hypothesis H_0 is rejected at the 5% level of significance if $|T| > t_{0.975,m-1}$, where

$$T = \frac{\sqrt{m}\left(\bar{x}_1 - \bar{x}_2\right)}{\hat{\sigma}_D} \tag{4.10}$$

and $\hat{\sigma}_D$ is the sample standard deviation based on the differences $x_{1j} - x_{2j}$, $j = 1,\ldots m$. Note that T has the noncentral t-distribution with $m - 1$ degrees of freedom and the noncentrality parameter

$$\theta = \frac{\sqrt{m}\left(\mu_1 - \mu_2\right)}{\sigma_D} \tag{4.11}$$

Consequently, the reproducibility probability obtained by using the estimated power approach is given by Equation 4.5 with T defined by Equation 4.10 and $n - 2$ replaced by $m - 1$.

Suppose that the study design is a 2 × 2 cross-over design in which n_1 patients receive the treatment at the first period and the placebo at the second period and n_2 patients receive the placebo at the first period and the treatment at the second period. Let x_{lij} be the normally distributed observation from the j-th patient at the i-th period and l-th sequence. Then the treatment effect μ_D can be estimated without bias by

$$\hat{\mu}_D = \frac{\bar{x}_{11} - \bar{x}_{12} - \bar{x}_{21} + \bar{x}_{22}}{2} \sim N\left(\mu_D, \frac{\sigma_D^2}{4}\left(\frac{1}{n_1} + \frac{1}{n_2}\right)\right)$$

where $\bar{x}_{li}$ is the sample mean based on x_{lij}, $j = 1,\ldots,m$, and An unbiased estimator of $\hat{\sigma}_D^2$ is

$$\hat{\sigma}_D^2 = \frac{1}{n_1 + n_2 - 2} \sum_{l=1}^{2} \sum_{j=1}^{m} (x_{l1j} - x_{l2j} - \bar{x}_{l1} + \bar{x}_{l2})^2$$

which is independent of $\hat{\mu}_D$ and distributed as $\sigma_D^2/(n_1 + n_2 - 2)$ times the chi-square distribution with $n_1 + n_2 - 2$ degrees of freedom. Thus, the null hypothesis H_0:$\mu_D = 0$ is rejected at the 5% level of significance if $|T| > t_{0.975,n-2}$, where $n = n_1 + n_2$ and

$$T = \frac{\hat{\mu}_D}{\frac{\hat{\sigma}_D}{2}\sqrt{\left(\frac{1}{n_1} + \frac{1}{n_2}\right)}} \tag{4.12}$$

Note that T has the noncentral t-distribution with n–2 degrees of freedom and the noncentrality parameter

$$\theta = \frac{\mu_D}{\frac{\sigma_D}{2}\sqrt{\left(\frac{1}{n_1} + \frac{1}{n_2}\right)}} \tag{4.13}$$

Consequently, the reproducibility probability obtained by using the estimated power approach is given by Equation 4.5 with T defined by Equation 4.12.

4.3.1.2 Confidence Bound Approach

Since $\hat{P}$ in Equation 4.5 or Equation 4.9 is an estimated power, it provides a rather optimistic result. Alternatively, we may consider a more conservative approach, which considers a 95% lower confidence bound of the power as the reproducibility probability. Consider first the case of the two-group parallel design with a common unknown variance σ^2. Note that $T(x)$ has the noncentral t-distribution with n–2 degrees of freedom and the noncentrality parameter θ given by Equation 4.4. Let $\Im_{n-2}(t|\theta)$ be the distribution function of $T(x)$ for any given θ. It can be shown that $\Im_{n-2}(t|\theta)$ is a strictly decreasing function of θ for any fixed t. Consequently, a 95% confidence interval for θ is given by$(\hat{\theta}_-, \hat{\theta}_+)$, where $\hat{\theta}_-$ is the unique solution of $\Im_{n-2}(T(x)|\theta) = 0.975$, and $\hat{\theta}_+$

is the unique solution of $\Im_{n-2}(T(x)|\theta) = 0.025$ (see, e.g., Shao, 1999, Theorem 7.1). Then, a 95% lower confidence bound for $|\theta|$ is

$$|\hat{\theta}|_- = \begin{cases} \hat{\theta}_- & \text{if } \hat{\theta}_- > 0 \\ -\hat{\theta}_+ & \text{if } \hat{\theta}_+ < 0 \\ 0 & \text{if } \hat{\theta}_- \le 0 \le \hat{\theta}_+ \end{cases} \tag{4.14}$$

and a 95% lower confidence bound for the power in Equation 4.3 is

$$\hat{P}_- = 1 - \Im_{n-2}(t_{0.975,n-2} \,||\hat{\theta}|_-) + \Im_{n-2}(-t_{0.975,n-2} \,||\hat{\theta}|_-) \tag{4.15}$$

if $|\hat{\theta}|_- > 0$ and $\hat{P}_- = 0$ if $|\hat{\theta}|_- = 0$. The lower confidence bound in Equation 4.15 is useful when the clinical result from the first trial is highly significant.

Table 4.2 contains values of the lower confidence bound $|\hat{\theta}|_-$ corresponding to $|T(x)|$ values ranging from 4.5 to 6.5. If $4.5 \le |T(x)| \le 6.5$ and the value of $|\hat{\theta}|_-$ is found from Table 4.2, the reproducibility probability $\hat{P}_-$ in Equation 4.15 can be obtained from Table 4.1. For example, suppose that $|T(x)| = 5$ was observed from a clinical trial with $n = 30$. From Table 4.2, $|\hat{\theta}|_- = 5$. Then, by Table 4.1, $\hat{P}_- = 0.709$.

Consider next the two-group parallel design with unequal variances σ_1^2 and σ_2^2. When both n_1 and n_2 are large, T given by Equation 4.7 is approximately distributed as $N(\theta,1)$ with θ given by Equation 4.8. Hence, the reproducibility probability obtained by using the lower confidence bound approach is given by

$$\hat{P}_- = \Phi(|T(x)| - 2z_{0.975})$$

with T defined by Equation 4.7.

4.3.1.3 Bayesian Approach

In practice, the reproducibility probability can be viewed as the posterior mean (see, e.g., Berger, 1985) of the power function $p(\theta) = P(|T| > c|\theta)$ for the future trial. Thus, under the Bayesian approach, it is essential to construct the posterior density $\pi(\theta|x)$ in Equation 4.2, given the data set observed from the previous trials.

Consider first the two-group parallel design with equal variances, that is, x_{ij}'s are independent and normally distributed with means μ_1 and μ_2 and a common variance σ^2. If σ^2 is known, then the power for testing hypotheses in Equation 4.3 is $\Phi(\theta - z_{0.975})$ with θ defined by Equation 4.4. A commonly

TABLE 4.2

95% Lower Confidence Bound

	Total Sample Size							
T(x)	10	20	30	40	50	60	100	∞
4.5	1.51	2.01	2.18	2.26	2.32	2.35	2.42	2.54
4.6	1.57	2.09	2.26	2.35	2.41	2.44	2.52	2.64
4.7	1.64	2.17	2.35	2.44	2.50	2.54	2.61	2.74
4.8	1.70	2.25	2.43	2.53	2.59	2.63	2.71	2.84
4.9	1.76	2.33	2.52	2.62	2.68	2.72	2.80	2.94
5.0	1.83	2.41	2.60	2.71	2.77	2.81	2.90	3.04
5.1	1.89	2.48	2.69	2.80	2.86	2.91	2.99	3.14
5.2	1.95	2.56	2.77	2.88	2.95	3.00	3.09	3.24
5.3	2.02	2.64	2.86	2.97	3.04	3.09	3.18	3.34
5.4	2.08	2.72	2.95	3.06	3.13	3.18	3.28	3.44
5.5	2.14	2.80	3.03	3.15	3.22	3.27	3.37	3.54
5.6	2.20	2.88	3.11	3.24	3.31	3.36	3.47	3.64
5.7	2.26	2.95	3.20	3.32	3.40	3.45	3.56	3.74
5.8	2.32	3.03	3.28	3.41	3.49	3.55	3.66	3.84
5.9	2.39	3.11	3.37	3.50	3.58	3.64	3.75	3.94
6.0	2.45	3.19	3.45	3.59	3.67	3.73	3.85	4.04
6.1	2.51	3.26	3.53	3.67	3.76	3.82	3.94	4.14
6.2	2.57	3.34	3.62	3.76	3.85	3.91	4.03	4.24
6.3	2.63	3.42	3.70	3.85	3.94	4.00	4.13	4.34
6.4	2.69	3.49	3.78	3.93	4.03	4.09	4.22	4.44
6.5	2.75	3.57	3.86	4.02	4.12	4.18	4.32	4.54

Source: Chow, S. C., J. Shao, and O. Y. P. Hu, *Journal of Biopharmaceutical Statistics*, 12, 385–400, 2002. With permission.

used prior for (μ_1, μ_2) is the noninformative prior $\pi\ (\mu_1, \mu_2) \equiv$ Consequently, the posterior density for θ is $N(T(x),1)$ where

$$T = \frac{\bar{x}_1 - \bar{x}_2}{\sigma\sqrt{\left(\frac{1}{n_1} + \frac{1}{n_2}\right)}}$$

and the posterior mean is

$$\int\left[\Phi(\theta - z_{0.975}) + \Phi(-\theta - z_{0.975})\right]\pi(\theta \mid x)d\theta = \Phi\left(\frac{T(x) - z_{0.975}}{\sqrt{2}}\right) + \Phi\left(\frac{-T(x) - z_{0.975}}{\sqrt{2}}\right)$$

When $T(x) > z_{0.975}$, this probability is nearly the same as

$$\Phi\left(\frac{|T(x)|-z_{0.975}}{\sqrt{2}}\right)$$

which is exactly the same as that in Goodman (1992, Equation 1).

For the more realistic situation where σ^2 is unknown, we need a prior for σ^2. A commonly used noninformative prior for σ^2 is the Lebesgue density $\pi(\sigma^2) = \sigma^{-2}$. Assume that the priors for μ_1, μ_2, and σ^2 are independent, the posterior density for (δ, u^2) is $\pi(\delta|u^2,x)\pi(u^2|x)$, where

$$\delta = \frac{\mu_1 - \mu_2}{\sqrt{\frac{(n_1-1)s_1^2+(n_2-1)s_2^2}{n-2}}\sqrt{\left(\frac{1}{n_1}+\frac{1}{n_2}\right)}}$$

$$u^2 = \frac{(n-2)\sigma^2}{(n_1-1)s_1^2+(n_2-1)s_2^2}$$

$$\pi(\delta \mid u^2, x) = \frac{1}{u}\phi\left(\frac{\delta - T(x)}{u}\right)$$

where ϕ is the density function of the standard normal distribution, T is given by Equation 4.2, and $\pi(u^2|x) = f(u)$ with

$$f(u) = \left[\Gamma\left(\frac{n-2}{2}\right)\right]^{-1}\left(\frac{n-2}{2}\right)^{(n-2)/2} u^{-n} e^{-(n-2)/(2u^2)}$$

Since θ in Equation 4.4 is equal to δ/u, the posterior mean of $p(\theta)$ is given by

$$\hat{P} = \int_0^{\infty}\left[\int_{-\infty}^{\infty} p\left(\frac{\delta}{u}\right)\phi\left(\frac{\delta - T(x)}{u}\right)d\delta\right]2f(u)du \tag{4.16}$$

which is the reproducibility probability under the Bayesian approach. It is clear that $\hat{P}$ depends on the data x through the function $T(x)$.

The probability, $\hat{P}$, can be evaluated numerically. A Monte Carlo method can be applied as follows. First, generate a variate γ_j from the gamma distribution with the shape parameter $(n-2)/2$ and the scale parameter $2/(n-2)$, and generate a variate δ_j from $N(T(x), u_j^2)$ where $u_j^2 = \gamma_j^{-1}$. Repeat this process independently N times to obtain (δ_j, u_j^2), $j = 1,\ldots,N$. Then $\hat{P}$ can be approximated by

$$\hat{P}_N = 1 - \frac{1}{N}\sum_{j=1}^{N}\left[\Im_{n-2}\left(t_{0.975,n-2} \mid \frac{\delta_j}{u_j}\right) - \Im_{n-2}\left(-t_{0.975,n-2} \mid \frac{\delta_j}{u_j}\right)\right]$$

Values of $\hat{P}_N$ for $N = 10{,}000$ and some selected values of $T(x)$ and n are given in Table 4.3. It can be seen that in assessing reproducibility, the Bayesian approach is more conservative than the estimated power approach but less conservative than the confidence bound approach.

Consider next the two-group parallel design with unequal variance and large n_i's. The approximate power for the second trial is

$$p(\theta) = \Phi(\theta - z_{0.975}) + \Phi(-\theta - z_{0.975})$$

$$\theta = \frac{\mu_1 - \mu_2}{\sqrt{\left(\frac{\sigma_1^2}{n_1} + \frac{\sigma_2^2}{n_2}\right)}}$$

Suppose that we use the noninformative prior density

$$\pi(\mu_1, \mu_2, \sigma_1^2, \sigma_2^2) = \sigma_1^{-2}\sigma_2^{-2}, \ \sigma_1^2 > 0, \sigma_2^2 > 0$$

Let $\tau_i^2 = \sigma_i^{-2}, i = 1, 2$, and $\varsigma^2 = (n_1\tau_1^2)^{-1} + (n_2\tau_2^2)^{-1}$. Then, the posterior density $\pi(\mu_1 - \mu_2 \mid \tau_1^2, \tau_2^2, x)$ is the normal density with mean $\bar{x}_1 - \bar{x}_2$ and variance ς^2 and the posterior density $\pi(\tau_1^2, \tau_2^2 \mid x) = \pi(\tau_1^2 \mid x)\pi(\tau_2^2 \mid x)$, where $\pi(\tau_i^2 \mid x)$ is the gamma density with the shape parameter (ni – 1)/2 and the scale parameter $2/\left[(n_i - 1)s_i^2\right], i = 1, 2$. Consequently, the reproducibility probability is the posterior mean of $p(\theta)$ given by

$$\hat{P} = \int\left[\Phi\left(\frac{\bar{x}_1 - \bar{x}_2}{\sqrt{2}\varsigma} - \frac{z_{0.975}}{\sqrt{2}}\right) + \Phi\left(-\frac{\bar{x}_1 - \bar{x}_2}{\sqrt{2}\varsigma} - \frac{z_{0.975}}{\sqrt{2}}\right)\right]\pi(\varsigma \mid x)d\varsigma$$

where $\pi(\varsigma|x)$ is the posterior density of ς constructed using $\pi(\tau_i^2 \mid x), i = 1, 2$. The Monte Carlo method previously discussed can be applied to approximate $\hat{P}$. Reproducibility probabilities under the Bayesian approach can be similarly obtained for the matched-pairs parallel design and the 2 × 2 crossover design.

Finally, consider the a-group parallel design where the power is given by

$$p(\theta) = 1 - \Im_{a-1,n-a}(F_{0.95;a-1,n-a} \mid \theta)$$

Under the noninformative prior

TABLE 4.3

Reproducibility Probability under the Bayesian Approach Approximated by Monte Carlo with Size 10,000

	Total Sample Size							
T(x)	10	20	30	40	50	60	100	∞
2.02	0.435	0.482	0.495	0.501	0.504	0.508	0.517	0.519
2.08	0.447	0.496	0.512	0.515	0.519	0.523	0.532	0.536
2.14	0.466	0.509	0.528	0.530	0.535	0.543	0.549	0.553
2.20	0.478	0.529	0.540	0.547	0.553	0.556	0.565	0.569
2.26	0.487	0.547	0.560	0.564	0.567	0.571	0.577	0.585
2.32	0.505	0.558	0.577	0.580	0.581	0.587	0.590	0.602
2.38	0.519	0.576	0.590	0.597	0.603	0.604	0.610	0.618
2.44	0.530	0.585	0.610	0.611	0.613	0.617	0.627	0.634
2.50	0.546	0.609	0.624	0.631	0.634	0.636	0.640	0.650
2.56	0.556	0.618	0.638	0.647	0.648	0.650	0.658	0.665
2.62	0.575	0.632	0.654	0.655	0.657	0.664	0.675	0.680
2.68	0.591	0.647	0.665	0.674	0.675	0.677	0.687	0.695
2.74	0.600	0.660	0.679	0.685	0.686	0.694	0.703	0.710
2.80	0.608	0.675	0.690	0.702	0.705	0.712	0.714	0.724
2.86	0.629	0.691	0.706	0.716	0.722	0.723	0.729	0.738
2.92	0.636	0.702	0.718	0.730	0.733	0.738	0.742	0.752
2.98	0.649	0.716	0.735	0.742	0.744	0.748	0.756	0.765
3.04	0.663	0.726	0.745	0.753	0.756	0.759	0.765	0.778
3.10	0.679	0.738	0.754	0.766	0.771	0.776	0.779	0.790
3.16	0.690	0.754	0.767	0.776	0.781	0.786	0.792	0.802
3.22	0.701	0.762	0.777	0.790	0.792	0.794	0.804	0.814
3.28	0.708	0.773	0.793	0.804	0.806	0.809	0.820	0.825
3.34	0.715	0.784	0.803	0.809	0.812	0.818	0.828	0.836
3.40	0.729	0.793	0.815	0.819	0.829	0.830	0.838	0.846
3.46	0.736	0.806	0.826	0.832	0.837	0.839	0.847	0.856
3.52	0.745	0.816	0.834	0.843	0.845	0.846	0.855	0.865
3.58	0.755	0.828	0.841	0.849	0.857	0.859	0.867	0.874
3.64	0.771	0.833	0.854	0.859	0.863	0.865	0.872	0.883
3.70	0.778	0.839	0.861	0.867	0.870	0.874	0.884	0.891
3.76	0.785	0.847	0.867	0.874	0.882	0.883	0.890	0.898
3.82	0.795	0.857	0.878	0.883	0.889	0.891	0.898	0.906
3.88	0.800	0.869	0.881	0.891	0.896	0.899	0.904	0.913
3.94	0.806	0.873	0.890	0.897	0.904	0.907	0.910	0.919

Note: Prior for with respect to the Lebesgue measure.
Source: Chow, S. C., J. Shao, and O. Y. P. Hu, *Journal of Biopharmaceutical Statistics*, 12, 385–400, 2002. With permission.

$$\pi(\mu_1,\ldots,\mu_a,\sigma^2)=\sigma^{-2},\ \sigma^2>0$$

the posterior density $\pi(\theta|t^2,x)$, where $\tau^2 = SSE/[n - a)\sigma^2]$ is the density of the noncentral chi-square distribution with $a - 1$ degrees of freedom and the noncentrality parameter $\tau^2(a - 1)T(x)$. The posterior density $\pi(\tau^2|x)$ is the gamma distribution with the shape parameter $(n - a)/2$ and the scale parameter $2/(n - a)$. Consequently, the reproducibility probability under the Bayesian approach is

$$\hat{P}=\int_0^{\infty}\left[\int_0^{\infty}p(\theta)\pi(\theta\mid\tau^2,x)d\theta\right]\pi(\tau^2\mid x)d\tau^2$$

The reproducibility probability based on the Bayesian approach depends on the choice of the prior distributions. The noninformative prior given above produces a more conservative reproducibility probability than that obtained using the estimated power approach but is less conservative than that under the confidence bound approach. If a different prior such as an informative prior is used, a sensitivity analysis may be performed to evaluate the effects of different priors on the reproducibility probability.

Let y be similar to x but is a response in a clinical bridging study conducted in the new region. Suppose the hypotheses of interest are $H_0{:}\mu_1 = \mu_0$ vs $H_a{:}\ \mu_1 \neq \mu_0.$

We reject H_0 at the 5% level of significance if and only if $|T| > t_{n-2}$, where t_{n-2} is the $(1 - \alpha/2)$th percentile of the t distribution with $n - 2$ degrees of freedom, $n = n_1 + n_2$

$$T=\frac{\bar{y}-\bar{x}}{\sqrt{\frac{(n_1-1)s_1^2+(n_0-1)s_2^2}{n-2}}\sqrt{\left(\frac{1}{n_1}+\frac{1}{n_0}\right)}}$$

and $\bar{x},\bar{y},s_0^2$ and s_1^2, are sample means and variances for the original region and the new region, respectively. Thus, the power of T is given by

$$p(\theta)=P\left(|T|>t_{n-2}\right)=1-\Im_{n-2}(t_{n-2}\mid\theta)+\Im_{n-2}(-t_{n-2}\mid\theta)$$

where

$$\theta=\frac{\mu_1-\mu_0}{\sigma\sqrt{\frac{1}{n_1}+\frac{1}{n_0}}}$$

and $\Im_{n-2}(\bullet|\theta)$ denotes the cumulative distribution function of the noncentral t distribution with $n-2$ degrees of freedom and the noncentrality parameter θ. Replacing θ in the power function with its estimate $T(x)$, the estimated power

$$\hat{p} = P(T(x)) = 1 - \Im_{n-2}(t_{n-2} \mid T(x)) + \Im_{n-2}(-t_{n-2} \mid T(x))$$

is defined as a reproducibility probability for a future clinical trial with the same patient population.

4.3.2 Evaluating the Generalizability Probability

When the ethnic difference is notable, Shao and Chow (2002) recommended assessing the generalizability probability for similarity between clinical results from a bridging study and studies conducted in the CCPD. The generalizability probability is defined as the reproducibility probability with the population of a future trial slightly deviated from the population of the previous trials. For simplicity, consider a parallel-group design for two treatments with population means μ_1 and μ_2 and an equal variance σ^2. Other designs can be similarly treated. Suppose that in the future trial, the population mean difference is changed to $\mu_1 - \mu_2 + \varepsilon$ and the population variance is changed to $C^2\sigma^2$, where $C > 0$. The signal-to-noise ratio for the population difference in the previous trial is $|\mu_1 - \mu_2|/\sigma$, whereas the signal-to-noise ratio for the population difference in the future trial is

$$\frac{|\mu_1 - \mu_2 + \varepsilon|}{C\sigma} = \frac{|\Delta(\mu_1 - \mu_2)|}{\sigma}$$

where

$$\Delta = \frac{1 + \varepsilon / (\mu_1 - \mu_2)}{C}$$

is a measure of change in the signal-to-noise ratio for the population difference. Chow et al. (2002) referred to as a sensitivity index when changing from a population to another. For most practical problems, $|\varepsilon| < |\mu_1 - \mu_2|$ and, thus, $\Delta > 0$.

If the power for the previous trial is $p(\theta)$, then the power for the future trial is $p(\Delta\theta)$. Suppose that Δ is known. Under the frequentist approach, the generalizability probability is $\hat{P}_\Delta$, which is $\hat{P}$ given by Equation 4.5 with $T(x)$ replaced by $\Delta T(x)$, or $\hat{P}_{\Delta-}$, which is $\hat{P}_-$ given by Equation 4.15 with $|\hat{\theta}|_-$ replaced by $\Delta|\hat{\theta}|_-$. Under the Bayesian approach, the generalizability probability is $\hat{P}_\Delta$, which is $\hat{P}$ given by Equation 4.16 with $p(\delta/u)$ replaced by

$p(\Delta\delta/u)$. When the value of Δ is unknown, we may consider a set of Δ– values to carry out a sensitivity analysis.

4.4 Assessing the Similarity-Based Sensitivity Index

4.4.1 Population Shift between Regions

In bridging studies, a commonly asked question is whether the foreign data can be extrapolated to a new region. To address this question, we may assess the similarity between populations in the original region and a new region. Denote the target population by (μ_y, σ_y). Assume that clinical data are collected from the target population. Thus, for the target patient population in the original region, $\mu_y = \mu_{original}$ and $\sigma_y = \sigma_{original}$ while for the target patient population in a new region, $\mu_y = \mu_{new}$ and $\sigma_y = \sigma_{new}$. Thus, we can link the target patient populations from the original region and the new region by the following:

$$\mu_{new} = \mu_{original} + \varepsilon$$

and

$$\sigma_{new} = C\sigma_{original}$$

In other words, we expect there are differences in population mean and population standard deviation due to possible difference in ethnic factors. As a result, the effect size adjusted for standard deviation in the new region can be obtained as follows:

$$\left|\frac{\mu_{new}}{\sigma_{new}}\right| = \left|\frac{\mu_{original} + \varepsilon}{C\sigma_{original}}\right| = |\Delta|\left|\frac{\mu_{original}}{\sigma_{original}}\right|$$

where $\Delta = (1 + \varepsilon/\mu_{original})/C$. Chow et al. (2002) referred to Δ as a sensitivity index when changing from a target population (the original region) to another (the new region). As it can be seen, the effect size in the new region is inflated (or reduced) by the factor of Δ. If $\varepsilon = 0$ and $C = 1$, we then claim that there is no difference between the original region and the new region. Thus, the new region is similar to the original region. Note that the shift and scale parameters (i.e., ε and C) can be estimated by

$$\hat{\varepsilon} = \hat{\mu}_{new} - \hat{\mu}_{original} \text{ and } \hat{C} = \frac{\hat{\sigma}_{new}}{\hat{\sigma}_{original}} \tag{4.17}$$

in which $(\hat{\mu}_{original}, \hat{\sigma}_{original})$ and $(\hat{\mu}_{new}, \hat{\sigma}_{new})$ are estimates of $(\mu_{original}, \sigma_{original})$ and $(\mu_{new}, \sigma_{new})$, respectively. Thus, the sensitivity index can be assessed as

$$\hat{\Delta} = (1 + \hat{\varepsilon} / \hat{\mu}_{original}) / \hat{C} \tag{4.18}$$

In practice, there may be a shift in population mean (i.e., ε) or in population standard deviation (i.e., *C*). Chow, Chang, and Pong (2005) indicated that shifts in population mean and population standard deviation can be classified into the following four cases: (1) both ε and *C* are fixed; (2) ε is random and *C* is fixed; (3) ε is fixed and *C* is random; and (4) both ε and *C* are random. Statistical methods for assessment of the sensitivity index under each of the aforementioned scenarios are briefly described in the subsequent sections.

To assess the sensitivity index under the four scenarios, assume the response variable x_i, $i = 1,\ldots,N_1$ for n_1 patients in the original region following a normal distribution, for convenience sake, denoting $N(\mu,\sigma^2)$, and the estimates of μ and σ^2 are obtained by the maximum likelihood estimates, that is,

$$\hat{\mu} = \frac{1}{N_1}\sum_{i=1}^{n_1} x_i \quad \text{and} \quad \hat{\sigma}^2 = \frac{1}{N_1 - 1}\sum_{i=1}^{n_1}(x_i - \bar{x})^2 \tag{4.19}$$

where

$$\bar{x} = \frac{1}{N_1}\sum_{i=1}^{n_1} x_i$$

4.4.2 Case Where Both ε and *C* Are Fixed

For the case of both ε and *C* are fixed, given the response variable in new region *y* be distributed as $N(\mu_{new}, \sigma^2_{new})$, as aforementioned $\mu_{new} = \mu + \varepsilon_0$ and $\sigma^2_{new} = C_0\sigma^2$, where ε_0 and C_0 are unknown constants. The maximum likelihood estimates of μ_{new} and σ^2_{new} are the sample mean and variance based on the data y_j, $j = 1,\ldots,N_2$ from n_2 patients in the new region:

$$\hat{\mu}_{new} = \frac{1}{N_2}\sum_{i=1}^{n_2} y_i \quad \text{and} \quad \hat{\sigma}^2 = \frac{1}{N_1 - 1}\sum_{i=1}^{n_1}(x_i - \bar{x})^2 \tag{4.20}$$

where

$$\bar{y} = \frac{1}{N_2}\sum_{i=1}^{n_2} y_i$$

Substituting Equations 4.19 and 4.20 into Equations 4.17 and 4.18, the sensitivity index can be assessed.

4.4.3 Case Where ε Is Random and *C* Is Fixed

Chow et al. (2005) derived statistical inference of Δ for the case where ε is random and *C* is fixed by assuming that *y* conditional on μ follows a normal distribution $N(\mu,\sigma^2)$. That is, $y|_{\mu-\mu_{new}} \sim N(\mu,\sigma^2)$, where μ is distributed as $N(\mu_\mu,\sigma^2_\mu)$. It can be verified that the unconditional distribution of *y* is a mixed normal distribution with mean μ_μ and variance $\sigma^2+\sigma^2_\mu$; that is, $y \sim N(\mu_\mu,\sigma^2+\sigma^2_\mu)$, where μ_μ, σ^2, and σ^2_μ are unknown constants given the observed response variables y_{ij}, $i = 1,\ldots,m$; $j = 1,\ldots,n_i$ and

$$\sum_{i=1}^{m} n_i = N_2$$

from N_2 patients in the new region, the observations satisfy the following conditions:

(i) $(y_{ji}|\mu_j,\sigma^2) \sim N(\mu_j,\sigma^2)$, $j = 1,\ldots m$; $i = 1,\ldots,n_j$ and given $\mu_j, y_{j1},\ldots,y_{jn_j}$ are iid;
(ii) $\{y_{ji}, i = 1,\ldots,n_j\}$, $j = 1,\ldots,m$ are independent; and
(iii) $\mu_j \sim N(\mu_\mu,\sigma^2_\mu)$, $j = 1,\cdots,m$.

The maximum likelihood estimates of unknown constants can be obtained by expectation maximum (EM) algorithm (see Dempster, Laird, and Rubin, 1977).

As is well-known, the EM algorithm is an iterative method back and forth between expectation (E) step and maximum (M) step. The E-step gets the expectation of the latent data given the observed data and the *t*-th iterative value of the unknown parameters, and the M-step takes the estimates of the unknown parameters by maximizing the expectation. For the sake of calculation, denote that $\theta = (\mu_\mu,\sigma,\sigma_\mu)$ and the latent data μ_j, $j = 1,\ldots m$, combining $y = (y_{11},\ldots,y_{mn_m})$ and $u = (\mu_1,\ldots,\mu_m)$ as the complete data $Z = (y,u)$, the log-likelihood function as follows:

$$\log f(Z\,|\,\theta) = \log f(y\,|\,u) + \log(u\,|\,\theta)$$

$$= -\frac{N_2}{2}\log\sigma^2 - \frac{m}{2}\log\sigma^2_\mu - \frac{\sum_{j=1}^{m}\sum_{i=1}^{n_j}(y_{ji}-\mu_i)^2}{2\sigma^2} - \frac{\sum_{j=1}^{m}(\mu_j-\mu_\mu)^2}{2\sigma^2_\mu}$$

4.4.3.1 E-Step

Assume that $\theta^{(t)} = (\mu_\mu^{(t)}, \sigma^{(t)}, \sigma_\mu^{(t)})$ is the t-th iterative estimate of unknown vector, θ, conditional on $\Omega^{(t)} = (y, \theta^{(t)})$; it is shown that $(\mu_j \mid \Omega^{(t)}) \sim N(\hat{\mu}_j^{(t)},\ \hat{V}_j^{(t)})$.

Let

$$\hat{y}_{j\cdot} = \frac{1}{n_j} \sum_{i=1}^{n_j} y_{ji}$$

where

$$\hat{\mu}_j^{(t)} = \left(\frac{\mu}{\left(\sigma_\mu^{(t)}\right)^{-2}} + \frac{n_j}{\left(\sigma^{(t)}\right)^2} \hat{y}_{j\cdot} \right) \Bigg/ \left(\frac{1}{\left(\sigma_\mu^{(t)}\right)^{-2}} + \frac{n_j}{\left(\sigma^{(t)}\right)^2} \right)$$

$$\hat{V}_j^{(t)} = \left(\frac{1}{\left(\sigma_\mu^{(t)}\right)^2} + \frac{n_j}{\left(\sigma^{(t)}\right)^2} \right)^{-1}$$

the expectation with regard to the latent data μ_j, $j = 1, \ldots m$ is as follows:

$$E\left[\left(\mu_j - c\right)^2 \mid \Omega^{(t)}\right] = \left(\hat{\mu}_j^{(t)} - c\right)^2 + \hat{V}_j^{(t)}$$

where c is an arbitrary constant. So the expectation of log-likelihood function is

$$Q(Z \mid \Omega^{(t)}) = -\frac{N_2}{2} \log \sigma^2 - \frac{m}{2} \log \sigma_\mu^2 - \frac{\sum_{j=1}^{m} \sum_{i=1}^{n_j} \left[(y_{ji} - \hat{\mu}_j^{(t)})^2 + \hat{V}_j^{(t)} \right]}{2\sigma^2} - \frac{\sum_{j=1}^{m} \left[(\hat{\mu}_j^{(t)} - \mu_\mu)^2 + \hat{V}_j^{(t)} \right]}{2\sigma_\mu^2}$$

4.4.3.2 M-Step

The MLE of unknown constant vector θ is

$$\hat{\mu}_{\mu}^{(t+1)} = \frac{1}{m}\sum_{j=1}^{m}\hat{\mu}_j^{(t)}$$

$$\hat{\sigma}^{(t+1)} = \left\{\frac{1}{N_2}\sum_{j=1}^{m}\sum_{i=1}^{n_j}\left[\left(y_{ji} - \hat{\mu}_j^{(t)}\right)^2 + \hat{V}_j^{(t)}\right]\right\}^{1/2}$$

$$\hat{\sigma}_{\mu}^{(t+1)} = \left\{\frac{1}{m+1}\sum_{j=1}^{m}\left[\left(\hat{\mu}_j^{(t)} - \hat{\mu}_{\mu}^{(t+1)}\right)^2 + \hat{V}_j^{(t)}\right]\right\}^{1/2}$$

The iteration is continued until $||\theta^{(t-1)} - \theta^{(t)}||$ is sufficiently small or some other convergence criterion is satisfied. The maximum likelihood estimates of $\theta = (\mu_\mu, \sigma, \sigma_\mu)$ can be obtained. Assume the $(t + 1)$-th iteration is convergent, then

$$\hat{\mu}_{new} = \hat{\mu}_{\mu}^{(t+1)} \tag{4.21}$$

$$\hat{\sigma}_{new}^2 = \left(\hat{\sigma}^{(t+1)}\right)^2 + \left(\hat{\sigma}_{\mu}^{(t+1)}\right)^2 \tag{4.22}$$

Thus, the sensitivity index between the original region and the new region can be obtained by

$$\hat{\varepsilon} = \hat{\mu}_{\mu}^{(t+1)} - \hat{\mu} \text{ and } \hat{C} = \sqrt{\frac{\left(\hat{\sigma}^{(t+1)}\right)^2 + \left(\hat{\sigma}_{\mu}^{(t+1)}\right)^2}{\hat{\sigma}^2}}$$

4.4.4 Case Where ε Is Fixed and C Is Random

We have discussed statistical inference in the case where ε is fixed and σ^2 is random. The data y from the new region are distributed as normal $N(\mu, \sigma^2)$, conditional on σ^2 following an inverse gamma distribution. That is,

$$y\,|_{\sigma^2=\sigma_{new}^2} \sim N(\mu, \sigma^2) \text{ and } \sigma^2 \sim IG(\alpha, \beta)$$

It is can be derived that y follows a noncentral t distribution with density function

$$f(y)=\frac{\Gamma(\alpha+1/2)}{\Gamma(\alpha)\sqrt{2\pi\beta}}\left[1+\frac{(y-\mu)^2}{2\beta}\right]^{-(\alpha+1/2)}$$

where θ = (μ,α,β) are the unknown constant vectors, the noncentral parameter is μ, the degrees of freedom is 2α, and the scale parameter is $\sqrt{\beta/\alpha}$.

Given the observed response variable y_{ij}, j = 1,...,m; i = 1,...,n_j from N_2 patients of the new region, where

$$\sum_{i=1}^{m} n_j = N_2$$

and the latent variable $\sigma^2=(\sigma_1^2,\cdots,\sigma_m^2)$, the response variable y_{ij} satisfies the following conditions:

(i) $(y_{ji}\mid\mu,\sigma_j^2)\sim N(\mu,\sigma_j^2), j=1,\cdots,m; i=1,\cdots n_j$, and given $\sigma_j^2 y_{j1},\cdots,y_{jn_j}$ are iid;

(ii) $\{y_{ji}, i=1,\cdots,n_j\}, j=1,\cdots,m$ are independent; and

(iii) $\sigma_j^2\sim IG(\alpha,\beta), j=1,\cdots,m$.

Combining $y=(y_{11},\ldots,y_{mn_m})$ and $\sigma^2=(\sigma_1^2,\ldots,\sigma_m^2)$ as the complete data $Z = (y, \sigma^2)$, resorting to the EM algorithm, we can derive the maximum likelihood estimates of θ = (μ,α,β). The log-likelihood function is given by

$$\log f(Z\mid\theta)=\log f(y\mid\sigma^2)+\log(\sigma^2\mid\theta)$$

$$=\sum_{j=1}^{m}\left(\frac{n_j}{2}+\alpha+1\right)\log\frac{1}{\sigma_j^2}+m\alpha\log\beta-m\log\Gamma(\alpha)-\sum_{j=1}^{m}\frac{2\beta+\sum_{i=1}^{n_j}(y_{ji}-\mu)^2}{2\sigma_j^2}$$

As mentioned already, the EM procedure is

$$E\left(\frac{1}{\sigma_j^2}\mid y,\theta^{(t)}\right)=\frac{\left(\alpha^{(t)}+n_j/2\right)}{\left(\beta^{(t)}+\sum_{i=1}^{n_j}(y_{ji}-\mu^{(t)})^2\Big/2\right)}$$

$$E\left(\log\frac{1}{\sigma_j^2}\mid y,\theta^{(t)}\right)=\varphi\left(\alpha^{(t)}+n_j/2\right)-\log\left(\beta^{(t)}+\sum_{i=1}^{n_j}(y_{ji}-\mu^{(t)})^2\Big/2\right)$$

$\phi(.)$ be digamma function, denoted that

$$\hat{V}_{1j}^{(t)} = E\left(\frac{1}{\sigma_j^2} \mid y, \theta^{(t)}\right),\ \hat{V}_{2j}^{(t)} = E\left(\log\frac{1}{\sigma_j^2} \mid y, \theta^{(t)}\right)$$

and the expectation of the log-likelihood function

$$E\left(\log f(Z \mid \theta^{(t)})\right) = Q(Z \mid y, \theta^{(t)})$$

Maximizing $Q(Z \mid y, \theta^{(t)})$, the (t + 1)-th iterative value can be obtained:

$$\hat{\mu}^{(t+1)} = \sum_{j=1}^{m}\sum_{i=1}^{n_j} y_{ji} \Big/ \sum_{j=1}^{m} n_j \tag{4.23}$$

$$\hat{\alpha}^{(t+1)} = \alpha^{(t)} + \frac{\sum_{j=1}^{m} \hat{V}_{2j}^{(t)} - m\varphi(\alpha) + m\log(\beta)}{m\varphi'(\alpha^{(t)})} \tag{4.24}$$

$$\hat{\alpha}^{(t+1)} = \alpha^{(t)} + \frac{\sum_{j=1}^{m} \hat{V}_{2j}^{(t)} - m\varphi(\alpha) + m\log(\beta)}{m\varphi'(\alpha^{(t)})} \tag{4.25}$$

without loss of generality, assume that the $(t + 1)$-th iteration is convergent, that is, that the estimates of θ can be addressed by

$$\hat{\mu}_{new} = \hat{\mu}^{(t+1)}, \hat{\alpha} = \hat{\alpha}^{(t+1)} \text{ and } \hat{\beta} = \hat{\beta}^{(t+1)}$$

Now we consider the variance of the response variable $(y_{ji} \mid \mu, \sigma_j^2) \sim N(\mu, \sigma_j^2)$, $j = 1,\ldots,i = 1,n_j$. Louis (1982) derived the observer information matrix when the EM algorithm is used to find maximum likelihood estimates in incomplete data problems. According to Louis's method, the information matrix of vector $\theta = (\mu,\alpha,\beta)$ could be given:

$$I_Y(\theta) = E_\theta\left\{B(Z,\theta) \mid Z \in R\right\} - E_\theta\left\{S(Z,\theta)S^T(Z,\theta) \mid Z \in R\right\} + S^*(y,\theta)S^{*T}(y,\theta) \tag{4.26}$$

where $S(Z,\theta)$ are the gradient vectors of log-likelihood function $\log f(Z|\theta)$ and $B(Z,\theta)$ are the negatives of the associated second derivative matrices. Of course, they need be evaluated only on the last iteration of the EM procedure, where $S^*(y,\theta) = E[S(Z,\theta) \mid Z \in R]$ is zero. Here,

$$S^T(Z,\theta) = \left(\sum_{j=1}^{m}\sum_{i=1}^{n_j}(y_{ji}-\mu)\Big/\sigma_j^2,\ \sum_{j=1}^{m}\log\frac{1}{\sigma_j^2}+m\log\beta-m\varphi(\alpha),\ \frac{m\alpha}{\beta}-\sum_{j=1}^{m}\frac{1}{\sigma_j^2} \right) \tag{4.27}$$

$$B(Z,\theta) = \begin{pmatrix} \sum_{j=1}^{m}\frac{n_j}{\sigma_j^2} & 0 & 0 \\ 0 & m\varphi'(\alpha) & -\frac{m}{\beta} \\ 0 & -\frac{m}{\beta} & \frac{m\alpha}{\beta^2} \end{pmatrix} \tag{4.28}$$

and

$$S^{*T}(y,\theta) = \left(\sum_{j=1}^{m}\sum_{i=1}^{n_j}\hat{V}_{1j}^{(t)}(y_{ji}-\mu),\ \sum_{j=1}^{m}\hat{V}_{2j}+m\log\beta-m\varphi(\alpha),\ \frac{m\alpha}{\beta}-\sum_{j=1}^{m}\hat{V}_{1j}^{(l)} \right) \tag{4.29}$$

Substituting equations (4.27) through (4.29) into equation (4.26), the information matrix $I_Y(\theta)$ of vector $\theta = (\mu,\alpha,\beta)$ can be obtained. $I_Y(\theta)$ can be inverted to find the covariance matrix of $\hat{\theta}$, that is,

$$Cov(\hat{\theta}) = I_Y^{-1}(\hat{\theta}) \text{ and } \hat{\sigma}_{new}^2 = Var(\hat{\mu}_{new}) = \left(I_Y^{-1}(\hat{\theta})\right)_{11}$$

Thus, the sensitivity index between the two regions could be estimated as $\hat{\Delta} = \hat{\sigma}^2[1+(\hat{\mu}_{new}-\hat{\mu})/\hat{\mu}]/\hat{\sigma}_{new}^2$.

4.4.5 Case Where Both ε and *C* Are Random

Due to the difference in ethnic factors between the original and new regions, it is possible there are differences in population mean and variance. Assuming that the clinical data based on the original region is distributed as $N(\mu, \sigma^2)$, in the new region the population Mμ and variance Σ^2 are random and follow a normal-scaled inverse gamma distribution $(\mu, \sigma^2) \sim N - \Gamma^{-1}(\mu_\mu, \nu, \alpha, \beta)$; that is, both ε and *C* are random. Given the data *y* from new region, we have

$$y\,|_{\mu=\mu_{new},\sigma^2=\sigma^2_{new}} \sim N(\mu,\sigma^2) \text{ and } \left(\mu,\sigma^2\right) \sim N-\Gamma^{-1}(\mu_\mu,\nu,\alpha,\beta)$$

Therefore, it could be proved that y follows a noncentral t distribution, its density distribution

$$f(y)=\frac{\Gamma(\alpha+1/2)}{\Gamma(\alpha)\sqrt{2\pi\beta(v+1)/v}}\left[1+\frac{v(y-\mu_\mu)^2}{2\beta(v+1)}\right]^{-(\alpha+1/2)}$$

with location parameter $\mu_\mu \in R$, scale parameter $\sqrt{\beta(v+1)/\alpha v}$, and the degrees of freedom 2α.

The observed response variable $y=\{y_{ji}, j=1,\cdots,m; i=1,\cdots,n_j\}$ from N_2 patients in the new region, where

$$\sum_{i=1}^{m} n_j = N_2$$

and the latent vector $(\mu,\sigma^2)=\{(\mu_j,\sigma_j^2), j=1,\cdots,m\}$, the response variable y_{ji} satisfies the following conditions:

(i) $(y_{ji}\,|\,\mu_j,\sigma_j^2)\sim N(\mu_j,\sigma_j^2)$, $j=1,\cdots,m; i=1,\cdots n_j$, and given (μ_j,σ_j^2) $y_{j1},\cdots,y_{jn_j}$ are iid;

(ii) $\{y_{ji}, i=1,\cdots,n_j\}$, $j=1,\cdots,m$ are independent; and

(iii) $(\mu_j,\sigma_j^2)\sim N-\Gamma^{-1}(\mu_\mu,v,\alpha,\beta)$, $j=1,\cdots,m$.

Let $Z = (y, \mu, \sigma^2)$ be the complete data. The maximum likelihood estimates of $\theta = (\mu_\mu, \nu, \alpha, \beta)$ can be derived by the EM algorithm. The log-likelihood function is as follows:

$$\log f(Z\,|\,\theta)=\log f(y\,|\,\mu,\sigma^2)+\log(\mu,\sigma^2\,|\,\theta)$$

$$=\sum_{j=1}^{m}\left(\frac{n_j+3}{2}+\alpha\right)\log\frac{1}{\sigma_j^2}-\sum_{j=1}^{m}\frac{2\beta+v(\mu_j-\mu_\mu)^2}{2\sigma_j^2}-m\ln\Gamma(\alpha)-\sum_{j=1}^{m}\sum_{i=1}^{n_j}\frac{\left(y_{ji}-\mu_j\right)^2}{2\sigma_j^2}$$

$$+\frac{m}{2}\ln v+m\alpha\ln\beta,$$

which is conditional on the observed data y and the t-th iterative estimates $\theta^{(t)}=(\mu_\mu^{(t)},v^{(t)},\alpha^{(t)},\beta^{(t)})$. The expectation with regard to latent data μ and σ^2 is given by

$$E\left\{\frac{1}{\sigma_j^2} \mid y,\theta^{(t)}\right\} = \frac{\Gamma\left(\frac{n_j}{2}+\alpha^{(t)}+1\right)}{\left(\beta^{(t)}+\frac{1}{2}\sum_{i=1}^{n_j}(y_{ji}-\bar{y}_{j\cdot})^2+\frac{v^{(t)}n_j}{2(n_j+v^{(t)})}(\bar{y}_{j\cdot}-\mu_\mu^{(t)})\right)\Gamma\left(\frac{n_j}{2}+\alpha^{(t)}\right)}$$

where

$$\bar{y}_{j\cdot} = \frac{1}{n_j}\sum_{i=1}^{n_j} x_{ji}$$

$$E\left\{\frac{(\mu_j-c)^2}{\sigma_j^2} \mid y,\theta^{(t)}\right\} = \frac{1}{n_j+v^{(t)}} + \left(\frac{\sum_{i=1}^{n_j} y_{ji}+v^{(t)}\mu_\mu^{(t)}}{n_j+v^{(t)}}-c\right)^2 \hat{W}_{1j}^{(t)}$$

$$E\left\{\log\frac{1}{\sigma_j^2} \mid y,\theta^{(t)}\right\} = \psi\left(\frac{n_j}{2}+\alpha^{(t)}\right) - \ln\left(\beta^{(t)}+\frac{1}{2}\sum_{i=1}^{n_j}(y_{ji}-\bar{y}_{j\cdot})^2+\frac{v^{(t)}n_j}{2(n_j+v^{(t)})}(\bar{y}_{j\cdot}-\mu_\mu^{(t)})\right)$$

denote that

$$\hat{W}_{1j}^{(t)} = E\hat{W}_{2j}^{(t)} = E\left\{\log\frac{1}{\sigma_j^2} \mid y,\theta^{(t)}\right\}, \left\{\frac{1}{\sigma_j^2} \mid y,\theta^{(t)}\right\}, \text{ and } \hat{W}_{3j}^{(t)} = E\left\{\frac{(\mu_j-c)^2}{\sigma_j^2} \mid y,\theta^{(t)}\right\}$$

The maximum likelihood estimates of the vector are

$$\hat{\mu}_\mu^{(t+1)} = \sum_{j=1}^{m}\left(\sum_{i=1}^{n_j} y_{ji}+v^{(t)}\mu_\mu^{(t)}\right)\Big/\left(n_j+v^{(t)}\right) \tag{4.30}$$

$$\hat{\gamma}^{(t+1)} = \frac{\gamma^{(t)}}{\gamma^{(t)}n_2+1} + \left(\frac{\gamma^{(t)}\sum_{j=1}^{n_2} y_j+\mu_\mu^{(t)}}{\gamma^{(t)}n_2+1}-\mu_\mu^{(t+1)}\right)^2 \hat{W}_1^{(t)} \tag{4.31}$$

$$\hat{v}^{(t+1)} = m \Big/ \sum_{j=1}^{m} \hat{W}_{3j}^{(t)} \tag{4.32}$$

$$\hat{\alpha}^{(t+1)} = \alpha^{(t)} + \frac{\frac{1}{m}\sum_{j=1}^{m} \hat{W}_{2j}^{(t)} - \varphi(\alpha^{(t)}) + \log\beta^{(t)}}{\varphi'(\alpha^{(t)})} \tag{4.33}$$

without loss generality. Assuming the $(t + 1)$-th iteration is convergent, the maximum likelihood estimate of the unknown constant vector θ is $(\hat{\mu}_{\mu}^{(t+1)}, \hat{v}^{(t+1)}, \hat{\alpha}^{(t+1)}, \hat{\beta}^{(t+1)})$.

The information matrix of θ is obtained by the method in Louis (1982), where

$$S^T(Z,\theta) = \left(\sum_{j=1}^{m} \frac{v(\mu_j - \mu_\mu)}{\sigma_j^2}, \; -\sum_{j=1}^{m} \frac{(\mu_j - \mu_\mu)^2}{2\sigma_j^2} + \frac{m}{2v}, \; \sum_{j=1}^{m} \log\frac{1}{\sigma_j^2} - m\varphi(\alpha) + m\log\beta, \; -\sum_{j=1}^{m} \frac{1}{\sigma_j^2} + \frac{m\alpha}{\beta} \right) \tag{4.34}$$

$$B(Z,\theta) = \begin{pmatrix} \sum_{j=1}^{m} \frac{v}{\sigma_j^2} & -\sum_{j=1}^{m} \frac{(\mu_j - \mu_\mu)}{\sigma_j^2} & 0 & 0 \\ -\sum_{j=1}^{m} \frac{(\mu_j - \mu_\mu)}{\sigma_j^2} & \frac{m}{2v^2} & 0 & 0 \\ 0 & 0 & m\varphi'(\alpha) & -\frac{m}{\beta} \\ 0 & 0 & -\frac{m}{\beta} & \frac{m\alpha}{\beta^2} \end{pmatrix} \tag{4.35}$$

and

$$S^*(y,\theta)=\begin{pmatrix} \sum_{j=1}^{m}\left(\dfrac{\sum_{j=1}^{n_2} y_{ji}+v^{(t)}\mu_\mu^{(t)}}{n_2+v^{(t)}}-\mu_\mu\right)v\hat{W}_{1j}^{(t)} \\ -\sum_{j=1}^{m}\dfrac{\hat{W}_{3j}^{(t)}}{2}+\dfrac{m}{2v} \\ \sum_{j=1}^{m}\hat{W}_{2j}^{(t)}-m\varphi(\alpha)+m\log\beta \\ -\sum_{j=1}^{m}\hat{W}_{1j}^{(t)}+\dfrac{m\alpha}{\beta} \end{pmatrix} \tag{4.36}$$

By substituting equations (4.34) to (4.36) into equation (4.26), the information matrix $I_Y(\hat{\theta})$ of vector $\theta = (\mu_\mu, v, \alpha, \beta)$ can be obtained, and the sample variance in new region is the (1,1)-th element in the inverse matrix of $I_Y(\hat{\theta})$, denoted $(I_Y^{-1}(\hat{\theta}))_{11}$.

As a result, when both ε and C are random, their estimates can be obtained:

$$\hat{\varepsilon} = \hat{\mu}_\mu^{(t+1)} - \hat{\mu} \text{ and } \hat{C} = \left(I_Y^{-1}(\hat{\theta})\right)_{11} \Big/ \hat{\sigma}^2$$

and the estimate of the sensitivity index is performed by Equation 4.18 between the original and the new regions, and the effect of ethnic factors resorting to sensitivity index will be measured. If it falls a prespecified interval, the result of similarity between the two regions can be confirmed; otherwise, similarity is denied.

4.5 Concluding Remarks

In clinical research, ethnic factors are often important facets to evaluate the efficacy and safety of study medicines under investigation, especially when the sponsor is interested in bringing an approved treatment agent from the original region to a new region, which has ethnic differences. To evaluate the influence of ethnic factors or to judge if clinical data generated from the original region are acceptable in the new region, testing the reproducibility or generalizability between the different regions is a very attractive problem for the statistical and medical researchers. Usually bridging studies are conducted to extrapolate the foreign efficacy data or safety data to the new region, deduce the foreign data if it shows that dose-response, safety, and efficacy in the original region are similar to those in the new region. Similarity is often interpreted as equivalence or comparability between two different regions. In the past, several criteria for assessing similarity have been proposed in the literature. In this article, we focus on the assessment of similarity by testing the reproducibility and generalizability probabilities and the sensitivity index.

In bridging studies for assessing similarity, Shao and Chow (2002) proposed the concepts of the reproducibility and generalizability probabilities. Reproducibility accounts for whether the clinical results in original region can be copied in the new region if the influence of ethnic factors is negligible. Otherwise, generalizibility will be considered to determine whether the clinical result in the original region can be generalized in a similar but slightly different patient population due to the influence of ethnic factors. Shao and Chow gave three methods for evaluating the reproducibility and generalizability probabilities: the estimated power approach, the confidence bound approach, and the Bayesian approach. The estimated power approach is based on a specified hypothesis test, such as the equality test between the test group and the control group, referring to the results of the original region, and getting a statistical reference on the data in new region, the power of test in new region is looked on as the reproducibility probability. The estimated power approach is a rather optimistic method. The confidence bound approach is more conservative and considers a 95% lower confidence bound of the power as the reproducibility probability. In practice the reproducibility probability can be viewed as the posterior mean for the future trial, which is the Bayesian approach. Actually the reproducibility probability depends on the choice of the prior distributions, at the same time; a sensitivity analysis should be performed to evaluate the effects of the different priors on reproducibility probability. Measuring the change

$$\Delta = \frac{1+\varepsilon/(\mu_1-\mu_2)}{C}$$

in the signal-to-noise ratio for the difference population aids in evaluating the generalizability probability; in addition, assessment of the sensitivity index resorts to the estimated power approach and Bayesian approach, which not only estimate reproducibility probability, but also the Bayesian approach is used to extrapolate the generalizability probability.

Actually to judge whether the foreign data can be extrapolated to a new region, assessment of the similarity between two regions can be performed using a more intuitive approach, that is, analysis of sensitivity index

$\Delta = (1 + \varepsilon/\mu_{original})/C$, which is a measure of change in the signal-to-noise ratio for two difference regions. The evaluation of sensitivity index can be classified into four cases in the light of the mean and variance shift. If the estimate of the sensitivity index falls into a prespecified interval, we claim that there is no difference between the original and the new region; otherwise, the result of similarity cannot be received. Of course further research is necessary for the method based on the sensitivity index, and it is worthwhile to determine the prespecified interval.

References

Berger, J. O. (1985). *Statistical decision theory and Bayesian analysis*. 2nd ed. New York: Springer-Verlag.

Chow, S. C., Chang, M., and Pong, A. P. (2005). Statistical consideration of adaptive methods in clinical development. *Journal of Biopharmaceutical Statistics*, 15: 575–591.

Chow, S. C. and Shao, J. (2006). On non-inferiority margin and statistical test in active control trials. *Statistics in Medicine*, 25: 1101–1113.

Chow, S. C., Shao, J., and Hu, O. Y. P. (2002). Assessing sensitivity and similarity in bridging studies. *Journal of Biopharmaceutical Statistics*, 12: 385–400.

Dempster, A. P., Laird, N. M., and Rubin, D. B. (1977). Maximum-likelihood from incomplete data via the EM algorithm. *Journal of the Royal Statistical Society Series B*, 39(1): 1–38.

Goodman, S. N. (1992). A comment on replication, p-values and evidence. *Statistics in Medicine*, 11: 875–879.

Hsiao, C. F., Hsu, Y. Y., Tsou, H. H., and Liu, J. P. (2007). Use of prior information for Bayesian evaluation of bridging studies. *Journal of Biopharmaceutical Statistic*, 17: 109–121.

Hsiao, C. F., Xu, J. Z., and Liu, J. P. (2003). A group sequential approach to evaluation of bridging studies. *Journal of Biopharmaceutical Statistics*, 13: 793–801.

Hsiao, C. F., Xu, J. Z., and Liu, J. P. (2005). A two-stage design for bridging studies. *Journal of Biopharmaceutical Statistics*, 15: 75–83.

Hung, H. M. J. (2003). Statistical issues with design and analysis of bridging clinical trial. Paper presented at the 2003 Symposium on Statistical Methodology for Evaluation of Bridging Evidence, Taipei, Taiwan.

Hung, H. M. J., Wang, S. J., Tsong, Y., Lawrence, J., and O'Neil, R. T. (2003). Some fundamental issues with non-inferiority testing in active controlled trials. *Statistics in Medicine*, 22: 213–225.

International Conference on Harmonisation. (ICH). (1998). Tripartite guidance E5 ethnic factors in the acceptability of foreign data. *U.S. Federal Register*, 83: 31790–31796.

International Conference on Harmonisation. (ICH). (2006). Technical requirements for registration of pharmaceuticals for human use. *Q&A for the ICH E5 Guideline on Ethnic Factors in the Acceptability of Foreign Data*. Available at: http://www.fda.gov/downloads/RegulatoryInformation/Guidances/ucm129323.pdf

Lan, K. K., Soo, Y., Siu, C., and Wang, M. (2005). The use of weighted Z-tests in medical research. *Journal of Biopharmaceutical Statistics*, 15: 625–639.

Liu, J. P., and Chow, S. C. (2002). Bridging studies in clinical development. *Journal of Biopharmaceutical Statistics*, 12: 359–367.

Liu, J. P., Hsueh, H. M., Hsieh, E., and Chen, J. J. (2002). Tests for equivalence or non-inferiority for paired binary data. *Statistics in Medicine*, 21: 231–245.

Louis, T. A. (1982). Finding the observed information matrix when using the EM algorithm. *Journal of the Royal Statistical Society. Series B (Methodological)*, 44(2): 226–233.

Shao, J. (1999). *Mathematical statistics*. New York: Springer-Verlag.

Shao, J., and Chow, S. C. (2002). Reproducibility probability in clinical trials. *Statistics in Medicine*, 21(12): 1727–1742.

Shih, W. J. (2001). Clinical trials for drug registration in Asian-Pacific countries: proposal for a new paradigm from a statistical perspective. *Controlled Clinical Trials*, 22: 357–366.

5

Combining Information in Clinical Drug Development: Bridging Studies and Beyond

Kuang-Kuo Gordon Lan and José Pinheiro
Janssen Pharmaceutical Companies of Johnson & Johnson PRD

5.1 Introduction

As the cost of developing new drugs keeps escalating and the chance of bringing them to market shows a worrisome decreasing trend, the efficient use of information in clinical drug development is increasingly critical to the success, and even survival, of the pharmaceutical industry. A variety of methods can be included under the broad *combination of information* class, such as meta-analyses, multiregional trials, and bridging studies. In this chapter, we'll focus on the last but will also discuss briefly the other two cited approaches in Section 5.4.

One important difference among the information combination methods is related to the type of data—existing versus new—that they employ. Meta-analytic methods (Borenstein, Hedges, Higgins, and Rothenstein, 2009; Whitehead, 2002) rely on data from previous studies, combining evidence on efficacy or safety endpoints under implicit assumptions of trial comparability (e.g., patient population, standard of care). The main goal of such analyses is to strengthen the evidence of a signal of interest by improving the precision of the associated estimates. Multiregional trials, on the other hand, combine information from different locations where the study was conducted (all data are new) to estimate average global effects in the patient population. One of the key questions they aim to address is the consistency of effect across regions, a necessary condition for the average treatment effect to be meaningful. Finally, bridging studies combine information from previous studies conducted in other parts of the world (e.g., United States and Europe) with new data from a study (or studies) conducted in the region where the sponsor is seeking registration (e.g., Japan). Their main goal is to leverage the existing information obtained from foreign studies to reduce the size of the domestic study needed for registration. All of these methods have in common the goal of increasing the information efficiency of drug development, and all rely on implicit assumptions on the combinability of different sources of information.

In the context of bridging studies, the amount of information that can be borrowed from previous studies conducted with a different patient population will typically be a matter of negotiations with the local health authorities. It can range from none, in which case the development program will need to be entirely reproduced in the new region (thus substantially delaying the availability of the drug in that market), to full, when the approval of the drug in a different country is considered sufficient to allow the compound to be marketed in the new country. Bridging studies are concerned with the intermediate cases of partial information from foreign studies being allowed.

The rest of this chapter is organized as follows. Section 5.2 describes two methods for leveraging previous information in bridging studies, the weighted Z-statistic and the discount factor (Lan, Soo, Siu, and Wang, 2005). Examples of the use of these methods are presented in Section 5.3. The last section briefly discusses meta-analytic and multiregional trial methods and proposes topics for future research in the area of combination of information.

5.2 Leveraging Existing Information in Bridging Studies

In the context of bridging studies, one wishes to leverage information obtained from foreign studies that resulted in a successful submission to reduce the resources needed to develop the compound in the new region—for example, using fewer patients or reducing the development program duration compared with what would be required if the sponsor were to rerun the entire clinical development in the new region. The use of existing favorable information, of course, poses technical difficulties from a traditional hypothesis testing point of view: it would not be possible to achieve the desired resource gains if one were required to control the type I error rate and power at conventional levels (e.g., 0.025 and 0.8 – 0.9). As discussed herein, some compromise is required, which will need to involve negotiations with local health authorities.

To make the problem more concrete, we need to introduce assumptions and notation about the scientific question of interest: the investigation of treatment effect associated with the drug. There are different ways to define treatment effect in a patient population being investigated in a clinical study. To keep the notation simple, while conveying the key ideas, we consider the simplest statistical model formulation, which involves a single treatment arm (one sample) and assumes that the individual responses are independent and identically distributed (i.i.d.) $N(\Delta, \sigma^2)$ random variables. The more realistic situations of two, or more, treatments can also be addressed in the context of bridging studies using the methods described in this section, but for now it suffices to say that conceptually Δ can represent the difference $\mu_1 - \mu_2$ between two treatment means. The normality assumption is not crucial for hypothesis testing, or estimation, when the sample size is large and the central limit theorem is applicable.

Without loss of generality, we assume that large values of Δ are associated with beneficial treatment effect, so that the null and alternative hypotheses of interest are specified as $H_0 : \Delta \le 0$ vs. $H_1 : \Delta > 0$, respectively. To further simplify the problem and focus on the key ideas, we assume that the standard deviation σ is known and, without loss of generality, will take it be equal to 1. Therefore, for a given clinical study of sample size N, we assume the primary endpoint measurements $X_1, X_2, \ldots, X_N$ re i.i.d. $N(\Delta,1)$.

Using this assumption and letting

$$\bar{X} = \sum_{i=1}^{N} X_i \,/\, N$$

represent the sample mean, the Z-statistic for testing the hypotheses on Δ is expressed as the B-value

$$Z = \sqrt{N}\bar{X} = \sum_{i=1}^{N} X_i \,/\, \sqrt{N}$$

As shown by Lan and Wittes (1988), the Z-statistic can be decomposed as the weighted sum of two independent B-values, corresponding to the Z-statistics for two subgroups of patients:

$$Z = \sum_{i=1}^{n} X_i \,/\, \sqrt{N} + \sum_{i=n+1}^{N} X_i \,/\, \sqrt{N} = \sqrt{n/N}\sum_{i=1}^{n} X_i \,/\, \sqrt{n} + \sqrt{(N-n)/N}\sum_{i=1}^{n} X_i \,/$$
$$\sqrt{N-n} = \sqrt{w}Z_1 + \sqrt{1-w}Z_2$$

where $w = n/N$.

5.2.1 Weighted Z-Test Approach

From the sponsor point of view, one appealing way of tackling the bridging data problem would be to combine the foreign and bridging studies data to produce a weighted Z-statistic similar to the one introduced previously, say, $Z = \sqrt{w}Z_B + \sqrt{1-w}Z_F$, where $w = N_B/(N_F + N_B)$, where Z_B and Z_F are the Z-statistics for the bridging and foreign studies, respectively, and N_B and N_F are the respective sample sizes. The key problem with this choice of w is that it assigns equal weight to patients in the foreign and bridging studies, which is unlikely to be acceptable to the local health authority (especially when Z_F is known to be significant). The local health authority needs to have sufficient evidence that the drug works in the local patient population but may be open to allowing some *borrowing* of information from the foreign study. The acceptable value for the weight w then becomes a negotiating point between the sponsor and the local health authority, with its value chosen based on other considerations beyond statistical properties (e.g., similarity between foreign and domestic patient populations, standard of care in the different regions).

For this type of negotiation, it is helpful to consider the statistical properties associated with the test based on the weighted Z-statistics, for a given fixed weight w. Assuming a nominal significance level α for the weighted Z-test, with corresponding critical value z_α, the actual significance level of the weighted Z-test is then equal to $\alpha_B = P\left(Z \geq z_\alpha \mid Z_F, \Delta = 0\right) = 1 - \Phi(z_\alpha - \sqrt{1-w}Z_F / \sqrt{w})$ Figure 5.1 presents the values of actual significance level for different values of w under a nominal $\alpha = 0.025$ and for $Z_F = 2.2$ and 3.2.

For values of w close to 0.5, the significance level for the bridging study is inflated considerably (28% for $Z_F = 2.2$ and 67% for $Z_F = 3.2$) and may not be acceptable to local health authorities. As part of the negotiations about the appropriate value of w, an acceptable value for α_B could need to be agreed upon. For example, if the local health authority required $\alpha_B \leq 0.1$, then one needs to have $w > 0.88$ for $Z_F = 2.2$ and $w > 0.95$ for $Z_F = 3.2$, so the borrowing of information from the foreign study would be fairly limited.

Figure 5.2 displays the minimum weight to be assigned to the bridging study for different values of Z_F to ensure $\alpha_B \leq 0.1$ under a nominal $\alpha = 0.025$. The minimum weight increases with the value of Z_F indicating that the more significant the result of the foreign study, the less contribution it can have to the weighted Z-test.

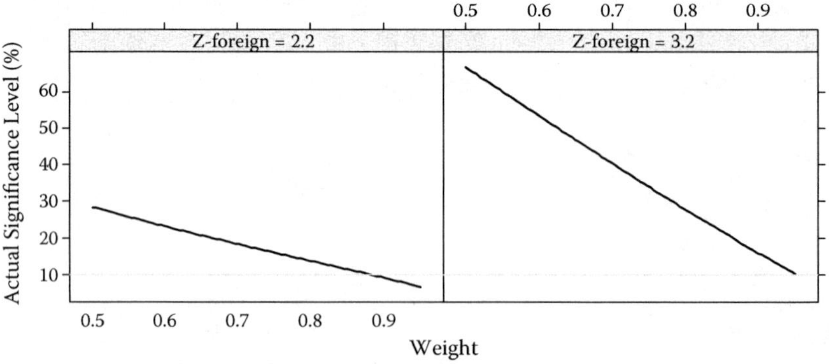

FIGURE 5.1
Actual significance level of bridging study, based on weighted Z-test, for different weights, under a nominal $\alpha = 0.025$ and for $Z_F = 2.2$ and 3.2.

5.2.2 Discount Factor Approach

An alternative approach to the evidence bridging problem is to consider a discount factor for the sample size that would be needed to conduct a properly powered study in the local population under a conventional nominal type I error rate α (typically 0.025, one-sided). The sample size N that would be needed to ensure $1-\beta$ power at a given treatment effect Δ at a significance level α, under the one-sample normally distributed endpoint established previously is given by the usual formula $N = \{(Z_\alpha + Z_\beta)/\Delta\}^2$. Suppose now that one negotiates a reduction in sample size for the bridging study according to a discount factor D, so that $N_B = D \bullet N$, but preserving the original power $1-\beta$. Of course, the only way this can be attained is by allowing the type I error rate of the bridging study to increase from the original nominal α level. It is easy to see in this case that the resulting significance level will be given by $\alpha_B = \Phi[Z_\beta - \sqrt{D}(Z_\alpha + Z_\beta)]$.

For example, to get a 40% reduction in sample size (i.e., $D = 0.6$ with 90% power and nominal significance level of 0.025), one would need to inflate the level of the bridging study to $\alpha_B = 0.1095$. Figure 5.3 displays the actual significance levels for different discount factors, under a nominal $\alpha = 0.025$, to ensure 80% and 90% power. As expected, α_B increases with discount factor, and it is highly unlikely that local health authorities would be willing

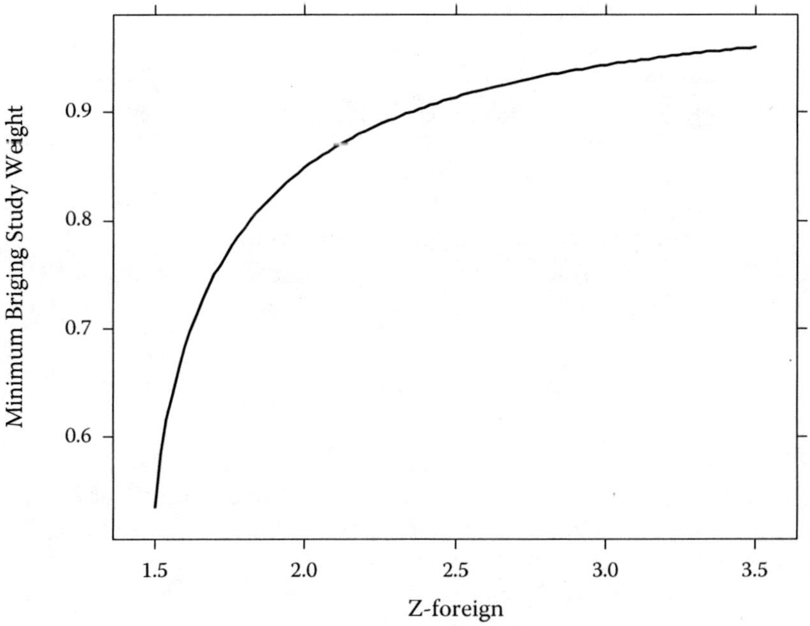

FIGURE 5.2
Minimum weight of bridging study in the weighted Z-test, to ensure an actual significance level of 0.1 under a nominal $\alpha = 0.025$ for varying values of Z_F.

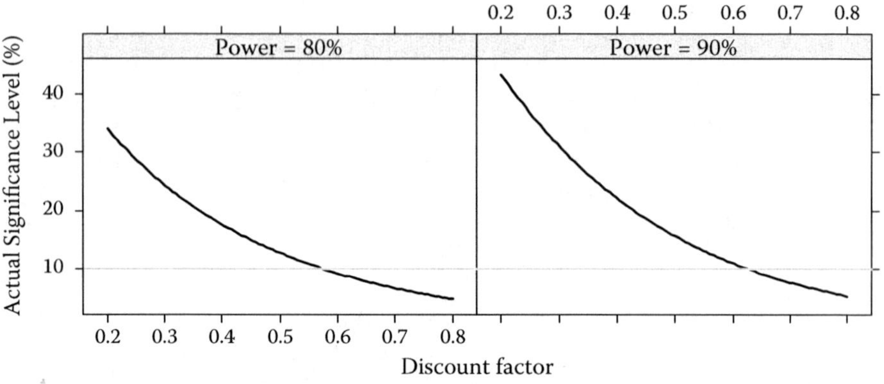

FIGURE 5.3
Actual significance level of bridging study for different sample size discount factors, under a nominal $\alpha = 0.025$, to ensure power values of 80% and 90%.

to accept the increase in type I error rate that would be necessary for large decreases in sample size. For example, if the local health authority requires $\alpha_B \leq 0.1$, then the maximum discount factors allowable for 80% and 90% power would be, respectively, 42% and 37%. Larger discount factors would be obtained under more lax significance level conditions.

The discount factor approach does not directly use the information from the foreign study—it just aims at obtaining a *credit* for the previous favorable result through a negotiated reduction in sample size obtained via an inflation of significance level for the bridging study. In particular, there is no direct association between the amount of evidence in favor of the treatment effect in the foreign study and the allowance in significance level increase in the bridging study. By contrast, the weighted Z-test approach directly incorporates the test statistic from the foreign study in the analysis. Both approaches require negotiations with local health authorities for their acceptance.

5.3 Application: Bridging of Blood Pressure Drug

To illustrate the weighted Z-test and discount factor approaches for bridging studies presented in the previous section, we consider a clinical program in the hypertension indication. A large randomized clinical study conducted in the United States and Western Europe produced a highly significant Z-statistic of 2.87 based on the change from baseline in systolic blood pressure endpoint. The study used a one-sided significance level of 0.025 and was designed to have 95% power to detect a mean difference of 0.1 standard deviation units, resulting in a sample size of 1300 patients. The company now wants to apply for approval of the drug in a different region and is planning to run a bridging study there. The local health authority is willing to allow the company to leverage the result from the previous study but has indicated that the maximum type I error rate that it will allow for the bridging study is 0.12. The company wants to ensure that the bridging study will have power of 80% at 0.1 standard deviation units.

Under these restrictions, the minimum sample size for the bridging study will need to be $N_B = [(Z_{0.12} + Z_{0.2})/0.1]^2 = 407$ patients, corresponding to a discount factor of $D = 407/1300 = 0.313$ with regard to the original foreign study. If one wants to keep the power at 95%, as in the foreign study, then the required sample size for the bridging study would need to increase to 796, for a discount factor of 0.612.

For comparison, we consider the weighted Z-test approach for the same trial. Figure 5.4 presents the actual significance level for the weighted Z-test, given the foreign study Z-value, for a range of combination weights.

To satisfy the local health authority requirement of a maximum significance level of 12% for the study, the minimum weight for the bridging study Z-statistic is $w = 0.915$. The power associated with the weighted Z-test at a standardized effect δ and bridging study sample size N_B under the assumptions and health authority requirements is then given by

$$\pi(\delta, N_B) = \Phi\left(\sqrt{N_B}\delta - \left[Z_{0.025} - \sqrt{1-w}Z_F\right]/\sqrt{w}\right) = \Phi\left(\sqrt{N_B}\delta - Z_{0.12}\right)$$

as w is such that the test has significance level 12%, that is,

$$\left[Z_{0.025} - \sqrt{1-w}Z_F\right]/\sqrt{w} = Z_{0.12}$$

It is then easy to see that, to ensure 80% at $\delta = 0.1$, one needs $N_B \geq 407$, and for 95% power, $N_B \geq 796$. It is not a coincidence that the sample size values for the weighted Z-test approach are the same as the ones obtained for the discount factor approach: under the assumptions and requirements (regulatory and from the sponsor), the two approaches give identical tests for the bridging study.

5.4 Discussion

We reviewed methods for leveraging information from foreign studies to reduce the resource requirements for bridging studies to get regulatory approval of a drug in a new region. One of these approaches, the weighted

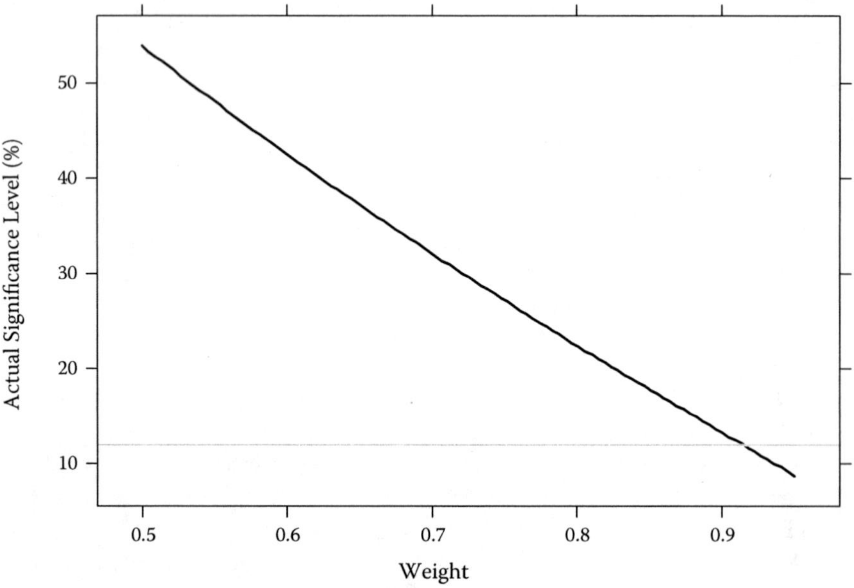

FIGURE 5.4
Actual significance level of bridging study in blood pressure drug example, based on weighted Z-test, for different weights, under a nominal $\alpha = 0.025$ and for $Z_F = 2.87$.

Z-test, can be generalized in different ways. First, in our application we considered only the combination of two Z-statistics: one for the foreign study and another for the bridging study under consideration. Often, in practice, more than one foreign study will be available, so multiple Z-tests will need to be combined with the bridging study. The extension of the weighted Z-test approach to the case of multiple Z-statistics is immediate:

$$Z = \sum_k \sqrt{w_k} Z_k$$

where

$$\sum_k w_k = 1$$

The key negotiating factor with the local health authorities will be the minimum weight to be given to the bridging study, which needs to be determined taking into account the actual significance level associated with the study.

As mentioned in Section 5.1, the weighted Z-test approach provides a framework for combining information from different data sources that transcends the bridging study case considered in this chapter. Two key areas in which similar approaches can be applied are meta-analysis investigations and multiregional studies.

In the context of meta-analysis, the summary Z-statistic is usually a weighted average of treatment effects for different studies of the same treatment or compound. These studies may not follow the same protocol, and important diversity or heterogeneity may exist. However, since the existing data are available, it is hard to argue not to combine the studies due to violation of statistical assumptions. Two main approaches have been proposed for combining information for the purpose of meta-analysis: the fixed-effects and random-effects approaches. The fixed-effects approach is the simplest and assumes that the treatment effect is the same for all studies under consideration. The mixed-effects approach assumes that the treatment effects vary with study, typically according to a normal distribution. It leads to more conservative results than the fixed-effects approach, such as larger confidence intervals for the overall treatment effect. The combination weights and overall treatment effects in the random-effects approach may depend on the between-study variation (such as in level II random-effects models; DerSimonian and Laird, 1986), making the interpretation of results more difficult. Level I random-effects models (Lan and Pinheiro, 2011), on the other hand, use weights that do not depend on variance parameters, allowing easier interpretation of overall treatment effects. Because meta-analysis deals only with existing data, it is not possible to control the (unconditional) significance level or prespecify the desired power for such an analysis.

A combination of information is also required in the context of multiregional clinical trials. As in bridging studies, health authority discussions may also play a role in the determination of the weights to be assigned to the information from each region (and multiple analyses may be required to satisfy different health authorities). One of the key differences with respect to bridging studies and meta-analyses is that all information to be combined in a multiregional study is new. Control of type I error rate and power considerations are typically critical in this type of study design and require prespecification of combination weights.

References

Borenstein, M., Hedges, L. V., Higgins, J. P. T., and Rothenstein, H. R. (2009). *Introduction to meta-analysis.* Chichester, UK: John Wiley and Sons.

DerSimonian, R. and Laird, N. (1986). Meta-analysis in clinical trials. *Controlled Clinical Trials*, 7: 177–188.

Lan, K. K. G. and Pinheiro, J. (2012). Combined estimation of treatment effect under a discrete random effects model. *Statistics and Biosciences.* doi: 10.1007/S12561-012-9054-9.

Lan, K. K. G., Soo, Y. W., Siu, C., and Wang, M. (2005). The use of weighted Z-tests in medical research. *Journal of Biopharmaceutical Statistics*, 15: 625–639.

Lan, K. K. G., and Wittes, J. (1988). The B-value: A tool for monitoring data. *Biometrics*, 44: 579–585.

Whitehead, A. (2002). *Meta-analysis of controlled clinical trials*. Chichester, UK: John Wiley and Sons.

6

A Bayesian Approach for Evaluation of Bridging Studies

Chin-Fu Hsiao and Hsiao-Hui Tsou
National Health Research Institutes

Jen-pei Liu
National Taiwan University

Yuh-Jenn Wu
Chung Yuan Christial University

6.1 Introduction

In 1998, the International Conference on Harmonisation (ICH) published a guidance on "Ethnic Factors in the Acceptability of Foreign Clinical Data" to facilitate the registration of medicines among ICH regions including European Union, the United States, and Japan by recommending a framework for evaluating the impact of ethnic factors on a medicine's effect such as its efficacy and safety at a particular dosage and dose regimen. This guideline is known as ICH E5 guideline. As indicated in the ICH E5 guideline, a bridging study is defined as a supplementary study conducted in the new region to provide pharmacodynamic or clinical data on efficacy, safety, dosage, and dose regimen to allow extrapolation of the foreign clinical data to the population of the new region. Therefore, a bridging study is usually conducted in the new region only after the test product has been approved for commercial marketing in the original region based on its proven efficacy and safety. Moreover, when a bridging study is conducted, the ICH E5 guideline directs the regulatory authority of the new region to assess if dose response, safety, and efficacy in the new region are similar to those in the original region. However, the ICH E5 does not clearly define the similarity.

Shih (2001) interpreted similarity as consistency among study centers by treating the new region as a new center of multicenter clinical trials. Under this definition, Shih proposed a method for assessment of consistency to determine whether the study is capable of bridging the foreign data to the new region. However, while the treatment effect by the bridging study in the new region is ineffective or effective with a similar magnitude of effectiveness to the original region, the approach developed by Shih can usually declare similarity between the new and the original region. On the other hand, if the magnitude of effectiveness of the bridging study is less than that of the original region but meets the minimal clinically meaningful requirement, Shih's approach might be disappointing. Alternatively, Shao and Chow (2002) proposed the concepts of reproducibility and generalizability probabilities for assessment of bridging studies. If the influence of the ethnic factors is negligible, then we may consider the reproducibility probability to determine whether the clinical results observed in the original region are reproducible in the new region. If there is a notable ethnic difference, the generalizability probability can be assessed to determine whether the clinical results in the original region can be generalized in a similar but slightly different patient population due to the difference in ethnic factors. In the assessment of sensitivity, the strategy proposed by Shao and Chow for determining whether a clinical bridging study is useful for regulatory authorities in making policy as to (1) whether a bridging study is recommended for providing substantial evidence in the new region based on the clinical results observed in the original region, and (2) what sample size of the clinical bridging study is needed for extrapolating the clinical results to the new region with desired reproducibility probability. Other methods such as those based on similarity in terms of equivalence and non-inferiority have also been proposed in the literature (Chow, Shao, and Hu, 2002; Hung, 2003).

For assessing the similarity between a bridging study conducted in a new region and studies conducted in the original region, the aforementioned methods may take only the observed bridging data into account. One of the crucial reasons for the ICH E5 guideline's emphasis on minimizing unnecessary duplication of generating clinical data in the new region is that sufficient information on efficacy, safety, dosage, and dose regimen has been already generated in the original region and is available in the complete clinical data package (CCDP). One should therefore borrow "strength" from the information on dose response, efficacy, and safety from the CCDP in the original region and incorporate it into the analysis of the additional data obtained from the bridging study. Liu, Hsiao, and Hsueh (2002) therefore proposed a Bayesian approach to synthesize the data generated by the bridging study and foreign clinical data generated in the original region for assessment of similarity based on superior efficacy of the test product over a placebo control. Lan, Soo, Siu, and Wang (2005) then focused on a combination of information of the type used in bridging studies, in which information is leveraged from previous foreign clinical studies to reduce the resource requirements (e.g., number of patients) for domestic registration of a new compound. The weighted Z-tests in which the weights may depend on the prior observed data for the design of bridging studies are introduced. However, the results of the bridging studies using Liu et al. and Lan et al. will be overwhelmingly dominated by the results of the original region due to an imbalance of sample sizes between the regions. In other words, it is very difficult, if not impossible, to reverse the results observed in the original region even the result of the bridging study is not consistent with those of the original region. However, this issue will occur for any methods for cross-study comparisons if the amount of information is seriously imbalanced between studies. Consequently, Hsiao, Hsu, Tsou, and Liu (2007) proposed a Bayesian approach with the use of mixed prior information for assessment of similarity between the new and original regions based on the concept of positive treatment effect.

This chapter introduces a Bayesian approach for evaluating bridging studies based on the results of Hsiao et al. (2007). In Section 6.2, a Bayesian approach with the use of a mixed prior information for assessment of similarity between the new and original region based on the concept of positive treatment effect will be described. The method for sample size determination is given in Section 6.3. Numerical examples are presented in Section 6.4 to illustrate the Bayesian approach. Discussion and final remarks are given in Section 6.5.

6.2 Mixture of Prior Information

For simplicity, we focus only on the trials for comparing a test product and a placebo control. We consider the problem for assessment of similarity between the new and original region based on superior efficacy of the test product over a placebo control. Let X_i and Y_j be some efficacy responses for patients i and j receiving the test product and the placebo control, respectively, in the new region. For simplicity, both X_i's and Y_j's are normally distributed with variance σ^2. We assume that σ^2 is known, although it can generally be estimated. Let μ_{NT} and μ_{NP} be the population means of the test product and the placebo, respectively, and let $\Delta_N = \mu_{NT} - \mu_{NP}$. The subscript N in μ_{NT}, μ_{NP}, and Δ_N indicates the new region. Because the test product has already been approved in the original region due to its proven efficacy against placebo control, if the data collected from the bridging study in the new region also demonstrate a superior efficacy of the test pharmaceutical over placebo, then the efficacy observed in the population of the new region is claimed to be similar to that of the original region. This concept of similarity is referred to as the similarity by the positive treatment effect.

One, of course, can directly conduct a bridging study in the new region with similar sample size to the phase III trials conducted in the original region to provide adequate power to test the previous hypothesis for confirmation of the efficacy observed in the original region. However, tremendous resources will be allocated to conduct this type of the confirmation bridging trial in the new region. Even when the sponsor is willing to conduct such a trial, recruitment and length of the trial may be serious problems due to insufficient number of patients available in some small new regions. In addition, the valuable information about the efficacy, safety, and dosage contained in the CCDP are not fully used in the design and analysis of the bridging study. Furthermore, it is extremely critical to incorporate the information of the foreign clinical data into evaluation of the positive treatment effect for the bridging study conducted in the new region. Liu et al. (2002) proposed a Bayesian approach to use a normal prior to borrow strength from CCDP for evaluation of similarity between the new region and the original region. However, as mentioned previously, their approach will be overwhelmingly dominated by the results of the original region if there is a serious imbalance in the information provided between the new and original regions.

Therefore, instead of the normal prior distribution used in Liu et al. (2002), we consider a mixture model for the prior information of Δ_N. If no information from the CCDP generated in the original region is borrowed, the statistical inference about Δ_N uses only the information generated by the bridging study conducted in the new region. This is equivalent to assuming a noninformative prior for Δ_N. On the other hand, most of primary endpoints in a majority of therapeutic areas such as hypertension, diabetes, and depression follow or approximately follow a normal distribution. Therefore, it is quite reasonable to use a normal prior for summarization of the results in CCDP of the original region. As a result, the proposed mixture model of the prior information for Δ_N is a weighted average of two priors and given as follows:

$$\pi(\Delta_N) = \gamma\pi_1(\Delta_N) + (1 - \gamma)\pi_2(\Delta_N) \tag{6.1}$$

where $0 \leqq \gamma \leqq 1$. In Equation 6.1, $\pi_2(.)$ is a normal prior with mean θ_0 and variance σ_0^2 summarizing the foreign clinical data about the treatment difference provided in the CCDP, whereas $\pi_1(.)$ has three choices:

Case I: $\pi_1(.) \equiv c$,

Case II: $\pi_1(.)$ is a normal prior with mean 0 and variance σ_0^2; and

Case III: $\pi_1(.)$ is a normal prior with mean 0 and variance 1000.

In Case I, $\pi(.)$ is a noninformative prior, so c can be any number. Our experience shows that changes in c will not have any influence on the conclusion. Here, for simplicity, c is set to be 1. In Case II, π_1 is a normal prior with mean representing the null hypothesis: no treatment difference assumed for the prior of Δ_N. In Case III, π_1 is a normal prior with very large variance, 1000, so it is very close to the noninformative prior considered in Case I. The proposed mixture model of the prior information for Δ_N in Equation 6.1 indicates that a γ value of 0 indicates that the prior π is equivalent to the prior used in Liu et al. (2002), while γ being 1 indicates that no strength of the evidence for the efficacy of the test product relative to placebo provided by the foreign clinical data in the CCDP from the original region would be borrowed. The choice of weight, γ, should reflect relative confidence of the regulatory authority on the evidence provided by the bridging study conducted in the new region versus those provided by the original region. It should be determined by the regulatory authority of the new region by considering the difference in both intrinsic and extrinsic ethnical factors between the new and original regions.

Let n_T and n_P represent the numbers of patients studied for the test product and the placebo, respectively, in new region. Based on the clinical responses from the bridging study in the new region, Δ_N can be estimated by

$$\hat{\Delta}_{\mathrm{N}} = \bar{x}_{\mathrm{N}} - \bar{y}_{\mathrm{N}}$$

where

$$\bar{x}_{\mathrm{N}} = \sum_{i=1}^{n_{\mathrm{T}}} x_i / n_{\mathrm{T}} \quad \text{and} \quad \bar{y}_{\mathrm{N}} = \sum_{j=1}^{n_{\mathrm{P}}} y_j / n_{\mathrm{P}}$$

For the choice of π_1 in Case I, the marginal density of $\hat{\Delta}_{\mathrm{N}}$ is

$$m(\hat{\Delta}_{\mathrm{N}}) = \gamma + (1-\gamma)\frac{1}{\sqrt{2\pi(\sigma_0^2 + \tilde{\sigma}^2)}}\exp\left\{-\frac{(\hat{\Delta}_{\mathrm{N}} - \theta_0)^2}{2(\sigma_0^2 + \tilde{\sigma}^2)}\right\} \tag{6.2}$$

where $\tilde{\sigma}^2 = \sigma^2/n_{\mathrm{T}} + \sigma^2/n_{\mathrm{P}}$. Given the bridging data and prior information, the posterior distribution of Δ_N is

$$\pi(\Delta_N \mid \hat{\Delta}_N) = \frac{1}{m(\hat{\Delta}_N)}\left\{\gamma\frac{1}{\sqrt{2\pi}\tilde{\sigma}}\exp\left[-\frac{(\Delta_N - \hat{\Delta}_N)^2}{2\tilde{\sigma}^2}\right] + \right.$$

$$\left.(1-\gamma)\frac{1}{2\pi\sigma_0\tilde{\sigma}}\exp\left[-\frac{(\Delta_N - \theta_0)^2}{2\sigma_0^2} - \frac{(\Delta_N - \hat{\Delta}_N)^2}{2\tilde{\sigma}^2}\right]\right\}$$

In both Case II and Case III, the marginal density of $\hat{\Delta}_{\mathrm{N}}$ is

$$m(\hat{\Delta}_N) = \gamma \frac{1}{\sqrt{2\pi(\sigma_1^2 + \tilde{\sigma}^2)}} \exp\left\{-\frac{(\hat{\Delta}_N)^2}{2(\sigma_1^2 + \tilde{\sigma}^2)}\right\} + (1-\gamma)\frac{1}{\sqrt{2\pi(\sigma_0^2 + \tilde{\sigma}^2)}} \exp\left\{-\frac{(\hat{\Delta}_N - \theta_0)^2}{2(\sigma_0^2 + \tilde{\sigma}^2)}\right\} \quad (6.3)$$

where $\tilde{\sigma}^2 = \sigma^2/n_T + \sigma^2/n_P$, and $\sigma_1^2 = \sigma_0^2$ in Case II, and $\sigma_1^2 = 1000$ in Case III. Given the bridging data and prior information, the posterior distribution of Δ_N is

$$\pi(\Delta_N \mid \hat{\Delta}_N) = \frac{1}{m(\hat{\Delta}_N)}\left\{\gamma \frac{1}{2\pi\sqrt{\sigma_1^2\tilde{\sigma}^2}} \exp\left[-\frac{(\Delta_N)^2}{2\sigma_1^2} - \frac{(\Delta_N - \hat{\Delta}_N)^2}{2\tilde{\sigma}^2}\right] + (1-\gamma)\frac{1}{2\pi\sqrt{\sigma_0^2\tilde{\sigma}^2}} \exp\left[-\frac{(\Delta_N - \theta_0)^2}{2\sigma_0^2} - \frac{(\Delta_N - \hat{\Delta}_N)^2}{2\tilde{\sigma}^2}\right]\right\}$$

For each choice of π_1, given the data from the bridging study and prior information, similarity on efficacy in terms of a positive treatment effect for the new region can be concluded if the posterior probability of similarity

$$\begin{aligned} P_{SP} &= P(\mu_{NT} - \mu_{NP} > 0 \mid \text{bridging data and prior}) \\ &= \int_0^\infty \pi(\Delta_N \mid \hat{\Delta}_N)\, d\Delta_N \\ &> 1-\alpha \end{aligned}$$

for some prespecified $0 < \alpha < 0.5$. However, α is determined by the regulatory agency of the new region and should generally be smaller than 0.2 to ensure that posterior probability of similarity is at least 80%.

6.3 Determination of Sample Size

Let n_N represent the numbers of patients studied per treatment in the new region. We now describe the method of determination of sample size for the choice of π_1 in Case I. The generalization to other choices of π_1 can be derived similarly. Based on the discussion in the previous section, the marginal density of $\hat{\Delta}_N$ in Equation 6.2 can be re-expressed as

$$m(\hat{\Delta}_N) = \gamma + (1-\gamma)\frac{1}{\sqrt{2\pi(\sigma_0^2 + 2\sigma^2/n_N)}}\exp\left\{-\frac{(\hat{\Delta}_N - \theta_0)^2}{2(\sigma_0^2 + 2\sigma^2/n_N)}\right\} \quad (6.4)$$

The posterior distribution of Δ_N is therefore given by

$$\pi(\Delta_N \mid \hat{\Delta}_N) = \frac{1}{m(\hat{\Delta})}\left\{\gamma\frac{1}{\sqrt{4\pi\sigma^2/n_N}}\exp\left[-\frac{(\Delta_N - \hat{\Delta}_N)^2}{4\sigma^2/n_N}\right] + \right.$$

$$\left.(1-\gamma)\frac{1}{2\pi\sqrt{2\sigma_0^2\sigma^2/n_N}}\exp\left[-\frac{(\Delta_N-\theta_0)^2}{2\sigma_0^2} - \frac{(\Delta_N - \hat{\Delta}_N)^2}{4\sigma^2/n_N}\right]\right\}$$

Given α, θ_0, σ_0^2, σ^2, and the estimate $\hat{\Delta}_N$, we can determine the sample size n_N by finding the smallest n_N such that the equation

$$P_{SP} = \int_0^\infty \pi(\Delta_N \mid \hat{\Delta}_N)\,d\Delta_N$$

$$> 1-\alpha$$

is satisfied.

One approach to determination of Δ_N for sample size estimation of the bridging study is to adopt the "worst outcome criteria" approach suggested by Lawrence and Belisle (1997). Assume that n_O represents the numbers of patients studied per treatment in the original region. The subscript O in n_O indicates the original region. We also assume that both efficacy endpoints of the test drug and the placebo group in the original region have the same variance σ^2. Consequently, θ_0 can be estimated by the difference in sample means of the original region, and $\sigma_0^2 = 2\sigma^2/n_O$ can be estimated by the pooled sample variance of mean difference. Hence, once θ_0 and σ_0^2 are determined, σ^2 in Equation 6.4 can be obtained by $n_O\sigma_0^2/2$. Because the test product has already been approved in the original region due to its proven efficacy against placebo control, the ratio of θ_0 to σ_0 is usually greater than 1.96. Following the "worst outcome criteria" approach by Lawrence and Belisle, the estimate of the treatment difference, $\hat{\Delta}_N$, is chosen to be the lower bound of a 95% confidence interval for Δ_N constructed from θ_0 and σ_0^2. Table 6.1 provides the ratio of the sample size per treatment group for the bridging study to that of the CCDP (n_N/n_O) for various combinations of θ_0 and variance σ_0^2 with $\alpha = 0.1$ and $\alpha = 0.2$.

From Table 6.1, the sample size required for the bridging study in the new region decreases as α or the ratio of θ_0 to σ_0^2 increase and γ decreases.

TABLE 6.1

The Ratio of the Sample Size per Treatment of the Bridging Study to That of the Clinical Trials in the CCDP at $\alpha = 0.1$ or $\alpha = 0.2$ Different Combinations of θ_0 and σ_0^2

	$\theta_0 = 3$, $\sigma_0^2 = 1$		$\theta_0 = 4$, $\sigma_0^2 = 1$		$\theta_0 = 4$, $\sigma_0^2 = 2$		$\theta_0 = 5$, $\sigma_0^2 = 2$	
γ	$\alpha = 0.1$	$\alpha = 0.2$	$\alpha = 0.1$	$\alpha = 0.2$	$\alpha = 0.1$	$\alpha = 0.2$	$\alpha = 0.1$	$\alpha = 0.2$
0	<.01	<.01	<.01	<.01	<.01	<.01	<.01	<.01
0.1	0.63	0.09	0.17	0.04	1.29	0.20	0.34	0.09
0.2	1.06	0.26	0.26	0.08	1.75	0.51	0.49	0.16
0.3	1.24	0.39	0.31	0.11	1.92	0.68	0.56	0.20
0.4	1.33	0.48	0.34	0.13	2.01	0.77	0.59	0.23
0.5	1.39	0.53	0.35	0.14	2.06	0.82	0.61	0.25
0.6	1.43	0.57	0.37	0.15	2.10	0.86	0.63	0.26
0.7	1.46	0.60	0.38	0.16	2.13	0.89	0.64	0.27
0.8	1.49	0.62	0.38	0.16	2.15	0.91	0.65	0.28
0.9	1.50	0.64	0.39	0.17	2.17	0.93	0.66	0.28
1.0	1.52	0.65	0.39	0.17	2.18	0.94	0.66	0.29
	$\theta_0 = 6$ $\sigma_0^2 = 2$		$\theta_0 = 6$ $\sigma_0^2 = 3$		$\theta_0 = 7$, $\sigma_0^2 = 3$		$\theta_0 = 8$, $\sigma_0^2 = 3$	
γ	$\alpha = 0.1$	$\alpha = 0.2$	$\alpha = 0.1$	$\alpha = 0.2$	$\alpha = 0.1$	$\alpha = 0.2$	$\alpha = 0.1$	$\alpha = 0.2$
0	<.01	<.01	<.01	<.01	<.01	<.01	<.01	<.01
0.1	0.17	0.05	0.42	0.11	0.22	0.07	0.14	0.05
0.2	0.24	0.08	0.57	0.19	0.30	0.11	0.18	0.07
0.3	0.26	0.10	0.63	0.24	0.33	0.13	0.20	0.08
0.4	0.28	0.11	0.66	0.26	0.35	0.14	0.21	0.09
0.5	0.29	0.12	0.68	0.28	0.36	0.15	0.22	0.09
0.6	0.30	0.12	0.70	0.29	0.36	0.15	0.22	0.09
0.7	0.31	0.13	0.71	0.30	0.37	0.16	0.23	0.10
0.8	0.31	0.13	0.72	0.30	0.37	0.16	0.23	0.10
0.9	0.31	0.13	0.72	0.31	0.38	0.16	0.23	0.10
1.0	0.32	0.14	0.73	0.31	0.38	0.16	0.23	0.10

Source: *Journal of Biopharmaceutical Statistics*, 17(1), 109–121.

Therefore, for a given value of θ_0/σ_0^2, with proper selection of γ and α, reduction of the total sample size for the bridging study is possible when a statistically significant evidence of efficacy for the test product against placebo is provided in the original region. In particular, when all information from the original region is used; that is, when $\gamma = 0$, the required sample size for the new region is always smaller than that of the original region. Also the required sample size per treatment for the bridging study in the new region increases as γ increases. For instance, when $\theta_0 = 4$, $\sigma_0^2 = 2$ (that is, two-side p-value = 0.0455 for the original region), and $\alpha = 0.2$, the sample size required per treatment for the bridging study increases from less than 1% of that required in the original region at $\gamma = 0$ up to 94% at $\gamma = 1.0$ with $\hat{\Delta}_N = 1.23$ (the lower bound of a 95% confidence interval for Δ_N constructed given that $\theta_0 = 4$ and $\sigma_0^2 = 2$). In other words, when less information borrowed from the original region is incorporated into the prior information, a larger sample size of the bridging study in the new region would be required. On the other hand, let n denote the total sample size for each group planned for detecting an expected treatment difference $\Delta_N = 1.23$ at the desired significance level 0.05 and with power 80% calculated by the traditional method for the two-sample problem. Thus,

$$n = \frac{2(1.96 + 0.84)^2}{(1.23 / \sqrt{n_O})^2} = 10.36 n_O$$

It is obvious that the sample size for the proposed Bayesian approach is much smaller than the total sample size required by the randomized trials with two parallel groups based on the traditional method.

6.4 Examples

Hypothetical data sets modified from our review experience of bridging studies are used to illustrate the proposed procedure. The CCDP provides the results of three randomized, placebo-controlled trials for a new antidepressant (test drug) conducted in the original region. The design, inclusion–exclusion criteria, dose, and duration of these three trials are similar, and hence the three trials are considered the pivotal trials for approval in the original region. The primary endpoint is the change from baseline of sitting diastolic blood pressure (mmHg) at week 12. Because the regulatory agency in the new region still has some concerns about ethnic differences, both intrinsically and extrinsically, a bridging study was conducted in the new region to compare the difference in efficacy between the new and original regions. Three cases with various π_1, which is described in the previous section, are considered in this example. For each case, there are three scenarios to be considered. The first scenario presents the situation where no statistically significant difference in the primary endpoint exists between the test drug and the placebo (two-sided p-value = 0.6430). The second situation is that the mean reduction of sitting diastolic blood pressure at week 12 of the test drug is statistically significantly greater than the placebo group (two-sided p-value < 0.0001). The third scenario is the situation where, due to the insufficient sample size of the bridging study, no statistical significance is found between the test drug and the placebo although the magnitude of

TABLE 6.2

Descriptive Statistics of Reduction from Baseline in Sitting Diastolic Blood Pressure (mmHg)

		Treatment Group	
Region	**Statistics**	**Drug**	**Placebo**
Original 1	N	138	132
	Mean	–18	–3
	Standard Deviation	11	12
Original 2	N	185	179
	Mean	–17	–2
	Standard Deviation	10	11
Original 3	N	141	143
	Mean	–15	–5
	Standard Deviation	13	14
New 1	N	64	65
(Example 1)	Mean	–4.7	–3.8
	Standard Deviation	11	11
New 2	N	64	65
(Example 2)	Mean	–15	–2
	Standard Deviation	11	11
New 3	N	24	23
(Example 3)	Mean	–11	–4
	Standard Deviation	13	13

Source: *Journal of Biopharmaceutical Statistics*, 17(1), 109–121.

the difference between the test drug and the placebo observed in the original region is preserved in the new region (two-sided p-value = 0.0716). The number of patients and mean reduction and standard deviations of sitting diastolic blood pressure are provided in Table 6.2. The three scenarios are denoted as new 1 (example 1), new 2 (example 2), and new 3 (example 3). The alternative hypothesis of interest is that the difference in change from baseline in sitting diastolic blood pressure at week 12 between the test drug and placebo is less than 0.

Using the technique of meta-analysis in Petitti (2000) to integrate the results from both the original and new regions, we derive that $\theta_0 = -13.91$ and $\sigma_0^2 = 0.59$. For the first two scenarios of the bridging studies considered here, $\hat{\sigma}^2 = 3.75$ for estimation of $\tilde{\sigma}^2$, while $\hat{\sigma}^2 = 14.39$ for estimation of $\tilde{\sigma}^2$ in the last scenario. Table 6.3 provides the values of P_{SP} with various values of γ for all three scenarios and all three choices of π_1.

For example 1, the difference in mean reduction of sitting blood pressure between the test drug and placebo is 0.9 mmHg, which is strikingly different from the figures obtained from three trials conducted in the original region. If the regulatory agency allows all information of the original region to be used for evaluation of similarity between the new and original region, γ is set to be 0 and hence $P_{SP} \approx 1.00$ regardless of the choice of π_1. That is the same

TABLE 6.3

Values of P_{SP} Derived from Examples 1, 2, and 3 with Various Values of γ

	P_{SP}								
	Example 1			**Example 2**			**Example 3**		
γ	**Case I**	**Case II**	**Case III**	**Case I**	**Case II**	**Case III**	**Case I**	**Case II**	**Case III**
0.0	≈1	≈1	≈1	≈1	≈1	≈1	≈1	≈1	≈1
0.1	0.6789	0.5680	0.6786	0.9999	≈1	≈1	0.9727	0.9656	0.9980
0.2	0.6789	0.5680	0.6786	0.9999	≈1	≈1	0.9700	0.9309	0.9957
0.3	0.6789	0.5680	0.6786	0.9999	≈1	≈1	0.9690	0.8960	0.9933
0.4	0.6789	0.5680	0.6786	0.9999	≈1	≈1	0.9685	0.8607	0.9906
0.5	0.6789	0.5680	0.6786	0.9999	≈1	≈1	0.9682	0.8252	0.9877
0.6	0.6789	0.5680	0.6786	0.9999	≈1	≈1	0.9680	0.7893	0.9844
0.7	0.6789	0.5680	0.6786	0.9999	≈1	≈1	0.9678	0.7532	0.9807
0.8	0.6789	0.5680	0.6786	0.9999	≈1	≈1	0.9677	0.7167	0.9766
0.9	0.6789	0.5680	0.6786	0.9999	≈1	≈1	0.9676	0.6800	0.9719
1.0	0.6789	0.5680	0.6786	0.9999	0.9934	≈1	0.9675	0.6429	0.9665

Source: *Journal of Biopharmaceutical Statistics*, 17(1), 109–121.

result obtained by Liu et al. (2002). Therefore, we conclude that the efficacy observed in the bridging study of the new region is similar to the efficacy from the original region even if there is no statistically significant difference in the primary endpoint between the test drug and the placebo. This phenomenon implies that when all information from the original region is used, the results of the bridging studies will be overwhelmingly dominated by those of the original region. On the other hand, if $\gamma \geqq 0.1$, then P_{SP} always drops to around 0.6789 in Case I, 0.5680 in Case II, and 0.6786 in Case III. Accordingly, we cannot conclude that the results of the new region are similar to those of the original region if $1 - \alpha$ is set to be greater than 80%. More specifically, P_{SP} drops to 0.8 when $\gamma = 1.0\text{E} - 0.8$ in Case I, $\gamma = 9.0\text{E} - 08$ in Case II, and $\gamma = 8.0\text{E} - 0.7$ in Case III. That is, even with use of very little information from the new region, our proposed procedure reaches a conclusion that is more consistent with the evidence provided by the new region.

For example 2, the difference in mean reduction of sitting blood pressure between the test drug and the placebo is 13 mmHg, which is quite consistent with those obtained from three trials conducted in the original region. As expected, the values of P_{SP} in example 2 appear to be close to 1.00 regardless of the choice of γ and π_1. We can therefore conclude similarity between the new and original regions. Again, our procedure obtains a conclusion that is consistent with the evidence provided by the results of the bridging study conducted in the new region.

For example 3, the magnitude of the mean difference is 7, which is similar to the original region. However, the difference is not statistically significant at the 5% level due to the smaller sample size and the larger variability in the new region. As seen from Table 6.3, the values of P_{SP} are all greater than 0.9665 for all values of γ between 0 and 1 when π_1 is chosen as in Case I and Case II. Hence, similarity between the new and original regions is concluded if α is less than 10%. With the strength of the substantial evidence of efficacy borrowed from the CCDP of the original region, our procedure can prove the similarity of efficacy between the new and the original region when a non-significant efficacy results but with a similar magnitude is observed in the bridging study. When π_1 is chosen as in Case II, the values of P_{SP} gradually decrease from around 1 to 0.6429 when the values of γ increase from 0 to 1. In particular, P_{SP} drops to be less than 0.80 if $\gamma > 0.50$. Therefore, we cannot conclude that the results of the new region are similar to those of the original region if $1 - \alpha$ is set to be greater than 80%. As indicated in Case II, π_1 is a normal prior, which represents the null hypothesis: no treatment difference assumed for the prior of Δ_N. Therefore, as γ increases, influence of the prior π becomes stronger toward the null hypothesis of no treatment difference. In this case, care should be exercised to choose γ.

This example demonstrates that with proper selection of γ by the regulatory agency of the new region, our Bayesian approach with the mixture prior in Equation 6.1 reaches a conclusion much more in line with the results of the bridging study in the new region. In addition, our approach can avoid the difficulty arising from imbalance amount of information between two regions, an issue suffered by the Bayesian procedure proposed by Liu et al. (2002).

In Case I, the prior is $\pi(\Delta_N) = \gamma c + (1-\gamma)\pi_2(\Delta_N)$. In fact, the prior is noninformative since

$$\int \pi(\Delta_N)d\Delta_N = \infty \text{ for any } c$$

We have therefore calculated P_{SP} under different values of c in examples 1 and 3. The results are shown in Table 6.4 and Table 6.5. As seen from the tables, the changes in c did not have a strong influence on the values of P_{SP}.

It should be noted, however, that we use a normal prior for summarization of the results in CCDP of the original region as described already. Nonetheless, it might be possible to use other prior distributions to borrow strength from CCDP. To see whether changes in the prior distribution cause any significant impact in conclusion, we repeat calculations of P_{SP} for the three examples shown in the preceding section using two other prior distributions for π_2 by choosing π_1 as in Case I. The first one is the double exponential distribution (a symmetrical distribution), and the other is the log-normal distribution (a skewed distribution). For the double exponential distribution, $P_{SP} = 0.9878$ for $\gamma = 0$ and is close to 0.6789 for other choices of γ in example 1. Also all the values of P_{SP} are greater than 0.9675 for all γ in both examples 2 and 3 with the double exponential prior. With respect to the log-normal distribution, the value of P_{SP} is equal to 1.00 for $\gamma = 0$ and is close to 0.6789 for other choices of γ

TABLE 6.4

Values of γ Corresponding to Various Values of P_{SP} in Example 1 under Different Values of c

	Case I in Example 1				
γ	$c = 1$	$c = 5$	$c = 10$	$c = 20$	$c = 50$
0.0	≈1	≈1	≈1	≈1	≈1
0.1	0.6789	0.6789	0.6789	0.6789	0.6789
0.2	0.6789	0.6789	0.6789	0.6789	0.6789
0.3	0.6789	0.6789	0.6789	0.6789	0.6789
0.4	0.6789	0.6789	0.6789	0.6789	0.6789
0.5	0.6789	0.6789	0.6789	0.6789	0.6789
0.6	0.6789	0.6789	0.6789	0.6789	0.6789
0.7	0.6789	0.6789	0.6789	0.6789	0.6789
0.8	0.6789	0.6789	0.6789	0.6789	0.6789
0.9	0.6789	0.6789	0.6789	0.6789	0.6789
1.0	0.6789	0.6789	0.6789	0.6789	0.6789

Source: *Journal of Biopharmaceutical Statistics,* 17(1), 109–121.

TABLE 6.5

Values of γ Corresponding to Various Values of P_{SP} in Example 3 under Different Values of c

	Case I in Example 3				
γ	$c = 1$	$c = 5$	$c = 10$	$c = 20$	$c = 50$
0.0	≈1	≈1	≈1	≈1	≈1
0.1	0.9727	0.9676	0.9681	0.9678	0.9676
0.2	0.9700	0.9676	0.9678	0.9676	0.9676
0.3	0.9690	0.9675	0.9677	0.9676	0.9675
0.4	0.9685	0.9675	0.9676	0.9676	0.9675
0.5	0.9682	0.9675	0.9676	0.9675	0.9675
0.6	0.9680	0.9675	0.9675	0.9675	0.9675
0.7	0.9678	0.9675	0.9675	0.9675	0.9675
0.8	0.9677	0.9675	0.9675	0.9675	0.9675
0.9	0.9676	0.9675	0.9675	0.9675	0.9675
1.0	0.9675	0.9675	0.9675	0.9675	0.9675

Source: *Journal of Biopharmaceutical Statistics,* 17(1), 109–121.

in example 1. Again, with the lognormal prior, all P_{SP}'s are greater than 0.9675 for all values of γ in both examples 2 and 3. In summary, three different distributions used for π_2 reach the same conclusion. Therefore, our proposed procedure is quite robust to choice of different prior distributions.

For sample size determination, to be conservative, we use the worst outcome criteria approach by Lawrence and Belisle (1997) with $\theta_0 = -8$, $\sigma_0^2 = 2.56$, and $\sigma^2 = 14.39$. Hence the lower limit of the 95% confidence interval is −11.136. When $\alpha = 0.1$, the required sample size for the bridging study in the new region is 26 per treatment group for $\gamma > 0$. The required sample size per group decreases to 11 if $\alpha = 0.1$ and $\gamma > 0$.

6.5 Concluding Remarks

Herein, a Bayesian method with a mixture prior information has been suggested to synthesize the data from both the bridging study and the original region to assess bridging evidence. The proposed prior information is a weighted average of a noninformative prior and a normal prior, or two normal priors. With an appropriate choice of weight γ, the evaluation of similarity based on the integrated results of the bridging studies in the new region and those from the original region will no longer be overwhelmingly dominated by the results of the original region due to an imbalance of sample sizes between the regions. Therefore, the proposed procedure can avoid the situation of concluding similarity between the new and original region when the efficacy result of the test drug observed in the bridging study of the new region is same as or even worse than that of the placebo group. However, as demonstrated in the examples, similarity between the new and original regions will be concluded when the difference in primary endpoint between the test drug and the placebo observed in the bridging study is of the same magnitude as that obtained from the original region although it is not statistically significant due to the small sample size of the bridging study. As a result, our proposed procedure not only can reach a conclusion that is more consistent with the results obtained from the bridging study but also can achieve the objective of minimizing duplication of clinical evaluation in the new region as specified in the ICH E5 guidance.

Selection of weight γ by the regulatory agency in the new region should consider all differences in both intrinsic and extrinsic ethnical factors between the new and original regions and at the same time should reflect their belief on the evidence of efficacy provided in the CCDP of the original region. As mentioned previously, a bridging study is conducted in the new region because of concerns on ethnic differences between the new and original regions; therefore, it is suggested that weight γ be greater than 0. However, from Table 6.1 and the examples, we can see the weight has a very minimal effect on the sample size of the bridging study and P_{SP} once it is greater than 0.2. For instance, in example 1, P_{SP} drops to 0.8 when $\gamma = 1.0E - 0.8$ in Case I, $\gamma = 9.0E - 08$ in Case II, and $\gamma = 8.0E - 0.7$ in Case III. That is, even with very little information from the new region, our proposed procedure reaches a conclusion that is more consistent with the evidence provided by the new region.

It should be noted that the concept of similarity we consider here is referred to as the similarity by the positive treatment effect, that is, $\Delta_N > 0$. In this regard, even if both regions have positive treatment effects, their effect sizes might in fact be different. That is, the aforementioned approach could not truly assess the similarity between two regions. One alternative approach is to select the similarity margin based on the treatment effect from the original region. More specifically, let Δ_O denote the treatment effect in the original region. We therefore can conclude similarity between the new and the original regions if $\Delta_N > \rho\Delta_O$ for some prespecified $\rho > 0$. Doing so may allow more flexibility on the assessment of similarity. Here ρ represents the magnitude of similarity. Again, selection of ρ should also reflect relative confidence of the regulatory authority on the evidence provided by the bridging study conducted in the new region versus that provided by the original region.

Another approach is to take the concept of noninferiority for assessment of similarity between the new and original region. Under the noninferiority concept, the efficacy observed in the bridging study in the new region can be claimed to be similar to that of the original region if it is no worse than the efficacy of the original region by some clinically acceptable limit, say, δ. In other words, the efficacy observed in the bridging study of the new region is similar if the posterior probability of similarity by the concept of noninferiority is at least $1 - \alpha$,

$$P_{SI} = Pr\{\mu_{NT} - \mu_{OT} > -\delta \,|\, \text{bridging data and prior}\} > 1 - \alpha$$

for some $\alpha > 0$. The equivalence limit δ can usually be expressed as a proportion of the relative efficacy of the test product against the placebo as

$$\delta = f(\mu_{OT} - \mu_{OP})$$

where f is a fixed prespecified constant, $0 < f < 1$, and μ_{OT} and μ_{OP} represent the population means of the test product and placebo, respectively. The details of a Bayesian noninferiority approach to evaluation of bridging studies are described in Liu, Hseuh, and Hsiao (2004).

Alternatively, the concept of average bioequivalence may also be applied for assessment of similarity between the new and original regions. Under the bioequivalence concept, the efficacy observed in the bridging study in the new region can be claimed to be similar to that of the original region if it is within the efficacy of the original region by some clinically acceptable limit, say, δ. In other words, the efficacy observed in the bridging study of the new region is similar if the posterior probability of similarity by the concept of bioequivalence is at least $1 - \alpha$,

$$P_{SB} = Pr\{-\delta < \mu_{NT} - \mu_{OT} < \delta | \text{bridging data and prior}\} > 1 - \alpha$$

for some $\alpha > 0$.

References

Chow, S. C., Shao, J., and Hu, O. Y. P. (2002). Assessing sensitivity and similarity in bridging studies. *Journal of Biopharmaceutical Statistics,* 12: 385–400.

Hsiao, C. F., Hsu, Y. Y., Tsou, H. H., and Liu, J. P. (2007). Use of prior information for Bayesian evaluation of bridging studies. *Journal of Biopharmaceutical Statistics,* 17(1): 109–121.

Hung, H. M. J. (2003). Statistical issues with design and analysis of bridging clinical trial. Paper presented at the 2003 Symposium on Statistical Methodology for Evaluation of Bridging Evidence, Taipei, Taiwan.

International Conference on Harmonisation. (ICH). (1998). Tripartite guidance E5 ethnic factors in the acceptability of foreign data. *U.S. Federal Register,* 83: 31790–31796.

Lan, K. K., Soo, Y., Siu, C., and Wang, M. (2005). The use of weighted Z-tests in medical research. *Journal of Biopharmaceutical Statistics,* 15(4): 625–639.

Lawrence, J., and Belisle, P. (1997). Bayesian sample size determination for normal means and differences between normal means. *Statistician,* 46: 209–226.

Liu, J. P., Hsiao, C. F., and Hsueh, H. M. (2002). Bayesian approach to evaluation of bridging studies. *Journal of Biopharmaceutical Statistics,* 12: 401–408.

Liu, J. P., Hsueh, H. M., and Hsiao, C. F. (2004). Bayesian non-inferior approach to evaluation of bridging studies. *Journal of Biopharmaceutical Statistics,* 14: 291–300.

Petitti, D. B. (2000). *Meta-analysis, decision analysis, and cost-effectiveness analysis.* New York: Oxford University Press.

Shao, J., and Chow, S. C. (2002). Reproducibility probability in clinical trials. *Statistics in Medicine,* 21: 1727–1742.

Shih, W. J. (2001). Clinical trials for drug registration in Asian-Pacific countries: Proposal for a new paradigm from a statistical perspective. *Controlled Clinical Trials,* 22: 357–366.

7

Issues of Sample Size in Bridging Trials and Global Clinical Trials*

Hsien-Ming James Hung, Sue-Jane Wang, and Robert O'Neill
U.S. Food and Drug Administration

Sample size is a critical design specification for a clinical trial to render a statistically meaningful interpretation of the trial's results. To plan the sample size or broadly the amount of statistical information for a randomized clinical trial to meet its objective, the concept of detecting a postulated treatment effect with a sufficient statistical power and the concept of estimating a treatment effect with a sufficient level of precision are commonly entertained. The key assumption behind these concepts is that the treatment effect parameter used in the hypothesis testing is constant and representative of the treatment effect in every subset of the study patient population. Under the global clinical trial strategy in which the same study protocol is implemented in two or more geographical regions, this assumption may be doubtful in the sense that the treatment effect may be heterogeneous across the geographical regions for a variety of plausible reasons. Such interregion heterogeneity will impact the sample size planning. The bridging trial strategy as described in the International Conference on Harmonisation (ICH, 1998) E5 document relies largely on the comparisons between the treatment effects in the foreign regions and the treatment effects in the new region. The across-trial comparisons will further impact the sample size planning.

7.1 Issues of Sample Size Planning for Bridging Trial

As noted earlier, the bridging trial strategy involves use of the trial results of the foreign (or original) region (herein the foreign region may consist of either one foreign region alone or multiple foreign regions in collection)

* This book chapter reflects the views of the authors and should not be construed to represent the FDA's views or policies.

for planning and analyzing a clinical trial of the so-called new region. The major utility stems from the spirit of extrapolation. More than one bridging trial may be needed. The bridging study may be a purely pharmacokinetic (PK)/pharmacodynamic (PD) trial or a regular clinical trial. The main objective of the bridging strategy is to reduce duplication of large phase III clinical trials in the new region, and thus extensive extrapolation from the foreign region to the new region in terms of interpretation of trial results would be required. We focus on the scenario where a bridging clinical trial is at issue.

Let Y be the clinical response variable of interest. Denote by θ the targeted treatment effect parameter of Y, such as the mean effect of the test medical product at a specific dose relative to a placebo, the slope of a linear dose response. Let θ_f and θ_1 denote the θ parameter for the foreign region and the new region, respectively. The statistical inference problem may be associated with testing the parameter θ_1 , given the fact that $\theta_f > 0$, which indicates that the test product's effectiveness has been concluded in the foreign region within the margin of false positive error no larger than one-sided 2.5%. A relevant hypothesis to test for the new region is H_{a1}: $\theta_1 > 0$, and the corresponding null hypothesis is H_{01}: $\theta_1 \le 0$. As usual, a test statistic can be constructed such that the maximum type I error occurs at the boundary point $\theta_1 = 0$.

The sample size implication for the new region can be investigated as follows. Let σ_f and σ_1 be the standard deviation of Y in the foreign region and the new region, respectively. For simplicity, assume that σ_f and σ_1 are known. Let H_{0f}: $\theta_f \le 0$ and H_{1f}: $\theta_f > 0$ for the foreign region. Denote $\theta_k^* = \theta_k / \sigma_k$, $k = f$, 1. Suppose that $4M$ patients are randomized with an equal proportion to receive either the test product or the placebo in the foreign region. Assume that the test statistics for testing H_{0f} and H_{01} are approximately normal under either the null hypotheses or the alternative hypotheses. The P-value associated with testing H_{0f} assumes the value

$$p_f = \Pr(\, P_f \le p_f \mid \theta_f = 0\,) < \alpha$$

where $\alpha \le 0.025$, p_f is associated with the realization, and z_{pf} of the test statistic for testing H_{0f}. The estimate of θ_f^* is then $\tilde{\theta}_f^* = z_{pf} / \sqrt{M}$. Likewise, the P-value associated with testing H_{01} has the power function evaluated at the observed p-value, given by

$$\Pr(\, P_1 \le p_1 \mid \theta_1^* = \lambda\theta_f^*\,)$$

$$= \Phi(-z_{p1} + \sqrt{n}\lambda\theta_f^*)$$

at $\theta_1^* = \lambda\theta_f^*$, for some $\lambda > 0$, where a total of $4n$ patients are randomized with an equal proportion to receive either the test product or the placebo in the new region. The value of λ reflects the degree of heterogeneity between the standardized treatment effect in the new region and that in the foreign trial. The degree of heterogeneity in the treatment effect or in the standard deviation of Y between the regions will determine the value of λ, which can be less than, equal to, or greater than 1. For instance, σ_1 can be smaller than σ_f, particularly when the ethnic factors are more homogeneous in the new region than in the foreign region; in this case, if $\theta_1 = \theta_f$, then $\theta_1^* > \theta_f^*$ and thus $\lambda > 1$. In practice, the value of λ can only be conjectured, provided that relevant prior experience is available to guide the choice.

Given the value of $\tilde{\theta}_f^*$, the sample size per treatment arm needed to detect $\theta_1^* = \lambda\tilde{\theta}_f^*$ at the α_1 level of statistical significance and power $1-\beta$ is $2n$, where

$$n = M\left[\frac{z_{\alpha_1} + z_\beta}{z_{p1}\lambda}\right]^2$$

Table 7.1 shows the sample size ratio n/M needed for the bridging clinical trial if the point estimate of the treatment effect is taken to plan the sample size of the new region and the level of statistical significance used is the same in the regions. The ratio depends on how significant the treatment effect is in the foreign region.

The potential difference in the treatment effect between the foreign region and the new region may arguably challenge the assumption that the treatment effect θ_f or θ_f^* is a fixed constant in the foreign region, particularly if the foreign region consists of multiple regions. As such, we may wish to view the treatment effect θ as a random variable with a limited variance and the variance should be a part of consideration in sample size planning. Under this paradigm, a conservative scenario is that the distribution of θ_f is noninformative for θ_1. Assume that conditional on θ_f, the estimator $\tilde{\theta}_f^*$ is approximately normal with mean θ_f^* and variance $1/M$. Then it can easily be shown that conditional on $\tilde{\theta}_f^*$, the posterior distribution of $\theta_1^* \equiv \lambda\theta_f^*$ is approximately normal with mean $\lambda\tilde{\theta}_f^*$ and variance λ^2/M. Therefore, given $\tilde{\theta}_f^*$,

TABLE 7.1

Ratio of Sample Size ($4n$) of New Region and Sample Size ($4M$) of Foreign Region

	P_f		
λ	**0.025**	**0.001**	**0.0001**
0.9	2.52	1.01	0.70
1.0	2.04	0.82	0.57
1.1	1.69	0.68	0.47

Note: $\alpha_1 = \alpha = 0.025$, $\beta = 0.20$, $\theta_1^* = \lambda\tilde{\theta}_f^*$.

TABLE 7.2

Ratio of Sample Size ($4n$) of New Region and Sample Size ($4M$) of Foreign Region

	P_f		
λ	**0.025**	**0.001**	**0.0001**
0.9	4.69	1.29	0.83
1.0	3.75	1.05	0.67
1.1	3.10	0.87	0.56

Note: $\alpha = 0.025$, $\beta = 0.20$, $\theta_1{}^* = \lambda\theta_f{}^*$. The prior distribution of θ_1 is noninformative.

$$\Pr(P_1 \le p_1 \mid \theta_1{}^* = \lambda\theta_f{}^*)$$

$$= \Phi([-z_{p1} + \sqrt{n}\lambda\tilde{\theta}_f{}^*] / \sqrt{\lambda^2 n / M + 1})$$

Then the n needed for detecting $\theta_1{}^* = \lambda\theta_f{}^*$ at significance level α_1 and power $1 - \beta$ is the solution to the equation

$$\Phi(-\sqrt{n / M}\lambda z_{p0} + z_\beta \sqrt{\lambda^2 (n / M) + 1}) = \alpha_1$$

Table 7.2 shows the sample size ratio (n/M) when the noninformative prior for θ_1 is used and $\alpha_1 = \alpha = 0.025$.

It seems clear that to demonstrate $\theta_1 > 0$ at the usual level of statistical significance and with reasonable power level for a bridging clinical trial, sample size will be demanding unless the standardized effect size in the new region is larger than that in the foreign region and the standardized effect size is estimated with great precision in the foreign region.

Testing to assert that $\theta_1 \approx \theta_f$ will unsurprisingly demand sample size even much more, as shown in Liu, Hsueh, and Chen (2002).

7.2 Issues of Sample Size Planning in Global Clinical Trial

In contrast to the bridging clinical trial strategy, the global clinical trial strategy embraces the premise that all regions participate in the trial under the same study protocol and that statistical inference is entirely based on within-trial comparisons. Hence, the inference paradigm is less complex than that of the bridging strategy. The global trial strategy dwells on the principle that simultaneous conduction of the trial with the same protocol will minimize the regional differences that may cause substantial heterogeneity in the treatment effect estimate among regions.

In the case where the treatment effect is internally consistent among the regions, estimation of θ_1 in a specific region becomes a subgroup estimation problem. Suppose that a global clinical trial of $2N$ subjects per treatment arm is planned to detect the global treatment effect $\theta = \delta$ at significance level α and power $1 - \beta$. Under the global trial strategy, each region may be considered as a subgroup. For the specific region of $2n$ subjects per arm that shares the same expected effect size $\theta = \delta$, the probability that the observed regional P-value (denoted by P_1) is less than or equal to α_1 is

$$\Pr(P_1 \le \alpha_1 \mid \theta_1 = \delta) = \Phi(-\Phi^{-1}(1-\alpha_1) + (z_\alpha + z_\beta)\sqrt{n/N})$$

The relationship between this probability and the ratio (n/N) is shown in Figure 7.1 when $\alpha_1 = 0.025$, following Hung and O'Neill (2003). If the global trial is tested at a one-sided 2.5% significance level, then the region has only about 63% chance of detecting the treatment effect equal to the global treatment effect. Even when the sample size for the global trial is planned for achieving ≤ 1% level of statistical significance and power 90%, the region will need to have at least 50% of the sample size of the entire trial to have a reasonably high probability of showing a p-value no larger than 0.025.

The ICH E5 document stipulates potential heterogeneity of treatment effect that may be caused by intrinsic factors or extrinsic factors. The quality of data and trial conduct may as well induce regional differences of treatment effect, as pointed out by Hung (2009a). In current practice, such heterogeneity is rarely taken into consideration in planning the sample size of the global trial and the global estimate of the treatment effect, which is the weighted average of regional estimates by weighting with regional sample size, is used to represent the treatment effect for each region. Suppose that a global trial

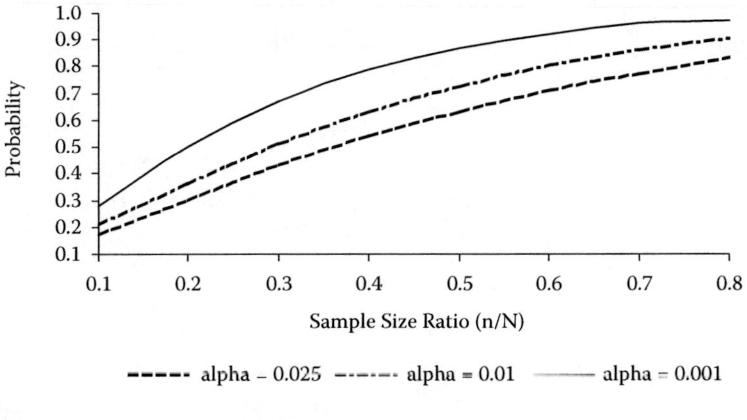

FIGURE 7.1
Probability that subgroup p-value is no greater than 0.025 (entire study planned with 90% power).

is planned on K regions. Let $2n_h$ be the per-arm sample size in region h, $N = \sum n_h$, θ_h the true effect size in region h, and $\hat{\theta}_h$ the estimated effect size of this region. A random-effect model can be used to explore the impact of regional differences on the efficiency of trial design. Assume, for simplicity, that each region has an equal variance, σ^2, in each treatment group. In the normal random-effect model, we assume that

$$\hat{\theta}_h \mid \theta_h \sim N(\theta_h, \sigma^2 / n_h)$$

$$\theta_h \sim N(\theta, \sigma_\theta^2)$$

where σ_θ is the between-region standard deviation of the regional effect sizes. If θ is interpretable for each region, it is usually estimated by the commonly used global effect estimate given by

$$\hat{\theta} \equiv \sum r_h \hat{\theta}_h$$

where $r_h = n_h / N$, which is a weighted average of the regional estimates, using the sample size proportion as the weight. However, if θ is not interpretable for each region, then the treatment effect in region h may have to be θ_h and the global trial will require a sufficient sample size for the region. Under the aforementioned random-effect model, the expectation and variance of $\hat{\theta}$ are

$$E(\hat{\theta}) = \theta$$

$$Var(\hat{\theta}) = \sigma^2 \left[\frac{1}{N} + \left(\frac{\sigma_\theta}{\sigma} \right)^2 \sum r_h^2 \right]$$

If θ is interpretable for each region with a nonzero σ_θ, we should plan N to detect $\theta = \delta > 0$ at significance level α and power $1 - \beta$, and the resulting per-arm sample size should be $2N$, where

$$N = \left[\left(\frac{\delta}{\sigma(z_\alpha + z_\beta)} \right)^2 - \left(\frac{\sigma_\theta}{\sigma} \right)^2 \sum r_h^2 \right]^{-1}$$

Note that since $N > 0$,

$$\frac{\sigma_\theta}{\delta} < \frac{1}{(z_\alpha + z_\beta)\sqrt{\sum r_h^2}}$$

If $\sigma_\theta = 0$, then N reduces to

$$N_0 = \left(\frac{\delta}{\sigma(z_\alpha + z_\beta)} \right)^{-2}$$

which is the usual sample size formula we are familiar with. If $\sigma_\theta \neq 0$, then N_0 underestimates N. The extent of underestimation can be evaluated by

$$\frac{N_0}{N} = 1 - \left(\frac{\sigma_\theta}{\delta} \right)^2 (z_\alpha + z_\beta)^2 \sum r_h^2$$

Assuming $\sigma_\theta \neq 0$ to plan N, the power for detecting treatment effect in region k at significance level α_k is

$$\begin{aligned} &\Pr(P_k \leq \alpha_k \mid \theta_k = \gamma_k \delta) \\ &= \Phi\left(-z_{\alpha_k} + (z_\alpha + z_\beta)\gamma_k \sqrt{r_k \left(1 + N \left(\frac{\sigma_\theta}{\sigma} \right)^2 \sum r_h^2 \right)} \right) \\ &> \Pr(P_k \leq \alpha_k \mid \theta_k = \gamma_k \delta, \sigma_\theta = 0) \end{aligned}$$

for any multiplier γ_k, where P_k is the p-value associated with the estimated treatment effect $\hat{\theta}_k$ in region k.

For illustrative purposes, suppose that a multiregional trial involves five regions with the sample size allocation ratio of (20%, 10%, 40%, 10%, 20%). The total sample size is planned to detect a common effect size δ at one-sided $\alpha = 0.025$ and 90% power. Figure 7.2 depicts the sample size ratio (N/N_0) as a function of (δ/σ) in the two situations, $\sigma_\theta/\sigma = 0.2$ and $\sigma_\theta/\sigma = 0.5$. It is clear that

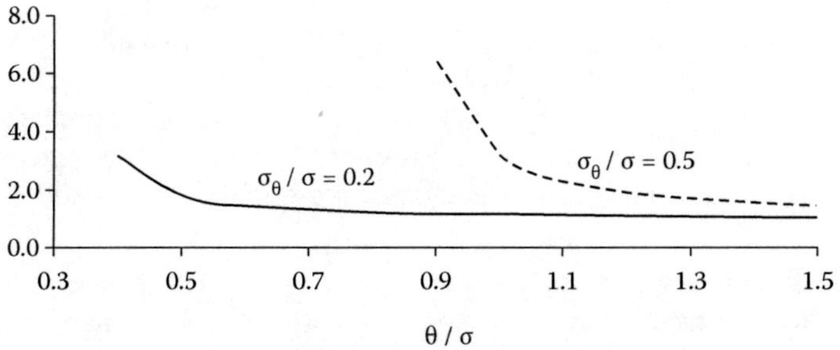

FIGURE 7.2
Sample size ratio (N/N_0) versus (θ/σ).

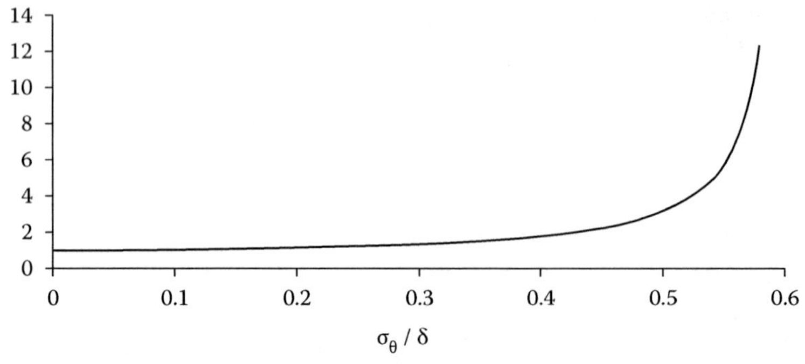

FIGURE 7.3
Sample size ratio (N/N_0) versus (σ_θ/δ).

when the between-region variability is small relative to the within-region variability, the extent of underestimation by N_0 for the N is not large for the most part unless the effect size (δ/σ) to detect is rather small. In contrast, when the between-region variability increases, the extent of underestimation by N_0 can be large. Figure 7.3 depicts the sample size ratio (N/N_0) as a function of (σ_θ/δ). It is clear that when the between-region variability is large relative to the effect size δ, the extent of underestimation by N_0 can be large. Therefore, at the design stage, it is important to project the extent of possible heterogeneity in the regional effect size.

7.3 Impacts of Consistency Assessment on Sample Size

As noted already, there is potential heterogeneity in treatment effect among the regions of a global clinical trial. Consistency assessment is important and should be routinely performed. Statistical methods for consistency assessment are abundant in statistical literature.

The Ministry of Health, Labor, and Welfare of Japan (2007) published a points-to-consider document for global drug development which stipulates that comparability in the results between the Japanese subpopulation and other populations must be taken into account in sample size planning. The following two methods of consistency assessment are introduced:

Method 1: The number of Japanese subjects should be set so that there is 80% or higher probability that the estimated treatment effect in Japanese, denoted by $\hat{\theta}_1$, is at least or greater than $100\pi\%$ of the global effect, $\hat{\theta}$, where $\pi \geq 0.5$ is generally recommended.

Method 2: If there are more than two regions involved in the global trial, then the trend should be similar with the estimated treatment effect $\hat{\theta}_h$ in all the regions. For example, if $\hat{\theta} > 0$, then the sample size should be set so that there is 80% or higher probability that the value of $\hat{\theta}_h$ will all exceed 0.

The points-to-consider document stimulated much research on sample size planning, specifically on sample size allocation to each region. Quan, Zhao, Zhang, Roessner, and Aizawa (2009) focused on Method 1 and derived the sample size formula, (6) in that article, for Japanese population necessary to achieve

$$\Pr(\hat{\theta}_1 / \hat{\theta} > \pi \mid \theta_1 = u\theta) \geq 1 - \gamma$$

where $\gamma \leq 0.20$, when the effect size of Japanese patients, θ_1, is a proportion of the global effect size, θ, that is, $\theta_1 = u\theta$, for some $u \leq 1$. For example, when the global sample size is planned to detect a global effect δ at one-sided 0.025 level of statistical significance and 90% power, the Japanese sample size must be at least 22.4% of the global sample size to achieve 80% probability for the estimated effect size in Japanese being larger than 50% of the estimated global effect, if in truth the treatment effect in Japanese is equal to the global treatment effect.

Kawai, Chuang-Stein, Komiyama, and Li (2007) considered the sample size partitioning such that there is a high probability of observing a consistent trend in treatment effect. Their work is certainly pertinent to Method 2. Assuming that the variance of the response variable is equal to σ^2 in all regions, the probability of observing a positive effect in all regions is

$$\Pr(\hat{\theta}_h > 0, \ \forall h = 1, \ldots, K \mid \theta_h = \theta, \ \forall h)$$
$$= \prod_{h=1}^{K} \Phi\left(\frac{\theta}{\sigma}\sqrt{n_h}\right)$$

which is maximized when all regions are equally represented, that is, $r_h = 1/K$, $h = 1, \ldots, K$. For unequal allocation, in the case of three regions, they demonstrated that if the total sample size is planned to provide 80% power for the global analysis, the sample size of the smallest region should be at least 21.3% of the global sample size so that the probability of observing consistently positive results across region is at least 80%, assuming that the effect size in truth is uniform across all regions.

Also considered by Kawai et al. (2007) is the probability of observing a positive effect for all regions conditional on the positive global treatment effect being statistically significant. According to their simulation studies, the smallest of three regions should contribute at least 15% of the total sample size for the conditional probability to be at least 80%.

Hung (2009b) raised an issue of applicability of either Method 1 or Method 2 to every region, when many regions are involved in the global trial. The sample size allocation proposed in these articles does not appear to be constrained by the condition that the total sample size of the global trial is fixed at the level dictated by the postulated global effect size, level of statistical significance, and level of statistical power.

Ko, Tsou, Liu, and Hsiao (2010) considered the following criteria for determining whether the test treatment is effective in a specific region, say, Region 1.

(i) $\theta_1 \geq u\theta_{1c}$, for some $0 < u < 1$
(ii) $\theta_1 \geq u\theta$, for some $0 < u < 1$
(iii) $u \leq \theta_1/\theta_{1c} \leq 1/u$, for some $0 < u < 1$
(iv) $u \leq \theta_1/\theta \leq 1/u$, for some $0 < u < 1$

where θ_{1c} is the effect size in the rest of regions combined. The sample size planning is made to ensure that the assurance probability associated with one of these criteria given $\theta = \delta$ is sufficiently high, say 80% or above. The assurance probability associated with criterion 1 is the probability that criterion 1 is met conditional on the global effect being statistically significantly positive at level of significance α and the total sample size being planned to detect $\theta = \delta$ at significance level α and power $1 - \beta$. Table 2 in their article shows that if $u = 0.50$, then Region 1 will need at least 30% of the total sample size to have the assurance probabilities associated with criterion 1 and criterion 2 no less than 80%. Criteria 3 and 4 are more of equivalence type. The behaviors of the assurance probabilities associated with these two criteria are quite different, as shown in their Table 2 and Figure 2. Choice of which consistency criterion to meet is therefore important.

Uesaka (2009) studied a more general framework where more than one treatment or dose group is compared with a control group. The parameters under study can be expressed as a linear contrast of the central tendency parameters of the comparative groups, such as dose-response contrast parameter. Similar consistency measures or efficacy measures are considered to meet a high threshold of assurance probability that is similarly defined in the work of Kawai et al. (2007) and the work of Quan et al. (2009). Depending on which contrast parameter is looked at and which sample size allocation rule is considered, the sample size allocation or the minimum sample size allocation for the specific region relative to the total sample size of the trial may differ largely. Consideration of whether the regional effects are homogeneous or heterogeneous also affects the assurance probability.

In contrast, particularly in the analysis stage, when some of the regions show an inconsistent trend in treatment effect relative to others, an issue with interpretability of the global treatment effect estimate arises. From this standpoint, Hung, Wang, and O'Neill (2010) considered inconsistency assessment across the regional estimates of treatment effect by examining directional inconsistency in the sense that the effect estimates are positive in some regions but negative in others. The probability of such a directional reversal can be computed, given a global effect size. Under the frequestist paradigm, the probability that $\hat{\theta}_h > 0$, given the true effect size θ, is

$$\Pr(\hat{\theta}_h > 0 \mid \theta) = \Phi([\theta / \sigma]\sqrt{r_h N})$$

assuming that normality approximation is applicable for each region, where N and σ are defined in Section 7.2. For each h, define the indicator variable $\pi_h = 1$ if $\hat{\theta}_h > 0$, and $\pi_h = -1$ if $\hat{\theta}_h \leq 0$. Then the probability that m of the K regions show a negative or nonpositive effect estimate is

$$P(\text{exactly } m \text{ of } K \text{ regions have } \hat{\theta}_h \leq 0 \mid \theta)$$

$$= \sum_{R_m} \prod_{h=1}^{K} \Phi(\pi_h \sqrt{r_h} \sqrt{N} (\theta / \sigma))$$

where

$$R_m = \{(\pi_1, \ldots, \pi_K) : \sum_{h=1}^{K} \pi_h = K - 2m\}$$

For illustration, suppose a multiregional (four regions) clinical trial is planned to detect a postulated global effect size $\delta > 0$ at one-sided 2.5% level of significance and 90% power, assuming all regions have an equal variance σ^2. Let p be the p-value associated with the statistically significant global estimate d of the treatment effect and $d > 0$. If the true global effect size is very close to d, we can compute the probability that m of the four regions show a reversal as a function of p, which is associated with d, since $d = [z_p/(z_\alpha + z_\beta)]\delta$, where z_α is the $(1 - \alpha)$-th percentile of the standard normal distribution. From Table 7.3, it can be seen that the probability that one out of the four regions shows a reversal is large. When $p = 0.05$, the probability that two of the four regions show a reversal is still substantial. For the fixed planned sample size, as the sample sizes allocated to the regions are more unbalanced, the probability of showing a reversal appears larger. When the global effect is highly significant (e.g., $p = 0.001$), the probability that two of the four regions show a reversal is small. The results of Table 7.3 also have ramifications on designing a multiregional clinical trial in terms of sample size allocation to each local region.

Figure 7.4 depicts the relationship between the probability of showing a nonpositive treatment effect in either one or two of four regions and the ratio

TABLE 7.3

Probability of Reversal (Assuming the True Global Effect Size Is Very Close to the Estimated Effect Size)

p	Probability That One Region Shows a Reversal	Probability That Two Regions Show Reversals
	$(r_1, r_2, r_3, r_4) = (0.25, 0.25, 0.25, 0.25)$	
.001	0.17	0.01
.01	0.29	0.05
.05	0.38	0.11
	$(r_1, r_2, r_3, r_4) = (0.20, 0.10, 0.30, 0.40)$	
.001	0.23	0.02
.01	0.33	0.06
.05	0.40	0.13
	$(r_1, r_2, r_3, r_4) = (0.10, 0.10, 0.10, 0.70)$	
.001	0.32	0.06
.01	0.39	0.11
.05	0.43	0.17

Source: Excerpted from Hung, H. M. J., S. J. Wang, and R. O'Neill, *Pharmaceutical Statistics*, 9, 173–178, 2010.

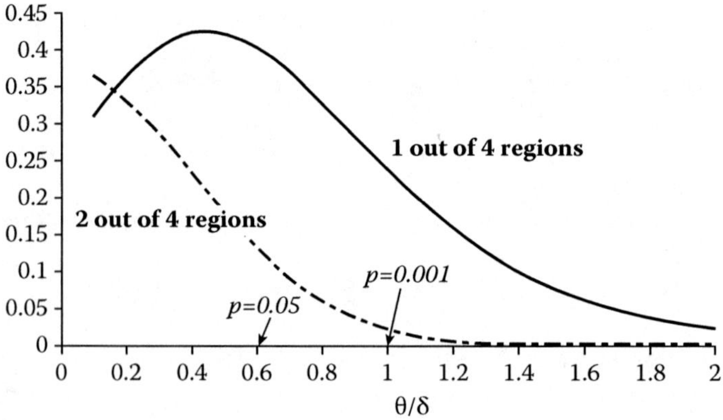

FIGURE 7.4
p (m of 4 regions show a nonpositive drug effect). Sample size allocation to 4 regions = (0.2, 0.1, 0.3, 0.4), δ is detected with 90% power.

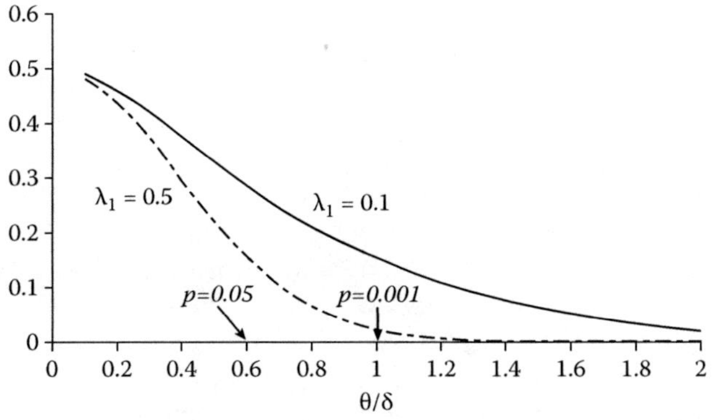

FIGURE 7.5
p (region 1 shows a non-positive drug effect). Sample size allocation for Region 1 vs. the rest = $(\lambda_1, 1 - \lambda_1)$, δ is detected with 90% power.

of true global effect size to the postulated effect size, given the sample size allocation is (20%, 10%, 30%, 40%). It is clear that one of four regions will yield a nonpositive effect with a large probability, particularly the true global effect size is small. From the previous formula, the larger the sample sizes are, the smaller the probability that m of K regions show nonpositive treatment effect.

At the analysis stage, it is also often necessary to look at a specific local region (called Region 1) versus the rest. Figure 7.5 depicts the probability that this region shows a nonpositive treatment effect.

Clearly, from the previous equation, this probability will depend inversely on the sample size allocation ratio for this region. The smaller the sample size allocated to this region, the larger the probability that this region shows a nonpositive treatment effect. In practice, it is important to take into account these probabilities and sample size allocation in the sample size planning of a multiregional clinical trial.

7.4 Discussion

Heterogeneity of regional treatment effects in a multiregional trial has appeared, at least, in many regulatory applications. Such heterogeneity can arise purely due to chance or with causes. Unfortunately, in practice, it is most often the case that the causes for such heterogeneity, if it occurs, are unknown. Thus, it is probably unwise to plan the sample size of the global trial using the assumption that the treatment effect is equal in all the regions. A difficult problem is to what extent the regional differences need to be anticipated and postulated for sample size planning. How to allocate sample size to each region also needs to be carefully considered in the planning. This makes the sample size planning even more difficult since there is no consensus as to what consistency measures need to be considered in all the regions. Regulatory authorities and regulated industries from all the regions need to engage in extensive discussions about these aspects. It is clear from Figures 7.4 and 7.5 that the probability of chance occurrence of such regional heterogeneity may be mitigated if the positive global treatment effect is highly statistically significant, which may imply a need for conservative sample size planning. On the other hand, research is definitely needed as to how to best present to the consumers the results of a global trial that show heterogeneity of the treatment effect among the regions. After all, when such heterogeneity appears, the chance occurrence may be a part of the cause and should be eliminated, if all possible, from the presentation.

References

Chow, S. C., Shao, J., and Hu, O. Y. P. (2002). Assessing sensitivity and similarity in bridging studies. *Journal of Biopharmaceutical Statistics*, 12: 385–400.

Hung, H. M. J. (2009a). Data quality in multi-regional clinical trial: A regulatory perspective. Paper presented at the Drug Information Association Annual Meeting, San Diego, CA, June 24.

Hung, H. M. J. (2009b). Discussion of papers presented in the session of considerations on design and analysis for multi-regional trials. Paper presented in American Statistical Association Joint Statistical Meetings, Washington, DC, August 16.

Hung, H. M. J. and O'Neill, R. (2003). Utilities of the *P*-value distribution associated with effect size in clinical trials. *Biometrical Journal*, 45: 659–669.

Hung, H. M. J., Wang, S. J., and O'Neill, R. (2010). Challenges in design and analysis of multi-regional clinical trials. *Pharmaceutical Statistics*, 9: 173–178. doi: 10.1002/pst.440.

International Conference on Harmonisation. (ICH). (1998). Tripartite guidance E5 ethnic factor in the acceptability of foreign data. *U.S. Federal Register*, 83: 31790–31796

Kawai, N., Chuang-Stein, C., Komiyama, O., and Li, Y. (2007). An approach to rationalize partitioning sample size into individual regions in a multiregional trial. *Drug Information Journal*, 42: 139–147.

Ko, F. S., Tsou, H. H., Liu, J. P., and Hsiao, C. F. (2010). Sample size determination for a specific region in a multiregional trial. *Journal of Biopharmaceutical Statistics*, 24: 870–885.

Liu, J. P., Hsueh, H. M., and Chen, J. J. (2002). Sample size requirement for evaluation of bridging evidence. *Biometrical Journal*, 44: 969–981.

Ministry of Health, Labour and Welfare of Japan. (2007). Basic principles on global clinical trials. Notification No. 0928010, September 28.

Quan, H., Zhao, P. L., Zhang, J., Roessner, M., and Aizawa, K. (2009). Sample size considerations for Japanese patients in a multi-regional trial based on MHLW guidance. *Pharmaceutical Statistics,* 8: 1–14.

Shih, W. J. (2001). Clinical trials for drug registrations in Asian-Pacific countries: Proposal for a new paradigm from a statistical perspective. *Controlled Clinical Trials*, 22: 357–366.

Uesaka, H. (2009). Sample size allocation to regions in a multiregional trial. *Journal of Biopharmaceutical Statistics*, 19: 580–594.

8

*Design and Sample Size Considerations for Global Trials**

Christy Chuang-Stein
Pfizer, Inc.

Yoichi Ii, Norisuke Kawai, Osamu Komiyama, and Kazuhiko Kuribayashi
Pfizer Japan Inc.

8.1 Introduction

ICH E9, finalized and adopted by the regulatory bodies of the European Union, Japan, and the United States on February 5, 1998, includes a section (Section 3.2) on multicenter trials. It acknowledges that the inclusion of multiple centers is necessary not only to complete a trial in a reasonable time frame but also to provide a broad patient base for inference. The need for large mortality and morbidity endpoint trials in the cardiovascular area started the trend for multinational trials in the 1980s. The majority of the nations in these early multinational trials were Western industrial countries. Data from these trials were used to support product registration in the United States and Europe initially and the rest of the world subsequently.

The year 1998 also marked the finalization of ICH E5, "Ethnic Factors in the Acceptability of Foreign Clinical Data." ICH E5 addresses the intrinsic characteristics of patients and extrinsic characteristics associated with environment and culture that could affect the results of clinical studies carried out in different regions. It also describes the concept of the "bridging study" that the regulatory agency in a new region may request to help determine if data from another region are applicable to its population.

ICH E5 was developed at a time when global pharmaceutical companies regularly used data from trials conducted in the developed world in the West to support registration in Japan and other Asian countries. The bridging

* The authors want to thank Dr. Bernadette Hughes and many colleagues at Pfizer who have contributed to the points raised in Section 8.2.

study could be a pharmacokinetic trial to demonstrate comparable drug concentration level in subjects between regions or a dose-response study to demonstrate a comparable dose-response relationship across regions. Much literature has been devoted to this topic (see, e.g., Chow, Shao, and Hu, 2002; Hsiao, Hsu, Tsou, and Liu, 2007; Hsiao, Xu, and Liu, 2005; Liu and Chow, 2002; Liu, Hsiao, and Hsueh, 2002; Shih, 2001). Because of the sequential drug development paradigm, some countries gained access to life-saving products years after the products had become available in other parts of the world. This phenomenon was referred to as drug lag in the affected countries.

Since the issuance of ICH E5, several questions have arisen. These questions and answers to them have been incorporated into a final Questions and Answers (Q&A) document by the E5 Implementation Working Group in 2006. Among the questions, the concept of a multiregional trial as a form of bridging came up in Question 11 (Q11). This concept was proposed by Japan Pharmaceutical Manufacturers Association, which had wanted to shift the paradigm from sequential drug development to a globally simultaneous one. Question 11 and its answer address the desire that in certain situations a sponsor could achieve the goal of bridging by conducting a multiregional trial under a common protocol that includes a sufficient number of patients from each of multiple regions to conclude about treatment effect in all regions.

During the first decade of the 21st century, the Pharmaceuticals and Medical Device Agency (PMDA) in Japan identified the reduction of drug lag as a top priority for the agency. To support this goal and to further articulate Q11 in the ICH E5 Q&A Addendum, the Ministry of Health, Labour and Welfare (MHLW) in Japan issued a guidance document on *Basic Principles on Global Clinical Trials* in September 2007.

Western European countries that were used to having multinational trials conducted in their countries faced a different type of product development challenge. For several years now, an increasingly higher percentage of subjects in multinational trials have been coming from developing countries. Investigators' clinical research experience and how trial results from developing countries could be translated to more medically established communities have been debated in recent years. In 2009, European Medicines Agency (EMA) finalized a reflection paper to highlight the need to include sufficient European population in confirmatory trials so that the trials could be used to support the application of a marketing authorization application (MAA) in Europe (CHMP, 2009).

Furthermore, during September 6–7, 2010, the EMA held an international workshop with broad participation to discuss a way forward to ensure a robust global framework of clinical trials. The workshop related to the consultation process for EMA's reflection paper on ethical and good clinical practice aspects of clinical trials of medicinal products for human use conducted in third countries and submitted in support of marketing authorization applications to the EMA (EMA, 2010). The new reflection paper signals regulators' concerns that the rights, safety, and well-being of trial subjects in third countries be protected and that all trials should follow the same and transparent standard.

Similar concerns have arisen in the United States. The U.S. Food and Drug Administration (FDA) has long been relying on data from subjects in Western European countries to supplement data obtained in the United States. For many years, the FDA has not made much distinction between the United States and Western European data. Nevertheless, recent multinational trials include Latin American, Eastern European, and Asian sites, often with the United States and Western Europe representing a minority of the patient populations. As Dr. Robert Temple stated at the FDA Pharmaceutical Research and Manufacturers of America (PhRMA) Workshop on Multiregional Trials in 2007, while the FDA continued to accept data from such trials it is looking closely at regional differences with a degree of nervousness, stimulated by a number of troubling examples.

The first highly visible case hinting at possibly different treatment effect in patients in the United States compared with patients outside of the United States is the MERIT-HF study (Anello, O'Neil, and Dubey, 2005). This study, conducted in the United States and the European Union, investigated the effect of Toprol-XL for the indication of congestive heart failure, when used in combination with the optimal standard treatment. The protocol specified two primary endpoints: time to all-cause mortality and time to the first event of all-cause death or hospitalization. A total of 3991 patients were randomized, with 1071 of them (about 27%) from the United States. When looking at subgroup results related to all-cause mortality, point estimates for the hazard ratio (Toprol-XL combined with optimal standard treatment vs. optimal standard treatment alone) for nearly all subgroups are less than 1 except for the U.S. subgroup. The point estimate for the hazard ratio for mortality for the EU population is 0.55 (95% confidence interval: 0.43–0.70), and the corresponding estimate for the U.S. population is 1.05 (95% confidence interval: 0.71, 1.56). This raised the question of whether the data suggest a lack of treatment effect among the U.S. subjects or whether what was observed was due to random chance. The previous question was hard to answer because the analysis was post hoc and there were many subgroup analyses.

This debate was renewed with the PLATO trial of ticagrelor (a blood thinner). Data from the PLATO trial were reviewed by the FDA's Cardiovascular and Renal Drug Advisory Committee (http://www.fda.gov/AdvisoryCommittees/CommitteesMeetingMaterials/Drugs/CardiovascularandRenalDrugsAdvisoryCommittee/ucm221382.htm) July 28, 2010. This single trial of 18,624 patients was used to support the application of ticagrelor for reduction of thrombotic events in patients with non-ST elevation myocardial infarction (NSTEMI) and ST segment elevation myocardia infarction (STEMI) acute coronary syndrome. It was designed as a superiority trial with clopidogrel as the comparator and the composite endpoint of cardiovascular death and myocardial infarction and stroke as the primary endpoint. Among the nearly 20,000 patients, 1,413 (< 8%) came from the United States and 17,211 came from outside the United States. The overall treatment effect was positive. As shown by the FDA at the advisory committee meeting, a 95% confidence interval for the hazard ratio (ticagrelor vs. clopidrogrel) for the composite endpoint in the U.S. population is (0.92, 1.75), while the corresponding confidence interval in the non-U.S. population is (0.74, 0.90). These two confidence intervals do not overlap. When discussing the results from PLATO, members of the AC were not convinced that the observed difference in the clinical outcome was due to chance alone. Instead, AC members speculated that differences in baseline characteristics of the patients and regional disparities in the practice of care such as aspirin dose might have contributed to the observed difference in treatment effect. On December 6, 2010, ticagrelor cleared European regulators. In the same month the FDA rejected ticagrelor and asked the sponsor for more information and additional analyses from the PLATO trial. On July 20, 2011, the FDA approved ticagrelor. The approved label includes a boxed warning about how the drug's effectiveness will be reduced if it is taken with higher doses of aspirin.

In this chapter, we define a multiregional study as a study conducted in multiple regions under a common protocol that includes a sufficient number of patients in each region to allow a decision about the treatment effect in that region. For convenience, regions are defined by regulatory jurisdictions in this chapter. Pharmaceutical industry has been conducting multinational trials for many years (see, e.g., Anello et al., 2005; Ho and Chow, 1998). What is new in our recent interest in multiregional trials stems from the desire to use such trials to fulfill the confirmatory requirement by health authorities in all the regions identified in the trials. Consequently, investigation of ethnic sensitivity and insensitivity, addressed in ICH E5, is more critical in multiregional trials than in multinational trials.

Returning to Q11 in the ICH E5 Q&A Addendum, it describes a hierarchy of persuasiveness of results from a multiregional trial. The most persuasive result

	Statistical significance in overall result	**Statistically significant result from Region of Interest**	**Similar trend among regions**
Stand Alone Regional Result	✓	✓	*
No Significant Regional Result but Similar Results across Regions	✓		✓

* "It will also be important to compare results across regions."

FIGURE 8.1
Hierarchy of persuasiveness.

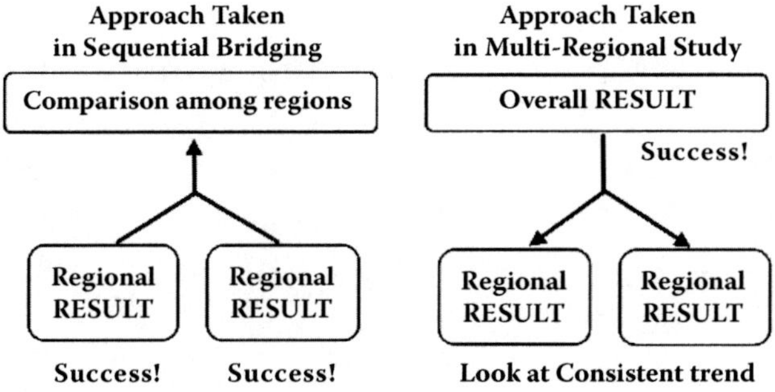

FIGURE 8.2
Viewing the results in the opposite direction.

is "Stand Alone Regional Result," and the next is "No Significant Regional Result but Similar Results across Regions," as displayed in Figure 8.1.

The "Stand Alone Regional Result" requires strong evidence for treatment effect in the region of interest. This level of requirement is close to what was often seen in a sequential bridging strategy, at least for Japan. For example, before comparing with foreign clinical data, a bridging study in Japan needed to show a statistically significant result in the primary analysis. By comparison, the second row in Figure 8.1 describes the usual expectation of a multiregional trial in that a sponsor would look at the overall result first and then investigate regional differences in the form of a prespecified subgroup analysis. As such, the "No Significant Regional Result but Similar Results across Regions" option allows for a more moderate evidential level for each region. Under this option, the overall result and the regional results would be viewed in the opposite direction between sequential bridging and multiregional trials, as displayed in Figure 8.2. A critical question then is how to determine if the treatment effect is similar across regions under the second option.

In the next section, we will discuss points to consider when designing a multiregional trial as a form of information bridging within a trial. The objective is to strengthen results observed in one region with results observed in another region within the same trial. (We are not interested in a separate bridging study in this chapter.) In Section 8.3, we will adopt one criterion in the MHLW guidance for deciding treatment effect consistency in determining sample size for different regions. We also acknowledge other criteria and offer additional references (Section 8.3.5). The approach in Section 8.3 is extended to a more complicated situation when the primary analysis is adjusted for important baseline covariates in Section 8.4. In Section 8.5, we discuss the importance of real-time monitoring in a multiregional trial since multiregional trials could be extremely complicated and represent substantial investment on the part of a sponsor. We will conclude this chapter with some additional comments and the story about IRESSA.

8.2 Points to Consider When Designing a Multiregional Trial

In this section, we will discuss points to consider from clinical, statistical, regulatory, commercial, and operational perspectives. Many of these issues are covered in the ICH E5 Q&A Addendum.

8.2.1 Clinical Considerations

These include intrinsic and extrinsic factors, choice of control group, choice of endpoints, inclusion and exclusion criteria, and concomitant therapies. Intrinsic factors include genetics, disease etiology, comorbidity, and drug metabolism, which could affect drug–drug interactions. Extrinsic factors include medical practice, disease diagnosis, and how health and comorbidity are managed. As for the choice of control group, different regions could have different attitudes toward the use of a placebo. Even if an active treatment is to be used as a control, different regions might have different preference for the active treatment. The gold standard in one region might not be approved and covered by the public health system in another region. If different comparators are to be used in different regions, a sponsor needs to consider how this might affect the assessment of treatment effect across regions.

Differences in disease criteria or diagnostic tools could lead to differences in patient populations from different regions. This could lead to questions by regulators on how information obtained in other regions might apply to patients in their own regions. Increasingly, a new treatment is being assessed on its effect when added to the standard background therapy. If the standard background therapy differs across regions, the added benefit of the new treatment could conceivably differ across regions. The latter was suspected to be a contributing factor to the observed differences in the ticagrelor case. Here, background disease management includes pharmacologic as well as nonpharmacologic disease management.

We have experienced situations where different health authorities demanded different primary endpoints. While this may be managed by a strategy under which every health authority is to spend its allowed two-sided 5% type I error rate on the endpoints of its choice, this could still lead to long discussions in cases where some health authorities disagree with this strategy.

If a patient reported outcome (PRO) is to be used to determine efficacy and to drive the language in the label, it is important that the PRO has been adequately validated in the target patient population to conform to relevant regulatory guidances (CHMP, 2006; FDA, 2009). The translations of the instrument used to record the PRO have to be developed in accordance with the gold standard process including forward–background, cognitive debriefing, and international harmonization. The development of a PRO instrument including translation and cultural adaptation to other languages for use in a multinational trial is given in the FDA (2009) "Guidance for Industry: Patient-Reported Outcome Measures: Use in Medical Product Development to Support Labeling Claims." An equally important consideration is whether payers will be receptive to the use of the PROs in pricing and reimbursement decisions.

8.2.2 Statistical Considerations

Statistical considerations could be discussed in the context of design, interim decision, and analysis. From the design perspective, a sponsor needs to do the following:

1. Determine the role of regions in the primary and key secondary analyses
2. Define how to assess the "consistency" of treatment effect across regions
3. Articulate the assumptions underlying sample size decision (e.g., uniform treatment effect and similar variability across regions)
4. Decide if the minimum clinically important difference (MCID) is the same across regions if MCID is the basis for sample size decision (Chuang-Stein, Kirby, Hirsch, and Atkinson, 2011)
5. Determine the overall sample size and regional sample sizes to support the primary objective on the overall treatment effect and a key secondary objective on treatment effects in prespecified regions
6. Decide if randomization will be stratified by regions
7. Decide if enrollment to a region will be stopped when enrollment into that region is completed

Additional comments on how consideration of regional difference may impact the design and analysis of a multiregional trial can be found in Hung, Wang, and O'Neill (2010).

Because of the complexity of a multiregional trial, it will be prudent to consider interim analyses to check design assumptions and take the necessary remediation actions. A sponsor needs to decide if an interim analysis should be conducted to check (1) if the design assumptions are appropriate, (2) if the trial (or some part of it such as randomization to a particular treatment group or recruitment from a region) should be stopped early for futility, and (3) if adaptations such as sample size reestimation or modifying the inclusion and exclusion criteria are necessary. Another important decision is whether the trial should be allowed to be terminated earlier for efficacy if some regions have not accumulated enough data to allow for a reasonable estimation of the treatment effect in those regions. There are also the usual decisions on who will perform the interim analysis, whether the sponsor will be involved in the interim decision in some fashion, and how regulators will be notified if there is a recommendation to stop the trial in a region. An example of an optimal adaptive design to address local regulations using global trials is given in Luo, Shih, Ouyang, and DeLap (2010).

As for the analysis, a sponsor needs to determine (1) how "region" will be handled in the primary and secondary analyses, (2) the analytical strategy if different regulatory agencies require different primary endpoints, (3) how to estimate treatment effect (overall and regional) if adaptations are part of the design, and (4) how to examine safety experience in different regions.

8.2.3 Regulatory Considerations

Since the multiregional trials are to provide pivotal information in support of product registration in multiple regions, it is important to seek regulatory input in all regions of interest. This is especially true for innovative concepts and novel indications with unprecedented mechanism of actions. If the development will deviate from existing key regulatory guidelines, it is important to have a scientifically justifiable rationale. In addition, it is important to understand key risks that could impact approvability and target label due to deviations. In the latter case, it will be crucial to have a mitigation strategy.

If the sponsor has previously sought regulatory advice on a similar compound, the sponsor needs to have a clear understanding on the outcome from the earlier interactions and decide whether to follow the prior regulatory advice. Some countries (e.g., European Union, China, Korea, Taiwan, India, Japan, Mexico) frequently require local clinical data such as pharmacokinetic data before allowing patients into a confirmatory global trial. A sponsor needs a strategy to obtain local data in these countries in a timely fashion to allow their patients to enroll in a multiregional trial. The process for obtaining clinical trial agreement as well as ethic committee approvals in some countries is longer than in other countries, leading to a need of advanced planning in the former so that enrollment into the global trial could start at approximately the same time at all sites. On the other hand, an extremely long review process might make some countries unsuitable to be part of the global trials.

In short, a sponsor needs to seek regulatory agreement on the protocol driving a multiregional trial. The sponsor also needs to be ready to make decisions to exclude some countries if the requirements from their regulatory authorities are not in general agreement with those from other countries. Regulatory input is especially critical if the interim data suggest terminating enrollment in some regions. The implications of this action to future development in the affected regions need to be fully explored before taking any action.

8.2.4 Commercial Considerations

Since the primary objective of a multiregional trial is to facilitate simultaneous registration in multiple regions, this objective needs to be first assessed in the context of market potential of selected regions/countries. This includes the value of the new medicine in the context of the standard of care and emerging new treatment options between now and the anticipated time of launch of the new investigational medicine. If the new medicine is considered to be of value by the medical thought leaders in the regions/countries, a sponsor needs to develop a strategy to highlight the value to the caregivers and possibly patients. The latter includes educational efforts on disease awareness and a plan to engage key opinion leaders from the regions and countries who could provide input to the development program from the region/country perspective.

Increasingly, pricing and reimbursement considerations are a major factor in launching a new medicine in a region/country. The latter depend on how the new medicine compares with other available treatments and whether results from the confirmatory trials are likely to apply more broadly to patients not included in the trials. Frequently asked questions include whether the economics and utility data collected can adequately support a reasonable assessment on cost-effectiveness and whether trial design such as the choice of the endpoints (including health-related quality of life assessment and PRO), duration of the trial, and the inclusion of a comparator meet payers' requirements or guidelines in a region.

Another important factor is the availability of the medical procedures needed to support a new medicine. For example, if the new medicine is indicated for patients with a particular genetic profile, a sponsor needs to decide if the countries have the scientific and commercial ability to genotype patients in the general population.

As a way to share risk and investment returns, many products are being codeveloped by partners through alliance arrangements. Alliance partners often divide marketing rights so partners own marketing rights in different parts of the world. Differences in regulatory and commercial needs in different countries could bring conflicting needs by the alliance partners to the negotiation table, further adding complexity to the planning of a global confirmatory development program.

8.2.5 Operational Considerations

In addition to clinical, statistical, regulatory, and commercial considerations, a sponsor needs to decide how to select clinical sites within a country and countries within a region. This needs to be a highly collaborative process involving program-level strategy at the headquarters and representatives in the countries/regions. Many global pharmaceutical companies have offices in many countries. The study team responsible for a global trial needs to collaborate with personnel in the country offices to seek input on incidence and prevalence of the disorder, standard of care, availability of comparators, regulatory process, and marketing strategy and access in the various countries.

Additional operational issues pertinent to a multiregional trial include decisions on the following:

1. Whether the drug will be dispensed centrally or by regional offices
2. Whether randomization will be done using an interactive voice randomization system
3. Whether a central laboratory will be used for safety, efficacy, or both
4. Whether all regions will use the same method (e.g., paper, remote data capture, Internet) to capture data
5. Whether enrollment can be initiated in all regions concurrently
6. How to conduct investigator training (and rater training, if relevant) to ensure consistent study conduct across regions
7. Whether PRO data will be collected by paper or electronically
8. What will be the remediation actions if a site does not deliver on enrollment or meet the quality requirement
9. How to conduct retraining if a site appears not to have understood the assessment procedure or not to have adhered to the protocol

In short, the highly complicated nature of a multiregional trial means that thorough planning is necessary to ensure that the trial has a chance to meet its objectives.

8.3 Determination of Regional Sample Size in a Multiregional Study

Q11 in the ICH E5 Q&A addendum states that a multiregional study should be designed with sufficient numbers of subjects so that there is adequate power to have a reasonable likelihood of showing an effect in each region of interest. As described earlier, the 11th Q&A introduces the concept of hierarchy of persuasiveness (see Figure 8.1) and suggests that the overall results should be of primary interest, supplemented by checking regions for consistency in treatment effect.

In the next section, we will describe in detail an approach proposed by Kawai, Chuang-Stein, Komiyama, and Ii (2008) to find the minimum sample size for the smallest region so that there is a high probability of observing a consistent trend in the estimated treatment effect across regions if the treatment effect is positive and uniform across regions. Assuming that high values on the primary endpoint represent a more favorable outcome, Kawai et al. define a consistent trend to have occurred if the point estimates for the treatment effect in different regions are all positive.

In Section 8.3.2 we extend regional sample size discussion to situations where the assumption of uniform treatment effect is relaxed to allow for possibly different treatment effect across regions. In Section 8.3.3 we expand the simple definition of consistency (i.e., the point estimates of treatment effect in all regions being positive) to a definition of the estimated treatment effects for all regions needing to be in a "consistency range."

8.3.1 Assumption That Treatment Effect Is Uniform across Regions

We assume that the study, which will be conducted in R regions, is a superiority trial to compare a new treatment with a control based on a continuous measurement. The primary endpoint is change from baseline at a preidentified time point, and positive change is indicative of a positive treatment effect. We underscore two premises in our discussion. The first one is that no region should proclaim itself to be the region of interest and demand the treatment to show a statistically significant result at the usual significance level (i.e., 0.05) in that region. Second, the study's primary objective is to demonstrate an overall treatment effect, and the overall sample size is determined by the primary objective.

In this section, we assume that the true (but unknown) mean treatment effect Δ is uniform across regions. We define a consistent trend to have occurred if the point estimates for the treatment effect in different regions are all positive. This is the consistency definition in Method 2 in the MHLW (2007) "Guidance on Basic Principles on Global Clinical Trials." Using this definition of consistency, Kawai et al. (2008) found the minimal sample size for the smallest region so that there is a high probability (80% or 90%) of observing the consistent trend.

Let D_r denote the estimated treatment effect in the r-th region and p_r the percentage of subjects from that region in the study, $r = 1,\ldots, R$. We assume that patients are to be randomized equally to the two treatment groups. Furthermore, we assume that D_r follows a normal distribution $N(\Delta; 2\sigma^2/n_r)$ where n_r is the number of subjects receiving each treatment in the r-th region and Δ and σ denote the true (common) treatment effect and the standard deviation of the primary endpoint.

Let N be the total number of subjects on each treatment, that is, $N = n_1 + \ldots + n_R$. Since the primary analysis is to test for the treatment effect using data from all regions, N can be computed using the following standard sample size formula:

$$N = \frac{2\sigma^2(z_{1-\alpha/2} + z_{1-\beta})^2}{\Delta^2} = \frac{2\sigma^2 C_{\alpha,\beta}^2}{\Delta^2} \tag{8.1}$$

where $C_{\alpha,\beta} = z_{1-\alpha/2} + z_{1-\beta}$, α is the significance level for a two-sided test, $100(1 - \beta)\%$ is the power to detect an effect size of Δ/σ, and z_r is the $100r$-th percentile of the standard normal distribution. Under these conditions, the probability of observing a positive result for all regions can be written as

$$\Pr(D_r > 0, \forall r = 1,\ldots R \mid \Delta, \sigma) = \prod_{r=1}^{R} \Pr(D_r > 0 \mid \Delta, \sigma)$$
$$= \prod_{r=1}^{R} \Phi\left(\sqrt{p_r}\, C_{\alpha,\beta}\right) \tag{8.2}$$

In Equation 8.2, Φ denotes the cumulative probability function of the standard normal distribution. The details of the derivation are given in Kawai et al. (2008).

The probability (Equation 8.2) is not conditional on whether the overall treatment effect is statistically significant. In practice, for a confirmatory trial, inference concerning regional results is relevant only if the overall treatment effect is statistically significant (see Figure 8.2). The probability of observing a positive result for all regions conditional on first concluding a significant overall treatment can be written as

Pr ($D_r > 0$ for all r|Concluding a significant overall treatment effect, Δ, σ)

= Pr ($D_r > 0$ for all r and concluding a significant overall treatment effect)/(1 – β)

$$= \frac{\Pr(z_1 < \sqrt{p_1}\, C_{\alpha,\beta}, z_2 < \sqrt{p_2}\, C_{\alpha,\beta}, \cdots, z_R < \sqrt{p_R}\, C_{\alpha,\beta}, z_{R+1} < z_{1-\beta})}{1-\beta} \tag{8.3}$$

where $(z_1, z_2, \ldots, z_R, z_{R+1})$ has multivariate normal distribution with the variance–covariate matrix in Equation 8.4, z_i represents the test statistic for treatment effect in region i ($i = 1, \ldots R$) and z_{R+1} represents the test statistic for treatment effect in the overall population.

$$\begin{pmatrix} 1 & 0 & \cdots & 0 & \sqrt{p_1} \\ 0 & 1 & \cdots & 0 & \sqrt{p_2} \\ \vdots & \vdots & \ddots & \vdots & \vdots \\ 0 & 0 & \cdots & 1 & \sqrt{p_R} \\ \sqrt{p_1} & \sqrt{p_2} & \cdots & \sqrt{p_R} & 1 \end{pmatrix} \tag{8.4}$$

Note that the correlation between D_r ($r = 1,\ldots R$) and the overall observed treatment effect can be expressed as $\sqrt{p_r}$. We can see from results in Equation

TABLE 8.1

Probability (%) of Observing Consistent Results across All Regions with or without Conditioning on a Statistically Significant Overall Positive Treatment Effect

	Unconditional		Conditional	
(p_1, p_2, p_3)	Power = 80%	Power = 90%	Power = 80%	Power = 90%
(0.05,0.05,0.9)	53.7%	58.6%	57.8%	60.8%
(0.1,0.1,0.8)	65.6%	71.7%	71.2%	74.6%
(0.15,0.15,0.7)	73.4%	79.9%	80.1%	83.3%
(0.2,0.2,0.6)	78.9%	85.3%	86.2%	88.9%
(0.25,0.25,0.5)	82.5%	88.8%	90.3%	92.6%
(0.3,0.3,0.4)	84.5%	90.7%	92.7%	94.6%

8.3 and Equation 8.4 that the probability depends only on the number of regions and the percentages of patients in different regions, assuming that the total sample size is calculated based on Equation 8.1.

For simplicity, we assume that the study will be conducted in three regions. For convenience, we assume that region 1 is the smallest region and region 2 is the second smallest one. In other words $p_1 \le p_2 \le p_3$ subject to $p_1 + p_2 + p_3 = 1$. The conditional probability in Equation 8.3 is the highest if all three regions are equally represented, that is, $p_1 = p_2 = p_3 = 1/3$. The probability is the smallest if p_1 and p_2 are equal for an admissible value of p_1. Thus, we need to investigate the probability only in the case of $p_1 = p_2$ to find the minimum p_1 that will produce an acceptable conditional probability in Equation 8.3 for all possible values of p_3. Table 8.1 shows the probabilities of observing consistent results across all regions with or without conditioning on a statistically significant overall positive treatment effect when the test for the overall treatment effect has a power of 80% or 90%.

First, we note that the unconditional and conditional probabilities for 90% power are generally above those corresponding to 80% power, by about 5% and 3%, respectively. This is as expected since the total sample size based on a 90% power is larger than that based on an 80% power.

The conditional probabilities are always higher than the unconditional ones, by about 2 to 8%. As stated previously, comparing results across regions would be of regulatory interest only when a statistically significant overall treatment effect has been concluded first. As a result, the conditional probabilities are more relevant than the unconditional ones when planning a confirmatory multiregional trial. When the total sample size is based on an 80% power for the overall treatment effect, Kawai et al. (2008) found that p_1 could be as low as 15% for the conditional probability to be at least 80%; p_1 needs to be around 25% for the conditional probability to be at least 90%. The findings for the case when the sample size is based on a 90% power are similar. In the latter case, $p_1 = 15\%$ will lead to a conditional probability around 83%, and $p_1 = 25\%$ will lead to a conditional probability around 93%.

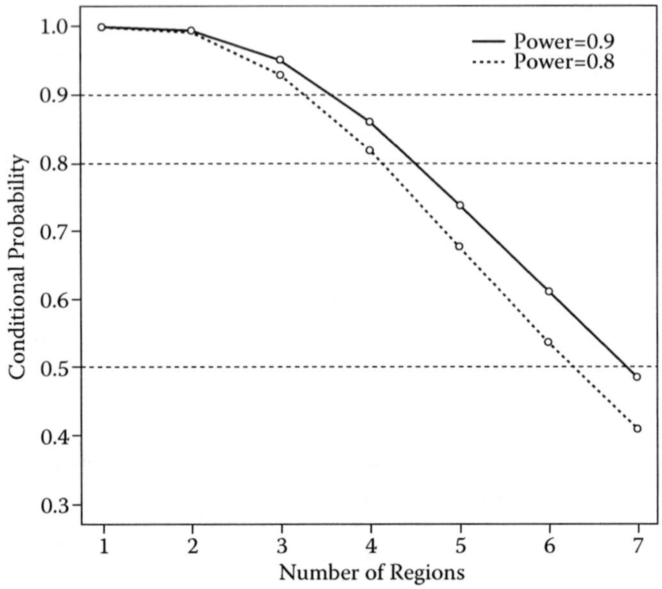

FIGURE 8.3
Conditional probability plotted against the number of regions R under $p_r = 1/R$ (for all r).

The decision to go with an 80% or a 90% conditional probability should be made with care. The probability of meeting both the primary objective and the consistency objective among regions is the product of the power for the primary analysis and that of the conditional probability. If the study is designed to have a 90% power for the primary analysis and the conditional probability is around 80%, then the power of meeting both objectives is 72% (0.9 times 0.8). Calling this power the "overall power," a sponsor needs to balance between the ability to recruit from the smallest region and the desire to have an acceptable overall power. If the intent is to have at least an 80% overall power and the power for the primary analysis is set at 90%, then the conditional probability needs to be close to 90%.

To investigate the impact of the number of regions on the conditional probabilities, plots of the conditional probabilities under the ideal case ($p_r = 1/R$ for all r) against the number of regions (from 1 to 7) are given in Figure 8.3. One can see that the probability dramatically decreases as the number of regions increases. In other words, the probability of observing at least one negative regional result becomes higher as the number of regions increases even though the true treatment effect is positive across regions.

8.3.2 Variation in True Treatment Effect across Regions

If there is strong evidence to suggest clinically meaningful differences in treatment effect across regions, then planning a multiregional trial in these regions will not be a wise action. Often, there is no strong evidence to suggest that the true treatment effect is the same across regions. In such cases, it might be prudent to consider relaxing the common true treatment effect assumption and allow for some variability across regions (Ii, Komiyama, and Kuribayashi, 2007). Such extension could be particularly useful to help assess the robustness and sensitivity of the trial plan and discuss expectations with members of the study team.

Variation in treatment effect among countries or regions is not uncommon. For example Weir, Sandercock, Lewis, Signorini, and Warlow (2001) reported variation among countries in post-stroke outcomes in the International Stroke Trial involving 19,435 subjects in 37 countries. They found that most of the variation could not be explained by measured factors and concluded that the variations "most likely reflect differences in unmeasured baseline factors," O'Neill (2007) reported an investigation of 16 major international cardiovascular outcome studies conducted in the previous 10 years. All 16 studies demonstrated a statistically significant overall treatment effect. However, 13 of these 16 studies had a negative point estimate for the treatment effect for the U.S. subjects. One study is the MERIT-HF trial of metoprolol discussed earlier.

There are situations when the mechanism by which regional differences in treatment effect are better understood. Consider treatment for major depression assessed by a change in HAM-D17 total score from baseline. For HAM-D17, lower baseline values offer less room for improvement. For example, if the baseline score is 20, the maximum improvement could only be 20. Thus, if an active treatment is truly effective, the difference between placebo and the active arm tends to be smaller at low baseline values compared with high baseline values. A similar phenomenon is observed in schizophrenia trials (Chen, Wang, Khin, Hung, and Laughren, 2010). Consequently, if there is a regional difference in the distribution of baseline values, this difference could potentially manifest as a region-by-treatment interaction. Methods to include such an interaction term to help "explain" regional differences are given in Section 8.4.2. While some researchers feel that such explanatory analysis could help provide evidence to consistency in treatment effect across regions, others feel that differences in baseline are an integral part of regional differences and should *not* be adjusted in the evaluation of consistency.

The previous discussions suggest that it may be worthwhile to consider various degrees of possible regional variations in treatment effect at the planning stage. In this section, we concentrate on using a random effect model to describe the variation. In some cases a fixed-effect approach might also be appropriate.

For simplicity, we will use the same hierarchical normal model as discussed by Ii, Komiyama, and Kuribayashi (2007). Under this model, the true treatment effect in a region is assumed to be normally distributed with mean δ_0 and standard deviation σ_δ as in Equation 8.5. The observed

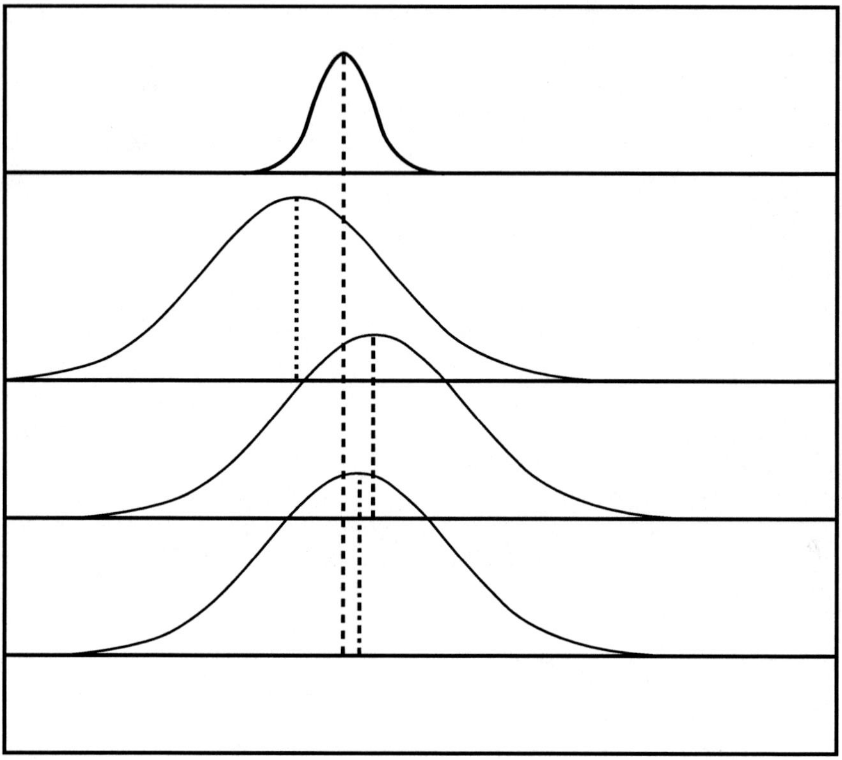

FIGURE 8.4
The top graph describes the interregional variability in the true treatment effect across regions and the bottom three graphs describe possible distributions of the observed treatment effect in each of three regions.

treatment difference, D_r conditional on the true regional effect is normally distributed with mean δ_r and variance $2\sigma^2/n_r$ as stated in Equation 8.6. This two-stage idea is pictured in Figure 8.4, where the top graph describes the interregional variability in the true treatment effect and the bottom three graphs describe possible distributions of the estimated treatment effect in each of the three regions.

$$\Delta \sim N\left(\delta_0, \sigma_\delta^2\right) \tag{8.5}$$

$$D_r \mid \Delta = \delta_r \sim N\left(\delta_r, \frac{2\sigma^2}{n_r}\right) \tag{8.6}$$

Under the random-effect assumptions, the unconditional probability P of observing a positive D_r in all regions is

$$P = \prod_{r=1}^{R} \Phi\left(\delta_0 \left(\frac{2\sigma^2}{n_r} + \sigma_\delta^2\right)^{-\frac{1}{2}}\right) \tag{8.7}$$

If we use the sample size based on the common true treatment effect assumption of δ_0 from Equation 8.1 (i.e., ignoring the additional variation introduced by the hierarchical structure), then the unconditional probability is

$$P = \prod_{r=1}^{R} \Phi\left(\left(\frac{1}{p_r C_{\alpha,\beta}^2} + \frac{\sigma_\delta^2}{\delta_0^2}\right)^{-\frac{1}{2}}\right) \tag{8.8}$$

Figure 8.5 displays the unconditional probability P as function of p_1 for four different values of interregional standard deviation for three regions, $p_1 = p_2$, $\alpha = 0.05$, $\beta = 0.1$, and $\delta_0 = 1.0$. It can be seen that P decreases with increasing interregional variability, whereas the case $\sigma_\delta = 0$ reduces to the previous case of a common true effect across regions in Equation 8.2. Specifically, at $p_1 = 0.15$, P is reduced from 0.8 to 0.76 as σ_δ increases from 0

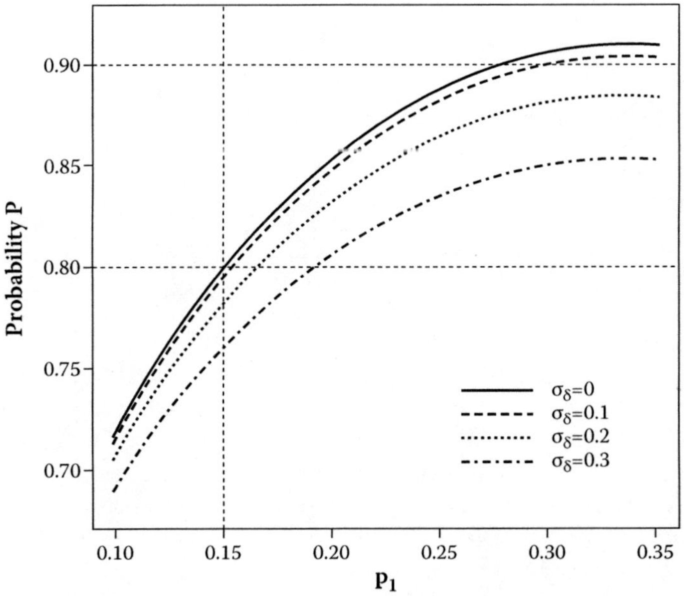

FIGURE 8.5
Unconditional probability P of observing $D_r > 0$ in all three regions as a function of p_1 (= p_2) when there is an interregional variation in the true regional treatment effect, for $\alpha = 0.05$, $\beta = 0.1$, $\delta_0 = 1$ and four different values of interregional standard deviation σ_δ.

to 0.3. Analogous probabilities conditional on statistically significant overall result can be computed.

One could determine the overall study sample size by taking into account the additional interregional variation. This can be done by computing the variance of an estimate for the overall treatment effect as in Equation 8.9.

$$Var(D) = Var\left(\sum_{r=1}^{R} p_r D_r\right) = \frac{2\sigma^2}{N} + \sigma_\delta^2 \sum_{r=1}^{R} p_r^2 \tag{8.9}$$

The last summation in Equation 8.9 ranges between $1/R$ and 1, and hence the maximum variance of D over all configurations of p_r is given by

$$\max_{p_r} Var(D) = \frac{2\sigma^2}{N} + \sigma_\delta^2 \tag{8.10}$$

Using the maximum variance, the required sample size is given by Equation 8.11.

$$N = 2\sigma^2 \left(\frac{\delta_0^2}{C_{\alpha,\beta}^2} - \sigma_\delta^2\right)^{-1} \tag{8.11}$$

When substituting Equation 8.11 into Equation 8.7, we arrive at Equation 8.12.

$$P = \prod_{r=1}^{R} \Phi\left(\left(\frac{1}{p_r}\left(\frac{1}{C_{\alpha,\beta}^2} - \frac{\sigma_\delta^2}{\delta_0^2}\right) + \frac{\sigma_\delta^2}{\delta_0^2}\right)^{-\frac{1}{2}}\right) \tag{8.12}$$

When $\sigma_\delta = 0$, the unconditional probability in Equation 8.12 again reduces to that in Equation 8.2. The unconditional probability in Equation 8.12 decreases as the coefficient of variation of Δ increases. This is reasonable, since a larger variability would mean that the true treatment effect in some regions might be closer to zero, thus driving down the probability P.

It is important to note that the quantity in Equation 8.11 needs to be positive. One could rewrite the expression on the right-hand side in Equation 8.11 as

$$\frac{\delta_0^2}{C_{\alpha,\beta}^2} - \sigma_\delta^2 = \delta_0^2\left(\frac{1}{C_{\alpha,\beta}^2} - \frac{\sigma_\delta^2}{\delta_0^2}\right) \tag{8.13}$$

What does it mean that the quantity in Equation 8.13 needs to be positive? Is this condition always met? Consider the scenario when $\alpha = 0.05$, $\beta = 0.1$. Under this scenario, $C_{\alpha\beta} \approx 3.24$ and the inverse of its square is approximately 0.1. In general, one would expect σ_δ to be much smaller than the intersubject variability σ. Assuming $\sigma_\delta = 0.05\,\sigma$ and the effect size (δ_0/σ) is 0.25, then $\sigma_\delta/\delta_0 = 0.2$ and its square is 0.04. Since $0.04 < 0.1$ (i.e., $\sigma_\delta^2/\delta_0^2 < 1/C_{\alpha,\beta}^2$) under this scenario, the quantity in Equation 8.13 is positive. However, if σ_δ is much larger in comparison with σ, then the inequality $\sigma_\delta^2/\delta_0^2 < 1/C_{\alpha,\beta}^2$ might not hold. When this happens, the extra variability, which does not depend on the sample size, cannot be compensated by increasing the sample size.

In some trials, the regional sample size proportions are subject to uncertainty due to, for example, competing enrollment at many study sites. In such situations, one may want to consider deviations from the planned regional sample size proportions. If one could approximate the sample size proportions by a probability distribution, one could explore its effect using, for example, Equation 8.8 or Equation 8.12.

It is important for the study team to gather information on sources and degrees of variations in true treatment effect across regions and discuss its consequences at the study planning stage. It is also important to discuss such information with regulatory authorities. The method introduced in this section could contribute to the discussion.

So far we define consistency as observing $D_r > 0$ in all regions. We design the study to have enough patients in each region so that the chance of observing a negative point estimate of treatment effect in any region is controlled at a prespecified level. In other words, this approach seeks to control the chance of observing an apparent qualitative region-by-treatment interaction when the treatment effect is positive and uniform across all regions. This approach does not focus on a quantitative region-by-treatment interaction. In the next section, we will expand the definition of consistency by requiring that the observed treatment effects in all regions fall within a "consistency range."

8.3.3 Consistency Range for Sample Sizing

The criterion of "$D_r > 0$" is simple and minimally addresses a regulatory agency's concerns that a treatment might bring no benefit to patients in their region. It is conceivable that such a simplistic criterion may not be enough and one needs to require something beyond simply the observed treatment effect being greater than 0. One such candidate is a "consistency range" within which all D_r's should lie. This criterion was considered by Ii et al. (2007). The "range" may be one-sided in which case the lower or upper limit is infinite. One could borrow the concept of a noninferiority margin as in a noninferiority study or a minimum clinically meaningful difference as in a placebo-controlled superiority study.

Following an analogous development as for the "$D_r > 0$" in Section 8.3.1, Ii et al. (2007) found that

$$P = \Pr\left(A_L < D_r < A_U,\ \forall r = 1,\ldots,R \mid H_1' : \Delta = \Delta_0 > 0\right)$$
$$= \prod_{r=1}^{R}\left\{\Phi\left(\left(\frac{A_U}{\Delta_0} - 1\right)\sqrt{p_r}C_{\alpha,\beta}\right) - \Phi\left(\left(\frac{A_L}{\Delta_0} - 1\right)\sqrt{p_r}C_{\alpha,\beta}\right)\right\} \tag{8.14}$$

where A_L and A_U are lower and upper limits of the consistency range. Setting

$$f_L = \frac{A_L}{\Delta_0} \leq 1, \quad f_U = \frac{A_U}{\Delta_0} \geq 1$$

the unconditional probability P can be expressed as

$$P = \prod_{r=1}^{R}\left\{\Phi\left((f_U - 1)\sqrt{p_r}C_{\alpha,\beta}\right) - \Phi\left((f_L - 1)\sqrt{p_r}C_{\alpha,\beta}\right)\right\} \tag{8.15}$$

When there is extra interregional variability as assumed in Section 8.3.2, the unconditional probability in Equation 8.15 becomes

$$P = \prod_{r=1}^{R}\left\{\Phi\left((f_U - 1)\left(\frac{1}{p_r C_{\alpha,\beta}^2} + \frac{\sigma_\delta^2}{\delta_0^2}\right)^{-\frac{1}{2}}\right) - \Phi\left((f_L - 1)\left(\frac{1}{p_r C_{\alpha,\beta}^2} + \frac{\sigma_\delta^2}{\delta_0^2}\right)^{-\frac{1}{2}}\right)\right\} \tag{8.16}$$

Figure 8.6 displays the unconditional probability P as a function of p_1 (= p_2), $R = 3$, $\alpha = 0.05$, $\beta = 0.1$, $\delta_0 = 1.0$, and $\sigma_\delta = 0$. The "$D_r > 0$" case corresponds to a consistency range of $(0, +\infty)$. It can be easily seen that P decreases with a tighter consistency range. For example, if the range is (0.5, 1/0.5), that is, 50% to 200% of δ_0, P is below 0.4 when the overall sample size is determined by Equation 8.1. Similarly, probabilities conditional on statistically significant overall results can be computed.

Introducing "consistency range" provides another tool to discuss, among the interested parties, the assumptions underlying trial planning and the expectations regarding the study outcomes. It should be pointed out that as the criteria become more stringent, it will become increasingly hard for a study to meet the criteria.

8.3.4 Other Approaches

Some researchers have proposed criteria that focus on consistency between a specific region and the overall results (instead of consistency across all regions). For example, Uesaka (2009) and Quan, Zhao, Zhang, Roessner, and Aizawa (2010) used the consistency requirement under Method 1 in the

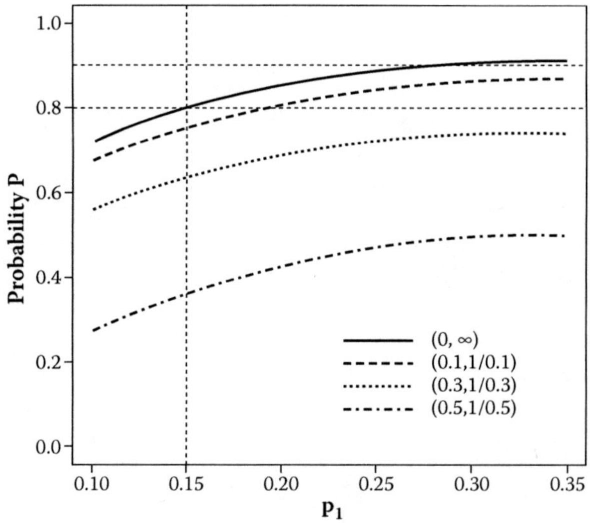

FIGURE 8.6
Unconditional probability P of observing all D_r's in the "consistency range" is plotted against p_1 $(= p_2)$ when the true treatment effect is the same across all three regions, $\alpha = 0.05$, $\beta = 0.1$, $\delta_0 = 1$ and four different ranges.

MHLW guidance to determine the sample size for a specific region (e.g., Japan). Method 1 requires that the observed treatment effect among the Japanese subjects be within a predefined percentage (e.g., 50%) of the observed treatment effect in all subjects in the trial. Focusing on a specific region, Ko, Tsou, Liu, and Hsiao (2010) expanded the aforementioned concept and considered four criteria for comparing results in a specific region with the overall results.

Increasing attention has been paid to other criteria of consistency (e.g., Chen, Quan, Binkowitz, Ouyang, Tanaka, Li et al. 2010; Quan, Li, Chen, Gallo, Binkowitz, Ibia et al., 2010). For any prespecified consistency definition, one could decide sample size for either a specific region or all regions so that the probability of passing the consistency requirement when the treatment effect is positive and uniform across all regions is at a desirable level. In most situations, one needs to rely on simulations to obtain the required sample size.

8.4 Additional Analysis to Estimate Treatment Effects in Different Regions

Chen, Quan et al. (2010) provided a systematic review of methods for assessing consistency of treatment effect across all regions. The methods are classified into three groups: global methods, multivariate quantitative methods, and multivariate qualitative methods. The global methods are based on one single global statistic combining data across all regions and may not directly apply to region-specific consistency assessment. Multivariate quantitative/qualitative methods consider all pair-wise differences simultaneously and can be easily extended to region-specific analysis. These methods require prespecified bounds/thresholds to conclude consistency of treatment effect. While prespecifying bounds/thresholds is possible for diseases with many treatment options, it might be difficult to do so in areas with very few successful treatments. Most of these approaches follow the frequentist philosophy.

We would like to point out that some researchers have also proposed Bayesian approaches to estimate regional treatment effect. For example, Liu and Chow (2002) and Liu et al. (2002) proposed a Bayesian approach to evaluate similarity on efficacy in the context of a separate bridging study. Chen, Wu, and Wang (2009) proposed a Bayesian approach to evaluate regional treatment effect in the context of a multiregional trial. The latter calculates the posterior distributions of regional treatment effects given study results and the assumption of a common prior for treatment effect in different regions. The posterior distributions yield an empirical Bayes estimator for regional effect size. Interested readers are encouraged to study these references.

Consistency assessment of treatment effect is not limited to the primary endpoint. Frequently, we also need to assess secondary endpoints to help assess ethnic sensitivity. In addition, analyses that adjust for pretreatment covariate measurements can also be conducted to help ascertain if differences in baseline covariate measurements might contribute to the observed treatment effect differences across regions. The latter are generally exploratory in nature and will be briefly discussed in this section.

8.4.1 Notations

Let Y_{rkis} denote the measurement on a continuous endpoint for subject s, $s = 1,\ldots, n_{rki}$, who is on treatment i, $i = 1,\ldots, I$, in center k, $k = 1,\ldots, K_r$, of region r, $r = 1,\ldots, R$. The experimental model for a continuous response Y_{rkis} is

$$Y_{rkis} = \mu + \alpha_r + \beta_{k(r)} + \delta_i + (\alpha\delta)_{ri} + (\beta\delta)_{k(r)i} + \varepsilon_{rkis} \tag{8.17}$$

where μ is the grand (overall) mean, α_r is the regional effect, $\Sigma_r\, \alpha_r = 0$, $\beta_{k(r)}$ is the center effect, $\Sigma_k\, \beta_{k(r)} = 0$, δ_i is the treatment effect, $\Sigma_i\, \delta_i = 0$, $(\alpha\delta)_{ri}$ is the region by treatment interaction, $\Sigma_r\, (\alpha\delta)_{ri} = \Sigma_i\, (\alpha\delta)_{ri} = 0$, $(\beta\delta)_{k(r)i}$ is the center by treatment interaction, $\Sigma_k\, (\beta\delta)_{k(r)i} = \Sigma_i\, (\beta\delta)_{k(r)i} = 0$, and ε_{rkis}'s are i.i.d. random variables with mean 0 and variance σ_e^2.

8.4.2 Estimation of Regional Effect Size

In multiregional trials, it is not always possible to enroll a large enough number of subjects within a center to estimate the center effect $\beta_{k(r)}$ in Equation 8.17. This means that the center effect $\beta_{k(r)}$ in Equation 8.17 is often not estimable. As a result, we will consider the reduced model in Equation 8.18 that leaves out the center effect.

$$Y_{ris} = \mu + \alpha_r + \delta_i + (\alpha\delta)_{ri} + \varepsilon_{ris} \tag{8.18}$$

In Equation 8.18, ε_{ris}'s are i.i.d. random variables with mean 0 and variance σ_c^2, $i = 1,\ldots, I$, $r = 1,\ldots, R$, $s = 1,\ldots, n_{ri}$ $(= \Sigma_k\, n_{rki})$. Note that the error variance includes between-center variation, and it is important to employ a standard approach to measure the endpoint across centers, investigators, and regions. If we assume a randomization scheme stratified by region (or center), we could expect approximately equal-sized treatment arms in a region, that is, $n_{ri} = n_r$ for $r = 1,\ldots, R$. To estimate the regional effect, we need to include α_r and $(\alpha\delta)_{ri}$ in the analytical models regardless of the consistency assumption made about the treatment effect at the planning stage. The least squares estimate of the effect of treatment i in region r is given by

$$\hat{\mu}_{ri} = \hat{\mu} + \hat{\alpha}_r + \hat{\delta}_i + \left(\widehat{\alpha\delta}\right)_{ri} \tag{8.19}$$

When $I = 2$ (i.e., two treatment groups), the regional difference in the treatment effects can be estimated as follows:

$$D_r = \hat{\mu}_{r2} - \hat{\mu}_{r1} = \left(\hat{\delta}_2 - \hat{\delta}_1\right) + \left(\widehat{(\alpha\delta)}_{r2} - \widehat{(\alpha\delta)}_{r1}\right) \tag{8.20}$$

There often exist some important covariates affecting treatment effect in multiregional trials. An example is the baseline value of the endpoint of interest. Let $\boldsymbol{x}$ be a covariate vector, $\boldsymbol{\theta}$ be the corresponding parameter vector, and $\boldsymbol{\gamma}$ be the parameter vector for the covariates by treatment interaction. The analytical model for $I = 2$ would be written as

$$Y_{ris} = \mu + \alpha_r + \delta_i + (\alpha\delta)_{ri} + \boldsymbol{x}_{ris}{}^T\boldsymbol{\theta} + (i-1)\boldsymbol{x}_{ris}{}^T\boldsymbol{\gamma} + \varepsilon_{ris} \tag{8.21}$$

A premise for planning a multiregional trial is the expectation that there is no substantial difference in treatment effect across regions. It is possible that distributions of baseline covariates that are prognostic for response are different among regions (Chen et al., 2010) and that these distributions characterize the populations in different regions. In other words, the regional effect in Equation 8.21 is subsumed by the covariates. When this happens, the analytical model Equation 8.21 is reduced to

$$Y_{ris} = \mu + \delta_i + \boldsymbol{x}_{ris}{}^T\boldsymbol{\theta} + (i-1)\boldsymbol{x}_{ris}{}^T\boldsymbol{\gamma} + \varepsilon_{ris} \tag{8.22}$$

Ii (2008) discussed this situation and provided the regional estimates of the effect of treatment i using the regional mean of the covariate as follows:

$$\hat{\mu}_{ri} = \hat{\mu} + \hat{\delta}_i + \bar{x}_r^T\hat{\theta} + (i-1)\bar{x}_r^T\hat{\gamma} \tag{8.23}$$

In the case of two treatments, the effect of the second treatment to the first one D_r in the r-th region can be estimated by

$$D_r = \hat{\mu}_{r2} - \hat{\mu}_{r1} = \left(\hat{\delta}_2 - \hat{\delta}_1\right) + \bar{x}_r^T\hat{\gamma} \tag{8.24}$$

The estimate in Equation 8.24, adjusted for covariates, could be used in assessing whether the data meet the consistency criterion. This needs to be prespecified in the analysis plan so that it is clear how the decision on consistency will be made.

While the estimate in Equation 8.24 can be obtained in the analysis, it will be challenging to use this estimate to plan for regional sample size since we often don't have adequate information on the distributions of the covariates in different regions. In the rare situations when the latter are available and there is a reasonable model describing the relationship between the covariates and the response, an estimate like that in Equation 8.24 could be used to plan the study based on modeling and simulation.

8.5 Real-Time Monitoring of Multiregional Trials

All challenges facing a multinational trial apply to a multiregional trial. The additional objective of simultaneous product registration in multiple regions adds another layer of complexity to multiregional trials. It requires greater regulatory interactions at the planning stage. When an unexpected event leads to the possibility of a protocol amendment, the amendment and its impact need to be brought back to the various regulatory agencies for further discussions. Disagreement among regulators and differences among clinical investigators are exacerbated in a multiregional trial due to the large number of players involved in the trial.

It is important to monitor a clinical trial in real time. It is even more so with a multiregional trial. We need to check enrollment regularly to ensure that the enrolled patients meet the expected patient mix. We need to take actions if the patient characteristics are not as planned. It is critical to monitor screen failures and dropout rates. If a region displays a much higher screen failure or dropout rate, we need to investigate the cause for this disparity. Is it because the presentation of the underlying disease is very different in the region, or is it because the toxicity management in that region is suboptimal? Have the investigators in the region received proper training in clinical research? Do they understand the importance of keeping patients in the trial as long as ethically possible? If the screen failure rate is high in general, we might want to reconsider inclusion–exclusion criteria. Similarly, if the dropout is high, we need to understand the reason and work with sites closely on patient retention strategy.

A sponsor needs to have a backup plan if the enrollment falls short of the expectation. Will the backup plan include recruiting additional centers in the same regions? If the enrollment to one region has reached the planned size while other regions are still enrolling, will the enrollment in the former be terminated? Because of the need for adequate numbers of patients in different regions, a sponsor does not have the luxury of making up the lack of patients in one region by recruiting additional patients in other regions. This, plus the longer time it takes to initiate trials in some regions, makes the alignment of enrollment across regions especially challenging in a multiregional trial.

Increasingly, interim data are being used to check design assumptions. For example, if sample size determination is based on the assumption of a uniform treatment effect across regions, a sponsor might want to check on this assumption using interim data. Because enrollment rate often differs across regions and the planned sample sizes in some regions might be appreciably lower than those in other regions, a sponsor needs to carefully determine the timing of the interim analysis to ensure that sufficient data are obtained in the smallest region to allow for a robust estimate on the treatment effect in that region. Data need to be collected in a timely manner to allow for the planned interim analysis. More importantly, timely data capture will allow a sponsor to spot potential problems early and take the necessary remediation actions. A fundamental assumption of using interim data to "project" future outcome is a stationary patient population. We have seen a suboptimal interim decision because of a population drift (Chuang-Stein and Beltangady, 2010). The issue of a population shift could be even more pronounced in a multiregional trial.

As discussed in Section 8.4, differences in the baseline covariates could contribute to an observed difference in treatment effect across regions. Thus, it is important to look at the distribution of covariates across regions. In areas where culture affects individual's perception of a condition such as pain, ensuring that patients are using the PRO instrument appropriately will help contribute to consistency in study conduct and results across sites.

8.6 Concluding Remarks

It is important to remember that the planning of a confirmatory trial relies on information obtained in phase 2 trials. If the phase 2 trials were conducted in a single region or, worse yet, in a single country, there will be much uncertainty about the treatment effect in other regions and countries. For conditions where patients in different regions are known to respond to treatments differently, planning a multiregional trial using data from a single region is extremely dangerous. CHMP (2009) provided examples (e.g., antithrombotics, antivirals, products for menopausal vasomotor symptoms and fibromyalgia) where past experience has suggested different treatment response among patients in different regions. Chen, Wang et al. (2010) reviewed data from 10 schizophrenia drug programs that included multiregional trials. They found that, on average, the observed treatment effect in the United States was generally smaller than in the non-U.S. region. Ando and Hamasaki (2010) discussed practical issues and lessons learned from multiregional clinical trials via case examples from the perspective of Japanese regulators. For disorders clearly exhibiting different treatment responses across regions, it will be better to plan regional trials instead. In general, a sponsor should have reasonable knowledge on how patients are likely to respond to a new treatment in major regions during the exploratory development stage before embarking on a multiregional confirmatory trial.

The interest on multiregional trials has been on the rise during the past decade. These trials are regarded by some product developers as an expedient pathway to get a valued medicine to patients in many parts of the world. As such, a sponsor could have very high expectations of these trials without realizing the underlying risks (O'Neill, 2007). Multiregional trials require thorough planning and involve many stakeholders. It takes time to obtain endorsement from many regulators on a common protocol. Even when all regions follow the same protocol, it is possible that the protocol allows different comparators or specifies different primary endpoints for different regions. When an instrument is used to record a patient reported outcome, the validation and translation of the instrument need to satisfy multiple regulatory requirements.

Another emerging challenge is the increasing demand of regulators wanting a certain percent of patients in a multiregional trial to come from their regions. Conflicting demands by different regulators create additional challenges to the trial, which could place the entire trial in jeopardy. Therefore, it is crucial for a sponsor who is considering a multiregional trial to carefully consider the advantages and disadvantages of such a trial in the overall product development strategy. It is quite possible that in some situations a multiregional trial may not be the most effective way to support product registration in multiple regions. Instead, conducting regional registration trials may be a better alternative.

The story of IRESSA (gefitinib) presents an interesting case to study. IRESSA is an epidermal growth factor receptor tyrosine kinase (EGFR-TK) inhibitor. It targets and blocks the activity of the EGFR-TK pathways implicated in cancer cell proliferation and survival. It is the first in the EGFR-TK class to gain market approval for non-small cell lung carcinoma (NSCLC) in some parts of the world. It was approved in Japan in 2002 and received conditional approval in the United States in May 2003.

The initial approvals were based on data from two pivotal phase 2 trials, which showed a positive effect of IRESSA in patients with previously treated NSCLC. Approximately 50% of the patients in the phase 2 studies experienced tumor shrinkage or had their disease stabilized with the IRESSA treatment. In December 2004, results from a pivotal global phase 3 survival trial (ISEL, abbreviation for IRESSA Survival Evaluation in Lung Cancer) comparing IRESSA with placebo in patients with advanced NSCLC who had failed one or more lines of chemotherapy, became available. The results were disappointing. The study showed that while IRESSA provided some benefit in the overall survival over the placebo, the increase did not reach statistical significance in the overall population. However, in patients of Oriental origin, IRESSA increased the median survival by 4 months. The hazard ratio (IRESSA to placebo) for survival in Asians is 0.66 with a 95% confidence interval of (0.48, 0.91). By comparison, the hazard ratio for non-Asians is 0.93 with a 95% confidence interval of (0.81, 1.08).

Following the release of the ISEL results, the sponsor voluntarily withdrew the European submission for IRESSA. A number of countries in the West (United States, Switzerland, and Canada) limited the use of IRESSA to patients already experiencing benefit from the drug. In the United States, patients who continued on IRESSA after September 15, 2005, had to fill their renewal prescriptions through a specialty mail-order pharmacy that administered the IRESSA Access Program.

An open-label phase 3 study was initiated in March 2004 by the sponsor to compare IRESSA with docetaxel in NSCLC patients who had been previously pretreated with platinum-based chemotherapy (Kim et al., 2008). The primary objective was to compare overall survival between the two treatment groups. There were two coprimary analyses. One was to assess noninferiority of IRESSA to docetaxel in the overall per-protocol population. The other was to assess superiority of IRESSA to docetaxel in patients with high EGFR-gene-copy number in the intent-to-treat (ITT) population. The study was completed in 2006. The noninferiority objective was confirmed. On the other hand, superiority of IRESSA over docetaxel in patients with high EGFR-gene-copy number in the ITT population was not confirmed.

Based on results in the Asian population in ISEL and the fact that the Asian populations have a relatively high incidence of somatic mutations in the region of the EGFR gene that encodes the tyrosine kinase domain, it was hypothesized that in a selected population, IRESSA could be an effective first-line treatment option. This led to the study IPASS (IRESSA Pan-Asia

Study) in Asia. IPASS was an open label and randomized study comparing IRESSA with the combination chemotherapy of carboplatin or paclitaxel as first-line treatment in clinically selected patients with advanced NSCLC. The study was designed as a noninferiority study with progression free survival (PFS) as the primary endpoint and overall survival as one of several secondary endpoints. The study was initiated in March 2006, and enrollment was completed in October 2007 in several Asian countries. IPASS showed a statistically significant longer PFS than the combination chemotherapy in the overall population. The estimated hazard ratio (IRESSA to combination chemotherapy) is 0.74 with a 95% confidence interval of (0.65, 0.85). The study also demonstrated a drastically different response in patients with EGFR mutation positive tumors from patients with EGFR mutation negative tumors (prespecified subgroups). Hazard ratio in the former population is 0.48 (95% confidence interval is 0.36 to 0.64), and hazard ratio in the latter population is 2.85 (95% confidence interval is 2.05 to 3.98). A similar pattern was observed with the overall survival endpoint (Mok et al., 2009).

In July 2009, the European Commission granted marketing authorization for IRESSA for the treatment of adults with locally advanced or metastatic NSCLC with activating mutations of EGFR-TK across all lines of therapy. The sponsor continues to work toward similar marketing authorizations in the United States.

The IRESSA case tells a story of how a multiregional trial provides critical information about differences in treatment effect across regions which are primarily due to differences in disease presentation across regions. The relationship between disease presentation and IRESSA's mechanism of action provides scientific explanations to the observed regional differences. The case highlights the need to investigate the impact of intrinsic and extrinsic ethnic factors when regional differences in treatment effect are observed. When we can identify such factors as in the IRESSA story, the finding contributes to our pursuit of personalized medicine by delivering the right medicine to the right patients.

References

Ando, Y. and Hamasaki, T. (2010). Practical issues and lessons learned from multiregional clinical trials via case examples: A Japanese perspective. *Pharmaceutical Statistics*, 9: 190–200.

Anello, C., O'Neil, R. T., and Dubey, S. (2005). Multicentre trials: A US regulatory perspective. *Statistical Methods for Medical Research*,14: 303–318.

Chen, J., Quan, H., Binkowitz, B., Ouyang, S. P., Tanaka, Y., Li, G. et al. (2010). Assessing consistent treatment effect in a multi-regional clinical trial: A systematic review. *Pharmaceutical Statistics* 9: 242–253.

Chen, Y. F., Wang, S. J., Khin, N. A., Hung, H. M. J., and Laughren, T. (2010). Trial design issues and treatment effect modeling in multi-regional schizophrenia trials. *Pharmaceutical Statistics*, 9: 217–229.

Chen, Y. H., Wu, Y. C., and Wang, M. A. (2009). Bayesian approach to evaluating regional treatment effect in a multiregional trial. *Journal of Biopharmaceutical Statistics*, 19: 900–915.

Committee for Medicinal Products for Human Use. (CHMP). (2006). Reflection paper on the regulatory guidance for the use of health-related quality of life (HRQL) measures in the evaluation of medicinal products. Available at: http://www.emea.europa.eu/pdfs/human/ewp/13939104en.pdf

Committee for Medicinal Products for Human Use. (CHMP). (2009). Reflection paper on the extrapolation of results from clinical studies conducted outside the EU to the EU-population. European Medicines Agency. Available at: http://www.emea.europa.eu/pdfs/human/ewp/69270208enfin.pdf

Chow, S. C., Shao, J., and Hu, O. Y. P. (2002). Assessing sensitivity and similarity in bridging studies. *Journal of Biopharmaceutical Statistics*, 12: 385–400.

Chuang-Stein, C., and Beltangady, M. (2010). FDA draft guidance on adaptive design clinical trials: Pfizer's perspective. *Journal of Biopharmaceutical Statistics*, 20(6): 1143–1149.

Chuang-Stein, C., Kirby, S., Hirsch, I., and Atkinson, G. (2011). The role of the minimum clinically important difference and its impact on designing a trial. *Pharmaceutical Statistics*, 10(3): 250–256.

European Medicines Agency. (EMA). (2010). Reflection paper on ethical and GCP aspects of clinical trials of medicinal products for human use conducted in third countries and submitted in marketing authorization applications to the EMA. Available at: http://www.ema.europa.eu/docs/en_GB/document_library/Regulatory_and_procedural_guideline/2010/06/WC500091530.pdf

Ho, H. T., and Chow, S. C. (1998). Design and analysis of multinational clinical trials. *Drug Information Journal*, 32: 1309S–1316S.

Hsiao, C. F., Hsu, Y. Y., Tsou, H. H., and Liu, J. P. (2007). Use of prior information for Bayesian evaluation of bridging studies. *Journal of Biopharmaceutical Statistics*, 17: 109–121.

Hsiao, C. F., Xu, J. Z., and Liu, J. P. (2005). A two-stage design for bridging studies. *Journal of Biopharmaceutical Statistics*, 15: 75–83.

Hung, H. M. J., Wang, S. J., and O'Neill, R. T. (2010). Consideration of regional difference in design and analysis of multi-regional trials. *Pharmaceutical Statistics*, 9: 173–178.

ICH E5. (1998). Ethinic Factors in the Acceptability of Foreign Clinical Data (R1). Available at http://www.ich.org/fileadmin/Public_Web_Site/ICH_Products/Guidelines/Efficacy/E5_R1/Step4/E5_R1_Guideline.pdf.

ICH E5. (2006). Implementation Working Group Questions & Answers (R1). Available at http://www.ich.org/fileadmin/Public_Web_Site/ICH_Products/Guidelines/Efficacy/E5_R1/Q_As/E5_Q_As_R5_.pdf.

ICH E9. (1998). Statistical Principles for Clinical Trials. Available at http://www.ich.org/fileadmin/Public_Web_Site/ICH_Products/Guidelines/Efficacy/E9/Step4/E9_Guideline.pdf.

Ii, Y. (2008). Some considerations in design and analysis of multi-regional trials. Presentation at the Joint Statistical Meetings, Denver, CO, August 3.

Ii, Y., Komiyama, O., and Kuribayashi, K. (2007). Issues in design of multi-regional trials. Presentation at the Joint Statistical Meetings, Salt Lake City, UT, July 29.

Kawai, N., Chuang-Stein, C., Komiyama, O., and Ii, Y. (2008). An approach to rationalize partitioning sample size into individual regions in a multiregional trial. *Drug Information Journal*, 42: 139–147.

Kim, E. S., Hirsh, V., Mok, T. S., Socinski, M. A., Gervais, R., Wu, Y.-L. et al. (2008). Gefitinib versus docetaxel in previously treated non-small-cell lung cancer (INTEREST): A randomised phase III trial. *Lancet*, 372(22): 1809–1818.

Ko, F. S., Tsou, H. H., Liu, J. P., and Hsiao, C. F. (2010). Sample size determination for a specific region in a multiregional trial. *Journal of Biopharmaceutical Statistics*, 24: 870–885.

Liu, J. P., and Chow, S. C. (2002). Bridging studies for clinical development. *Journal of Biopharmaceutical Statistics*, 12: 357–369.

Liu, J. P., Hsiao, C. F., and Hsueh, H. M. (2002). Bayesian approach to evaluation of bridging studies. *Journal of Biopharmaceutical Statistics*, 12: 401–408.

Luo, X., Shih, W. J., Ouyang, P., and DeLap, R. J. (2010). An optimal adaptive design to address local regulations in global clinical trials. *Pharmaceutical Statistics*, 9: 179–189.

Ministry of Health, Labour and Welfare of Japan. (2007). Basic principles on global clinical trials. Available at: http://www.pmda.go.jp/operations/notice/2007/file/0928010-e.pdf

Mok, T. S., Wu, Y., Thongprasert, S., Yang, C.-H., Chu, D.-T., Saijo, N. et al. (2009). Gefitinib or carboplatin-paclitaxel in pulmonary adenocarcinoma. *New England Journal of Medicine*, 361(3): 947–957.

O'Neill, R. (2007). Multi-regional clinical trials: Why be concerned? A regulatory perspective on issues. Paper presented at the PhRMA-FDA Workshop on Challenges and Opportunities of Multi-Regional Clinical Trials. Washington, DC, October 29–30.

Quan, H., Li, M., Chen, J., Gallo, P., Binkowitz, B., Ibia, E. et al. (2010). Assessment of consistency of treatment effects in multiregional clinical trials. *Drug Informational Journal*, 44: 617–632.

Quan, H., Zhao, P. L., Zhang, J., Roessner, M., and Aizawa, K. (2010). Sample size consideration for Japanese patients in a multi-regional trial based on MHLW guidance. *Pharmaceutical Statistics*, 9(2): 100–112.

Shih, W. J. (2001). Clinical trials for drug registration in Asian-Pacific countries: Proposal for a new paradigm from a statistical perspective. *Controlled Clinical Trials*, 22: 357–366.

Tsou, H. H., Chow, S. C., Lan, K. K. G., Liu, J. P., Wang, M., Chern, H. D. et al. (2010). Proposals of statistical consideration to evaluation of results for a specific region in multi-regional trials—Asian perspective. *Pharmaceutical Statistics*, 9(3): 201–206.

U.S. Food and Drug Administration. (FDA). (2009). Guidance for industry: Patient-reported outcome measures: Use in medical product development to support labeling claims. Available at: http://www.fda.gov/downloads/Drugs/GuidanceComplianceRegulatoryInformation/Guidances/UCM193282.pdf.

Uesaka, H. (2009). Sample size allocation to regions in a multiregional trial. *Journal of Biopharmaceutical Statistics*, 19: 580–594.

Weir, N., Sandercock, P., Lewis, S. C., Signorini, D. F., and Warlow, C. P. (2001). Variations between countries in outcome after stroke in the international stroke trial (IST). *Stoke*, 32: 1370–1377.

9

Application of Genomic Technologies for Bridging Strategy Involving Different Race and Ethnicity in Pharmacogenomics Clinical Trials*

Sue-Jane Wang
U.S. Food and Drug Administration

9.1 Introduction

A properly powered-controlled trial, if it included patients from only a single clinical site or center, would be challenged regarding its ability to capture sufficiently variable responses of patients with the disease defined by their clinical phenotype due to site-to-site or center-to-center variability. Baseline factors that are prognostic of disease, such as age, gender, race/ethnicity, and disease severity, are important factors for trial design consideration. This is because variability is the law of life, and as no two faces are the same, so no two bodies are alike, and no two individuals react alike, or behave alike under the abnormal conditions we know as disease (Sir William Osler, 1849–1919). Single-center controlled trials are therefore discouraged as the sole basis for providing substantial and persuasive evidence to conclude that treatment would be effective for the indication sought.

The well-known conventional clinical trials are multicentric by design where the variability of observed clinical outcomes provides data information on differences among individual patients and captures reasonably center-to-center or site-to-site variability. In a broader scope, clinical trials have advanced from a multicenter controlled trial conducted within a country that is for the most part predominately one race (e.g., Japan, Canada) or a

* I thank Dr. Chin-Fu Hsiao of National Health Research Institute, Taiwan, Dr. Jen-pei Liu of Taiwan University, Taiwan and Dr. Shein-Chung Chow of Duke University, USA, for the kind invitation. The research work was supported by the RSR funds #02-06, #04-06, #05-2, #05-14, #08-48 awarded by the Center for Drug Evaluation and Research, U.S. Food and Drug Administration. The research views expressed in this article are the author's professional views and are not necessarily those of the U.S. Food and Drug Administration.

country with a mixture of ethnic backgrounds (e.g., United States) to within a geographical region covering multiple countries that may be primarily of the same ethnicity (known as multinational controlled trial) or multiple ethnicities to the more obvious ethnically diverse population in multiregional clinical trials (MRCTs) enrolling patients from different regions defined by a mixture of ethnicities and geographical regions. In the mid '90s, prior to the release of the International Conference on Harmonisation's ICH E5 (ICH, 1998) titled "Ethnic Factor in the Acceptability of Foreign Clinical Data," a multicenter controlled trial covering different ethnicity was called a multicenter multiethnic controlled trial (see, e.g., Chan et al., 2004). The concept of *center* evolves. Many clinical development programs for pharmaceutical drug products have gradually incorporated multiregional or global strategies since the late '90s to also enroll patients from the rest of the world in addition to the U.S.-based and West Europe regions.

Ethnic sensitivity may have major influences on the interpretability of clinical trials. Prior to the emerging trend of globalization, confirmatory trials in original regions were considered *foreign trials* to regions that had limited participation at the time the experimental therapy was approved. We will call them *foreign trials in the original region* when an external bridging strategy is considered or *original region trials* with a global strategy. To this end, trials conducted in the "local" regions are known as bridging trials. We will call them *bridging trials in the new region*. When the new region trials are designed to study the same or similar clinical endpoint, the external bridging strategy (Wang 2009, 2010) relies mainly on cross-trial comparisons between the foreign trials in the original regions and the bridging trials in the new region.

In contrast, a global strategy could embrace MRCTs to cover a wide range of ethnicities from different geographical regions under the common protocol. However, the level of complexity of trial conduct and the potentially much larger variability impacted by ethnic sensitivity may have increased to a large scale, though the statistical inference may look much easier because it is based on within-trial comparisons.

Ethnic sensitivity may pertain to two general levels: intrinsic and extrinsic. The intrinsic ethnic factors are those factors relating to genetic (gender, race, genetic polymorphism of the drug metabolism, and genetic diseases), physiologic and pathological conditions (age, organ functions, diseases), and those in between genetic and physiological/pathological conditions (height and body weight of patients, absorption, discretion, metabolism, excretion, and receptor sensitivity of drug therapy). The extrinsic ethnic factors are those factors associated with environment (e.g., climate, sunlight, pollution), culture (e.g., socioeconomic factors, educational status, language, regional medical practice, disease definition/diagnostic, therapeutic approach, and drug compliance), regional regulatory practice, good clinical practice, and methodology of clinical endpoints collections, as was laid out in Appendix A of ICH E5 (1998). It is obvious that geographical regions as defined using global strategy are confounded with both intrinsic and extrinsic ethnic factors (ICH E5 Q&A, 2006).

In this chapter, we consider the treatment effect that is evaluated in a controlled clinical trial setting. We will focus on genomics considerations for bridging treatment effects in global drug development with an emphasis of intrinsic ethnic influences due to the variability of genomic/genetic factors.

9.2 Pharmacogenomics and Pharmacogenetics

With the advent of newer biotechnologies for further clinical research, the recent genomic technology is centered around intermediate to high throughput biotechnology. This includes reverse transcriptase-polymerace chain reaction (rt-PCR), microarray, single nucleotide polymorphisms (SNPs) array (known as SNP array), proteomic array, metabonomics, and the next-generation sequencing tools, among others.

Following the completion of the human genome project and the International HapMap Consortium (2005) in the early 21st century, pharmacogenetics as a field has evolved into studies of whole genome SNPs scanning or screening for identifying important genetic associations with diseases or therapeutics. Around the same time, transcription profiling using microarray biotechnology aiming at similar objectives has also been actively pursued and is known as pharmacogenomics. In fact, pharmacogenetics, which involves investigating single genes that have major effect on the action of a therapeutic drug, was originally introduced in the late '50s and early '60s and was coined by Vogel (1959) and used by several others, such as Kalow (1962).

9.2.1 Definition

Simon and Wang (2006) defined pharmacogenomics as the science of determining how the benefits and adverse effects of a drug vary among a target population of patients based on genomic features of each patient's germ line and diseased tissue. As science evolves, there is a need to harmonize across regions internationally and globally on the meaning of pharmacogenomics, especially in a bridging trial or bridging strategy. Pharmacogenomics is defined as the investigation of variations of DNA and RNA characteristics as related to drug response. As for pharmacogenetics, it is the influence of variations in DNA sequence on drug response, which is a subset of pharmacogenomics (ICH E15, 2007). In this chapter, we will use the general term *genomics* or *pharmacogenomics* to include molecular, genetic, or pharmacogenetics where appropriate.

It has become increasingly apparent that treatment effects between different genomic patient subsets can be dissimilar, and the value and need for genomic biomarkers to help predict therapeutic effects, particularly in cancer clinical studies, have become issues of paramount importance. Pharmacogenomics has thus become intensely focused on the search for genomic biomarkers for use as classifiers to select patients in randomized controlled trials.

9.2.2 Genomic (Composite) Biomarker

Parallel to biomarker definition (2001), a genomic biomarker is defined as a DNA or RNA characteristic that is an indicator of normal biologic processes, pathogenic processes, or response to therapeutic or other intervention (ICH E15, 2007). Naturally, a genomic biomarker as an indicator in a pharmacogenomics clinical trial can be viewed in the context of classifying patients as likely versus unlikely to predict therapeutic response before treatment intervention (Simon and Wang, 2006; Wang, 2005) and used to assess its predictiveness of treatment effect. The more traditional approach considers single biomarkers, such as the HER2/NEU biomarker in Herceptin drug development (Baselga, 2001; Eiermann, 2001). When multiple genes are to be used collectively, a genomic composite biomarker (GCB; Wang, 2005) can be developed aiming for a targeted therapy that includes efficacy or safety at molecular, cellular, or genomic levels.

A genomic composite biomarker is generally developed by first combining many individual genes, SNPs, or peptides via a prediction algorithm to form a risk score, which is then used to classify patients into good versus poor signatures depending on the risk score being "greater than or equal to" versus "less than" a prespecified cutoff threshold value. The classifier so developed may predict patients' therapeutic outcomes or guide drug treatment. A genomic composite biomarker as a classifier has its appeal over a single biomarker when it provides much higher sensitivity and specificity or when it adds much value to the existing clinical criteria to classifying patients prior to treatment intervention.

9.2.3 Clinical Utility

Clinical utility of a genomic (composite) biomarker can be categorized into prognostic utility, predictive utility, and prognostic-predictive utility. Wang, O'Neill, and Hung (2007) presented these three scenarios of clinical utility of a genomic (composite) biomarker in the setting of a two-arm pharmacogenomics controlled trial, which can be either a bridging trial or a global trial:

Scenario A: predictive of drug effect relative to its comparator

Scenario B: prognostic of disease mechanism

Scenario C: prognostic of disease state and predictive of drug effect relative to its comparator

When there are potential genomic subsets defined a priori, which is postulated to have major impacts (efficacy or toxicity) on treatment intervention, we consider the positive genomic subset, denoted by $g+$.

9.2.3.1 Prognostic

In what follows, if a genomic biomarker is incorporated in a controlled trial, the genomic biomarker might be used as a classifier to determine the treatment effect in a specific $g+$ genomic subset (see Figure 9.1). To illustrate, we use response rate as the primary endpoint. In Figure 9.1, disease state is abbreviated as Dx and treatment is abbreviated as *T*. To investigate if there is a significant treatment effect, clinical outcomes in patients from both *T* and *P* groups are compared. Graph (iii) shows that the genomic biomarker is prognostic of disease mechanism and has no impact on treatment (also Scenario B of Wang et al., 2007), and, Graph (iv) depicts a prognostic genomic biomarker for disease mechanism and the treatment effect exists but is not impacted by the biomarker status. In other words, a prognostic genomic

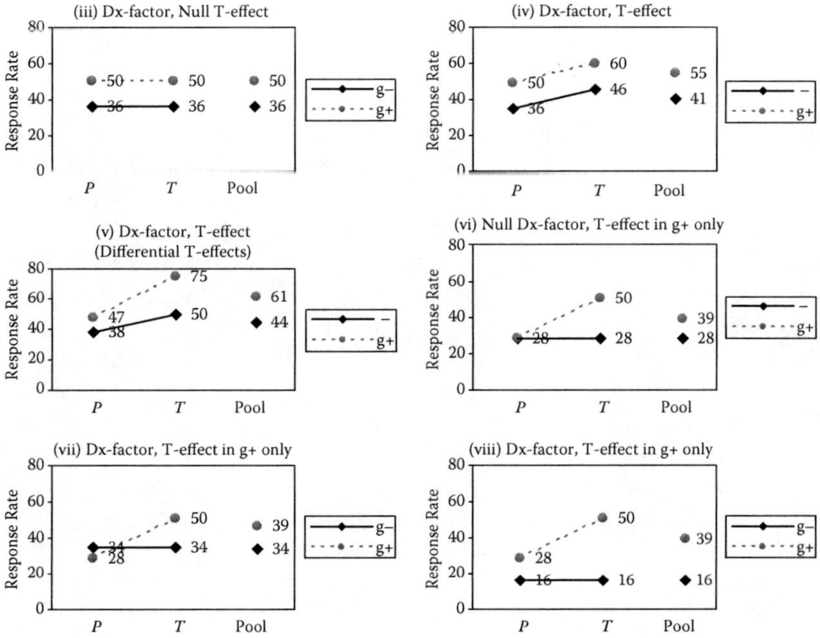

FIGURE 9.1
Utility of genomic biomarker as a classifier in therapeutic drug trial.

biomarker is independent of treatment administration and does not influence treatment effect.

9.2.3.2 Predictive

Strictly speaking, a genomic biomarker is said to be a predictive factor of treatment effect if in truth there are two distinct treatment effects ($\Delta_- = 0$ and $\Delta_+ > 0$): a null effect in the *g*– genomic subset, and a positive treatment effect in the *g*+ genomic subset as shown in Graphs (vi), (vii), and (viii). That is, the therapy is effective only in patients who are classified as *g*+. The implicit treatment-by-biomarker qualitative interaction not formally tested signifies the *predictive* utility of the genomic biomarker to select patient subset for an effective therapy (also Scenario A of Wang et al., 2007). In the extreme case the treatment effect can be inferior in the *g*– genomic subset, that is, $\Delta_- < 0$ and $\Delta_+ > 0$).

Sometimes the predictivity defines sensitivity of a tumor to a distinct therapeutic agent, then Graphs (v) to (viii) satisfy the definition of predictivity. For power consideration, Wang et al. (2007) distinguished between quantitative treatment-by-biomarker interaction (Graph (v)) and qualitative interaction (Graphs (vi)–(viii)) anticipated in designing a clinical trial.

9.2.3.3 Prognostic and Predictive

With a potential quantitative interaction, a genomic biomarker may be prognostic of treatment effects that are different in magnitude between the *g*+ and *g*– biomarker subsets, such as those shown in Graph (v). Here, the biomarker is prognostic of disease state and predictive of differential treatment effects, where ($\Delta_+ > \Delta_- > 0$) numerically. In such cases, the role of a genomic biomarker can be to differentiate treatment effects and its clinical utility could be considered *prognostic-predictive of drug effect* (also Scenario C of Wang et al., 2007).

When the prognostic utility is evaluated in the placebo arm alone, the clinical utility of a genomic biomarker shown in Graph (viii) might be considered prognostic-predictive in the sense of prognostic of disease state and predictive of treatment effect. That is, the genomic (composite) biomarker for assessing drug effect can be defined as a measurable characteristic serving as an indicator for differential response or predictive of response to therapy, such as between patients diagnostically classified as *g*+ or *g*– (ICH, 2007).

9.2.4 Assessment of Clinical Utility and Therapeutic Effect

Once a genomic (composite) biomarker is developed, say, from among plausible exploratory biomarkers, the genomic *in vitro* diagnostic (IVD) assay of an established biomarker classifier should be analytically validated with acceptable analytical performance characteristics. The analytically validated genomic IVD diagnostic assay can then be used in prospectively planned trials to classify patients into biomarker positive or biomarker negative status prior to its commercialization. Suppose these prospective clinical trials are placebo controlled trials. The preliminary clinical validation of the genomic IVD assay can be assessed in the placebo treated patients. In addition, the clinical utility of the genomic IVD assay can be evaluated based on the treatment effect estimated in the biomarker positive patient subset and the biomarker negative patient subset. A genomic biomarker to be used at this stage of its drug development may pursue the regulatory path to qualify the biomarker for its context of use in drug development.

When a GCB is developed using microarray or SNP array biotechnology, its clinical utility as a diagnostic, prognostic, predictive, or prognostic/predictive tool for patient selection needs to be demonstrated for commercial use. The same process applies to single genomic biomarkers. Following the analytical validation and if the result from the preliminary clinical validation is promising, diagnostic trials can be formally conducted to assess the performance characteristics of a genomic IVD classification including sensitivity, specificity, positive predictive value, and negative predictive value. Some examples follow. For a single genomic biomarker, HER2 testing was mentioned in the Herceptin drug labeling update in 2008. As an example, HercepTest is an IVD diagnostic test for detecting the presence or absence of HER2/Neu protein biomarker, which was approved only in 2010 (http://www.fda.gov/MedicalDevices/ProductsandMedicalProcedures/DeviceApprovalsandClearances/Recently-ApprovedDevices/ucm234142.htm), but the treatment Herceptin was initially approved in 1998 (http://www.accessdata.fda.gov/scripts/cder/drugsatfda/index.cfm?fuseaction=Search.Label_ApprovalHistory#apphist). For a genomic composite biomarker, examples include AmpliChip CYP450 test (Jain, 2005) for diagnosing the presence of specific CYP450 gene variants and MammaPrint (Glas et al., 2006) as a prognostic genomic biomarker for identifying patients whose breast cancer prognosis is poor or good.

It is worth noting that the predictive values of a genomic IVD assay may be influenced by region if the disease prevalence differs among regions in an MRCT. When the disease prevalence is known to differ dramatically among regions, regional strategies may be pursued in lieu of an MRCT. A nongenomic example is the investigation of rectal treatment given to malaria patients before referring to clinics at which oral injections can be given. Since most malaria deaths occur in rural areas, a global strategy consisting of patients from two ethnically and geographically distinct regions was used to investigate the treatment effect. That is, the investigation of the treatment effect was conducted in two Africa countries and one Asia country (Gomes et al., 2009). In Section 9.3.1, a genomic example is given, which led to the study of three regional pharmacogenomics trials.

Assessment of treatment effects by genomic classifier status should be performed in a drug trial also known as a pharmacogenomics clinical trial. The genomic IVD assay used in a pharmacogenomics trial should be either analytically validated or commercially available. The requirement of a commercially available diagnostic test differs depending on the region of an MRCT. In the United States, a risk-based approach is used. That is, an IVD test depending on the risk level is either cleared or approved by the U.S. regulatory health authority. In Europe, however, a genomic diagnostic is commercially available if it is marked as Conformite Europeene (in French; CE, meaning European Conformity). The marking CE on a product indicates to governmental officials that the product may be legally placed on the market in their country (http://www.ce-marking.org/what-is-ce-marking.html). In addition, the genomic samples of the intent-to-treat patients, such as blood, specimen, or tissue samples, should have been taken at study baseline. In such controlled therapeutic trials, multiple clinical hypotheses of treatment effects in prespecified patient subsets, nested or nonnested, can be evaluated. To assess these clinical hypotheses, statistical inferential paradigm in late phase drug development is unlikely to change.

9.3 Bridging

The impact of ethnic factors on a treatment effect may vary depending on the drug's pharmacologic class and indication and on age and gender of the patients. Characterization of a drug on its pharmacokinetic, pharmacodynamic, and therapeutic effects may be useful to determine what type of bridging study is needed in the new region (ICH, 1998). On the other hand, to what extent bridging clinical studies separate from original clinical development are needed for external bridging strategy due to differences in ethnic composition by countries or by regions may be debatable given that globalization of medical drug product development is more attractive and potentially more cost-effective. To minimize duplication of clinical data in the new region and with the emerging trend of conducting MRCTs, an alternative approach known as internal bridging strategy may simply be prespecification of what constitutes regions or countries of interest at the design stage. Such design consideration would allow prospective assessment of the treatment effect that may be relatively more favorable to the region/country of ultimate interest (Wang, 2009, 2010).

9.3.1 New Region Trial—External Bridging Strategy

Conventionally, an external bridging strategy of regional trials is to conduct a small study in the new region when the treatment effect in the original region trial has been demonstrated with evidential rigor to avoid duplicating efforts but to raise confidence level that the treatment effect found in the original region trial would be applicable to the new region. The premise of the external bridging strategy in the conventional one-size-fits-all approach lies in the belief that the treatment is effective on average in a disease patient population irrespective of ethnic sensitivity, and the source of variability due to intrinsic and extrinsic ethnic factors should be within the level of variability typically observed accounting for known prognostic factors (see, e.g., Polanczyk et al., 2008).

With an external bridging strategy, unlike the conventional approach, there may be a need to conduct a more rigorous new region pharmacogenomics trial possibly much larger than 40 patients. Note that to accept foreign clinical data the conventional approach adopts the bridging study results, which is often faced with small sample sizes as small as 40 patients required by some regulators, such as the Taiwan Center for Drug Evaluation (Hsiao, Chern, Chen, and Lin, 2003). We will use the current practice found in the recent literature as a way of introducing the interest level and the importance of new region pharmacogenomics trials. Specifically, the regional pharmacogenomics approach in the development of gefitinib as first-line treatment in chemonaive non-small cell lung cancer (NSCLC) patients will be used to highlight the attempt of "regional" clinical trials conducted to evaluate gefitinib effect in Asia using the genomic biomarker status.

9.3.1.1 External Bridging Strategy

In 2004, two large phase 3 placebo-controlled outcome trials—INTACT1 (Giaccone et al., 2004) and INTACT2 (Herbst et al., 2004)—failed to show an overall survival benefit (the primary efficacy endpoint) in 1093 (INTACT1) and 1037 (INTACT2) chemonaive NSCLC patients. Both studies included a placebo arm, a low dose (250 mg/day) and a high dose (500 mg/day) arm with cisplatin/gemcitabine as the background therapy in INTACT 1 and carboplatin/paclitaxel in INTACT2. These two large phase 3 trials are considered the original region trials recruiting patients mainly from Europe (e.g., 75% in INTACT1) and U.S. regions (e.g., 80% in INTACT2). Approximately 90% of the NSCLC patients from these regions are Caucasian with only 1–2% Asian (3 placebo) in INTACT1 and less than 5% Asian (10 placebo) in INTACT2. Given the limited number of patients of Asian ethnicity in INTACT1 and INTACT2, it was not possible to study whether the gefitinib effect could be applied to Asian patients.

Around the same time, Lynch et al. (2004), Paez et al. (2004), and Pao et al. (2004) showed that the presence of somatic mutations in the kinase domain of epidermal growth factor receptor (EGFR) strongly correlates with increased responsiveness to EGFR tyrosine kinase inhibitors (TKIs) in patients with NSCLC. It was later found that subgroups of patients with NSCLC who had sensitivity to gefitinib had a high incidence of EGFR mutation. Thus, EGFR mutation as a genomic biomarker may serve as an indicator for therapeutic response to TKIs, such as gefitinib and erlotinib, in patients with NSCLC. The predictiveness of EGFR mutation to select genomically prone patient subpopulation for medical treatment can be tested in well-controlled pharmacogenomics trials whereby the gefitinib effect in the EGFR mutation positive and the EGFR mutation negative patient subsets could be formally evaluated.

Researchers have also reported that East Asian ethnicity, no smoking history, adenocarcinoma histology, and female gender are factors predictive of response to gefitinib and erlotinib (Chang et al., 2006; Yang et al., 2006) TKI agents. Three regional phase 3 trials for first-line treatment in chemonaive NSCLC patients all conducted in East Asia were just recently completed and published (Maemondo et al., 2010; Mitsudomi et al., 2010; Mok et al., 2009). These new region trials assessed if gefitinib would be effective in chemonaive NSCLC patients whose ethnicity is East Asian or who are classified as EGFR mutation positive (EGFR+).

9.3.1.2 NSCLC Patient Composition in Regional Pharmacogenomics Trials

Study IPASS (Iressa Pan-Asia Study) was an open-label trial comparing gefitinib with carboplatin plus paclitaxel (Armour and Watkins, 2010; Mok et al., 2009). A total of 1217 advanced NSCLC patients were recruited in 2006–2007 from 87 centers in Hong Kong, China, Indonesia, Japan, Malaysia, the Philippines, Singapore, Taiwan, and Thailand with approximately 51% Chinese and 19% Japanese, among others. The analysis population included 609 gefitinib treated patients and 608 carboplatin plus paclitaxel treated patients.

Study NEJ002 was a multicenter Japanese trial comparing gefitinib with carboplatin plus paclitaxel (Maemondo et al., 2010) in EGFR mutation enriched patient population. A total of 230 EGFR+ NSCLC patients were recruited at 43 institutions in Japan in 2006–2009. The analysis was based on 114 patients in each treatment arm.

The West Japan Thoracic Oncology Group Study (WJTOG 3405) was an open-label trial comparing gefitinib with cisplatin plus docetaxel in EGFR mutation enriched patient population (Mitsudomi et al., 2010). A total of 177 EGFR+ patients were recruited at 36 centers in Japan in 2006–2009. The efficacy analysis was based on 86 patients receiving cisplatin/docetaxel and 86 patients receiving gefitinib.

The predictive factors reported in the literature for these regional trials are summarized in Table 9.1. Specifically, we are interested in region/ethnicity, EGFR mutation biomarker positivity, never smoker, female gender, and prevalence of adenocarcinoma histology. As shown, the original trials (INTACT1 and INTACT2) recruited a very limited number of patients of East Asian ethnicity (fewer than 20 patients per arm) lacking the ability

TABLE 9.1

Summary of Predictive Factors for NSCLC Treatment Reported from the Literature

First Line Treatment	Original Region Trial (gefitinib)		New (Asia) Region Trial (gefitinib)			Original Trial (erlotinib)
Study	**INTACT1**	**INTACT2**	**IPASS**	**NEJ002**	**WJTOG3405**	**Rosell et al. (2009)**
N	1093	1037	1217	228	172	217[1]
% Asia	5%	4%	100%[2]	100%[3]	100%[3]	< 2%
Region	Multiple	Multiple	Asia	Asia	Asia	Spain
% EGFR+	na	na	**60%**	100%	100%	100%
% never smoker	na	na	94%	62%	69%	67%
% female	26%	40%	80%	63%	69%	70%
% adenocarcinoma	46%	55%	96%	93%	98%	81%

[1] EGFR+ with 113 first-line patients.
[2] 19% Japanese.
[3] 100% Japanese.

to properly describe the gefitinib effect in this region. There was no report of EGFR biomarker data in the original trials in Giaccone et al. (2004) and Herbst et al. (2004).

In the three new region trials, only study IPASS can assess the estimated prevalence of EGFR mutation. In IPASS, although 85% (n = 1038) of patients consented for EGFR biomarker testing, 56% (n = 683) provided EGFR samples, and only 36% (n = 437) were patients whose EGFR biomarker could be classified as mutation positive (n = 261) or mutation negative (n = 176). Thus, the estimated EGFR mutation prevalence was 60% obtained from predominately never smoker female NSCLC patients who had adenocarcinoma and lived in East Asia. It is obvious that patient population in the three new region trials is very different from those in the original region trials.

As a contrast, Rosell et al. (2009) reported an estimated EGFR mutation prevalence of only 17% (i.e., 350/2105) in the NSCLC patient population from 129 institutions in Spain seeking TKI treatment of erlotinib (another TKI). Among the 350 patients, 217 were eligible for erlotinib treatment, of which 113 received first-line treatment. There were differences in patient composition in that the majority of NSCLC patients in this single arm trial (Rosell et al.) were Caucasians (98%), whereas the three regional gefitinib trials (IPASS, NEJ002, and WJTOG3405) recruited patients only from East Asia. These differences imply that the EGFR prevalence may be race/ethnicity dependent.

9.3.1.3 Results Observed in Regional Pharmacogenomics Trials

The primary efficacy endpoint was progression free survival (PFS) for the three regional trials. Table 9.2 presents the analysis results on the primary

TABLE 9.2

Results Using Gefitinib as First-Line Therapy in Patients with Advanced NSCLC

Study	# of pts	OTR (%)	PFS (mon)	HR_g/o *p* or 95%CI	OS (mon)	HR_g/o *p* or 95%CI
			Original Region Trial			
INTACT1	365	50	5.5	$p = .763$	9.9	$p = .456$
c/g/g500md/d	365	51	5.8		9.9	
c/g/g250mg/d	363	47	6.0		10.9	
c/g/placebo						
INTACT2	347	30	4.6	$p = .056$	8.7	$p = .639$
c/p/g500mg/d	345	30	5.3		9.8	
c/p/g250mg/d	345	29	5.0		9.8	
c/p/placebo						
		New Region Trial—Regional Intended or Country Intended Trial				
IPASS	608	32.2	5.8	0.74[1,2]	17.3	0.91
car/pac (ITT)	609	43.0[1]	5.7	(0.65,0.85)	18.6	(0.76, 1.10)
gef250mg/d ITT	129	47.3	6.3	0.48[1]	19.5	0.78
car/pac (+)	132	71.2[1]	9.5	(0.36, 0.64)	nr	(0.50, 1.20)
gefitinib (+)	85	23.5	5.5	2.85[1]	12.6	1.38
car/pac (–)	91	1.1[1]	1.5	(2.05, 3.98)	12.1	(0.92, 2.09)
gefitinib (–)	394	29.2	—	0.68[1,2]	—	0.86
car/pac (uk)	386	43.3[1]	—	(0.58, 0.81)	—	(0.68, 1.09)
gefitinib (uk)						
NEJ002[3]	114	30.7	5.4	0.30[1]	23.6	$p = 0.31$
car/pac (+)	114	73.7[1]	10.8	(0.22, 0.41)	30.5	
gef250mg/d(+)						
WJTOG3405	86	33.2	6.3	0.49[1]	n/a	1.64
cis/doc (+)	86	62.1[1]	9.2	(0.34, 0.71)	30.9	(0.75, 3.58)
gef250mg/d(+)						
		Reference of a TKI for the Same First-Line Indication				
Rosell et al.	113&	14m[4]	53%[5]	—	28	95%CI
erl150mg/d (+)						(22.7, 33.0)

[1] $p \le 0.001$; INTACT1 (Giaccone et al., 2004); INTACT2 (Herbst et al., 2004); IPASS (Mok et al., 2009); NEJ002 (Maemondo et al., 2010); WJTOG3405 (Mitsudomi et al., 2010).

[2] Survival curve crossed at around median and resulted in more total events in car/pac arm than in gefitinib arm.

[3] Early terminated for superior efficacy; & 52% of 217 are first line EGFR evaluable patients.

[4] Median duration of response.

[5] % progressed.

na, not available; nr, not reached.

efficacy endpoint along with objective tumor response (OTR) and overall survival (OS). For comparison, the results of OS (the primary efficacy endpoint in the original region trials) were also summarized. Both INTACT1 and INTACT2 showed no dose response on OTR, PFS, or OS in a population with 90% Caucasian.

9.3.1.4 Consistent Observation between OTR and PFS in EGFR+ NSCLC Patient Subset

In the EGFR+ patient subset, gefitinib was shown to prolong the time to progression compared with its active comparator carboplatin plus paclitaxel (IPASS and NEJ002) or cisplatin plus docetaxel (WJTOG3405) with $p < 0.001$ (see Table 9.2). The hazard ratios (HRs) reported were 0.48 (95%CI: 0.36, 0.64) in IPASS, 0.30 (95%CI: 0.22, 0.41) in NEJ002, and 0.49 (95%CI: 0.34, 0.71) in WJTOG3405. Among the three regional pharmacogenomics trials, the PFS was longest with gefitinib and shortest with carboplatin plus paclitaxel in study NEJ002, which was terminated early per the recommendation from the data monitoring committee due to a superior efficacy at approximately 88% information time when 88% of the ITT patients completed the study (Maemondo et al., 2010). The finding of OTR tracked the finding of PFS in all three trials.

9.3.1.5 Inconsistent Observation of OS in EGFR+ NSCLC Patient Subset

Given the primary efficacy endpoint of OS in the original trial and that EGFR biomarker was thought to be associated with better outcome, it is of interest to explore if there was survival advantage with gefitinib in the enriched EGFR+ patient subset. As summarized in Table 9.3, EGFR+ patients receiving gefitinib appeared to show a numerically favorable 22% hazard reduction yielding as good as 50% hazard reduction to as bad as 20% hazard increase. The numerically favorable overall survival trend in EGFR+ patients was also reported in NEJ002. The median time to death was 6.9 month (NEJ002) to at least 9 months (IPASS) longer in EGFR+ patients treated with gefitinib than with carboplatin/paclitaxel. However, it was disturbing that the favorable

TABLE 9.3

Survival Analysis Based on % Death in NSCLC Patients with EGFR Mutation in Rosell et al. (2009)

Study	IPASS		NEJ002		WJTOG3405		Rosell
Treatment	gefi	cntl[1]	gefi	cntl[1]	gefi	cntl[2]	erlotinib
n	132	129	114	114	86	86	113
% death	29%	33%	39%	53%	20%	12%	53%
% death	31%		46%		16%		53%

[1] carboplatin plus paclitaxel.
[2] cisplatin plus docetaxel.

trend with gefitinib was reversed in WJTOG3405 of at least 9 months shorter than with cisplatin/docetaxel, the estimated hazard ratio was 1.64. Mitsudomi et al. (2010) noted that data for OS were immature because only 27 patients (16%) had died at the data cutoff.

To explore the inconsistent observation in overall survival, we compared the death rate across the three Asia region trials. From Table 9.3, it appeared that the death rate of 16% may be immature in WJTOG3405 compared with 31% in IPASS and 46% in NEJ002. The more interesting observations was that if the trend of lower death rate in a different control in WJTOG3405 persists, the inferior mortality with gefitinib might be directly related to the differences between the two standard doubly chemotherapies. Per personal communication with Mitsudomi (2011), survival data in WJTOG3405 are to be updated shortly.

The numerical, but not statistically significant, survival advantage with gefitinib over carboplatin/paclitaxel may be arguably an underpowering issue. We note that the number of patients who are EGFR+ was 114 in NEJ002 and approximately 130 receiving either gefitinib (n = 132) or carboplatin plus paclitaxel (n = 129) in IPASS. If it is believed that the mortality effect with cisplatin/docetaxel should be the same as with carboplatin/paclitaxel, a study with twofold more than 86 patients per arm in WJTOG3405 may be needed.

9.3.2 Original Region Trial—Internal Bridging Strategy

Acute coronary syndrome (ACS) exists across geographical regions (WHO, 2000). To date, several ACS large trials have demonstrated significant regional variation in clinical outcomes and treatment effect (see, e.g., Chang et al., 2005; Wallentin et al., 2009). Reasons attributed to these differences include variable disease epidemiology such as subjects' baseline risk, regional differences in medical practices including the clinical care processes, and statistical chance finding due to post hoc subgroup analyses (see, e.g., O'Shea and Califf, 2000).

With the more recent development for ACS treatment specifically in TRITON TIMI38, prasugrel therapy was shown superior to clopidogrel in reducing the risk of ischemic events including stent thrombosis (HR = 0.81 with 95% CI of 0.73 to 0.90, $p < 0.001$) but with an increased risk of major bleeding, including fatal bleeding (1.4% vs. 0.9%, $p = 0.01$; Wiviott et al., 2007). TRITIN TIMI 38 was a multiregional clinical trial in which 13,608 recruited ACS patients from 30 countries across 5 continents were undergoing percutaneous intervention (PCI).

9.3.2.1 Internal Bridging Strategy

Given the regional variation reported in the literature, Ruff et al. (2010) reanalyzed the data from TRITON TIMI-38 comparing the effect of prasugrel with clopidogrel by dividing the enrollment into five prespecified geographical regions: 32% (n = 4310) subjects enrolled in North America; 4% (534) in South America; 26% (3553) in West Europe; 24% (3322) in East Europe; and 14% (1889) in Africa/Asia Pacific/Middle East. A secondary measure of the Human Development Index (HDI) was also used as a composite measure of social and economic development (Mahbub ul Haq, 1990), which resulted in 71% (9688) subjects enrolled in developed countries and 29% (3920) in developing countries. Ruff et al. concluded that, despite differences in patient demographics, procedural techniques, and adjunctive medications, consistent reduction in ischemic events and increased bleeding were seen with prasugrel compared with clopidogrel across all regions.

9.3.2.2 Potential Genomics Factors Explored

In TRITON TIMI 38, use of a GP IIb/IIIa inhibitor was at the physician's discretion. To address the potential heterogeneity between patients with versus without use of a GP IIb/IIIa inhibitor, O'Donogue et al. (2009) reanalyzed data and concluded no heterogeneity between the two strata (HR of 0.76; 95% CI of 0.64 to 0.90 with use, and HR of 0.78; 95% CI of 0.63 to 0.97 without use, respectively). The analysis was performed using 30 days outcome and was stratified by use of GP IIb/IIIa inhibitor.

Other recent reports included exploratory analyses using 21.5% of 13,608 intent-to-treat ACS patients who voluntarily consented for pharmacogenomics substudy of TRITON TIMI 38 (Mega et al., 2010). The authors suggested a pharmacogenomics association between genetic variants (ABCB1 3435 gene and CYP2C19 gene) and clopidogrel; that is, individuals with these genetic variants are at increased risk of major cardiovascular events (MACE) including cardiovascular death, myocardial infarction, and stroke.

9.3.2.3 Absence of Patients from East Asia

Given a consistent benefit of prasugrel over clopidogrel for reducing risk of recurrent ischemic events (or MACE) in ACS patients reported in TRITON TIMI 38 trial, the observed superior prasugrel therapy would seem reasonably applicable to ACS patient population in general. However, a closer look at those reported by Ruff et al. (2010), countries grouped into Africa/Asia Pacific/Middle East (14% of ITT patients) included Australia, Israel, New Zealand, and South Africa. It was obvious that an East Asia region pharmacogenomics trial could be envisioned to confirm the clinical benefit of reducing recurrent ischemic events and to replicate the finding of pharmacogenetic association with genetic variants reported in Mega et al. (2010).

A literature search resulted in one phase 3 regional trial designed to study ACS patients of Asian ethnicity undergoing PCI. Specifically, Ge et al. (2010) considered an East Asia region trial of 3 dose regimens of prasugrel and one dose of clopidogrel for 90 days (n = 715 or approximately 180 patients per arm). The primary objective of this East Asia region trial was to confirm superior inhibition of platelet aggregation with prasugrel versus clopidogrel, a pharmacodynamic comparison.

Although Mega et al. (2010) did not suggest the association study with prasugrel, additional key endpoints not statistically powered included genetic analyses of cytochrome P450 polymorphisms. In this context, this East Asia region pharmacodynamic trial is designed to select the prasugrel dose based on inhibition of platelet aggregation to inform which doses of prasugrel would be appropriate for patients of Asian ethnicity. Essentially, it is hypothesized that the superior prasugrel effect shown in TRITON TIMI 38 could be extrapolated to East Asia patients with ACS, but the dose regimen suitable was to be investigated in a much smaller trial of approximately 2.6% of the sample size per arm used in TRITON TIMI 38.

9.4 Bridging Study Evaluation

Conventionally, bridging trials are conducted only when the foreign trials have demonstrated treatment efficacy. For an external bridging strategy, bridging trials may be of small trial size for short-term pharmacodynamic investigation to identify the appropriate dose regimen for the bridging region (see, e.g., Ge et al., 2010) following the finding in TRITON TIMI 38. A bridging study not of large size also allows exploration of pharmacogenomics association (see, e.g., Ge et al.).

In some cases, a pharmacogenomics bridging trial alone can be an adequate and well-controlled outcome trial that is conducted in a prespecified new region where genomic data are also collected prior to treatment intervention in addition to the usual clinical data, such as IPASS (Mok et al., 2009). In this context, the objective of an external bridging strategy in a confirmatory pharmacogenomics trial addresses a bigger genomic question that might be specific to or confounded with intrinsic ethnic factors.

9.4.1 Treatment Effect Demonstrated in Original Region

To assess ethnic sensitivity, an external bridging strategy can be viewed as an approach to demonstrate treatment effect in the bridging region through strength by borrowing foreign clinical data. Let θ_f be the treatment effect in a foreign clinical trial, and θ_b be the effect in the bridging region. When a significant treatment effect is concluded in the foreign clinical trial, the clinical hypothesis of no treatment difference to the placebo is rejected, that is, concluding $\theta_f > 0$. A bridging clinical study could be to demonstrate $\theta_b > 0$ given $\theta_f > 0$.

In the following sections we summarize Wang's (2009) work on statistical methods for evaluating the external bridging trials, and Wang et al.'s (2007) and Wang, Hung, and O'Neill's (2009) studies on the statistical designs for evaluating the internal bridging effect. Specifically, Wang (2009) considered two statistical formulations of the problem, an indirect approach and a direct approach with an external bridging.

9.4.1.1 Indirect Evaluation of Bridging Effect

Let λ_0 be the strength of treatment effect borrowing parameter. The bridging effect is defined as *treatment effect in the bridging region is in the neighborhood of that shown in the foreign clinical trial,* which can be smaller than, the same as, or larger than the effect in the foreign trial. Namely,

$$H_0: \quad \theta_b \le \lambda_0\, \theta_f \text{ vs. } H_1: \quad \theta_b \ge \lambda_0\, \theta_f \tag{9.1}$$

where $\lambda_0 > 0$. Treatment effect θ_f can be estimated using the foreign clinical data, $\tilde{\theta}_f + C_\gamma\, \sigma_f / \sqrt{N}$ for some fixed γ-level > 0, which is (1 − 2γ) 100% the confidence interval estimate. Note that, $\tilde{\theta}_f$ is the point estimate of the treatment effect θ_f, the assumed standard deviation σ_f, and $2N$ the per-group sample size in the foreign trial.

An indirect method aims to address the following working hypotheses at conventional level α. That is,

$$K_0: \quad \theta_b \le \lambda_0 \left(\tilde{\theta}_f + C_\gamma\, \sigma_f / \sqrt{N}\right) \text{ vs. } K_1: \quad \theta_b > \lambda_0 \left(\tilde{\theta}_f + C_\gamma\, \sigma_f / \sqrt{N}\right) \tag{9.2}$$

Let σ_b be the assumed variability in the bridging trial with per-group sample size of $2M$. If the data from the new region satisfies the following condition:

$$\hat{\theta}_b - z_\alpha \sigma_b / \sqrt{M} > \lambda_0 (\tilde{\theta}_f + C_\gamma\, \sigma_f / \sqrt{N})$$

then the working null hypothesis, K_0 (Equation 9.2) is rejected. The decision rule can be written as

$$\begin{aligned} & p\{\hat{\theta}_b - z_\alpha \sigma_b / \sqrt{M} > \lambda_0 (\tilde{\theta}_f + C_\gamma\, \sigma_f / \sqrt{N}) \mid \partial H_0\} \\ & = p\{\hat{\theta}_b - \lambda_0\, \tilde{\theta}_f > z_\alpha\, \sigma_b / \sqrt{M} + \lambda_0\, C_\gamma\, \sigma_f / \sqrt{N}) \mid \partial H_0\} \\ & = \Phi(-\frac{\lambda_0\, C_\gamma \sigma_f / \sigma_b \sqrt{M/N} + z_\alpha}{\sqrt{\lambda_0^2 (\sigma_f^2 / \sigma_b^2)(M/N) + 1}}) \end{aligned} \tag{9.3}$$

9.4.1.2 Type I Error Assessment

Let $C_\gamma = h\,Z_\alpha, \upsilon = M/N$. Suppose $\sigma_f = \sigma_b$, then under the original H_0 (Equation 9.1), the type I error probability (Equation 9.3) is controlled for $h \geq 1$. That is,

$$\Phi\left(-Z_\alpha \frac{\lambda_0\, h\sqrt{\nu}+1}{\sqrt{\lambda_0^2\,\nu+1}}\right) \leq \Phi(-Z_\alpha) = \alpha \qquad (h \geq 1)$$

However, if $h = 0$ corresponding to using the point estimate for the treatment effect, θ_f, in the foreign clinical trial, then the type I error probability is anticonservative.

$$\Phi\left(-Z_\alpha \frac{1}{\sqrt{\lambda_0^2\,\nu+1}}\right) > \Phi(-Z_\alpha) = \alpha$$

Figure 9.2 depicts the type I error probability for the indirect assessment method on the interplay of the relative sample size (*N/M*) and the relative variability (σ_f^2/σ_b^2) between the foreign trial and the bridging trial, and the level of strength borrowing (λ_0) from the foreign trial. The larger the ratio

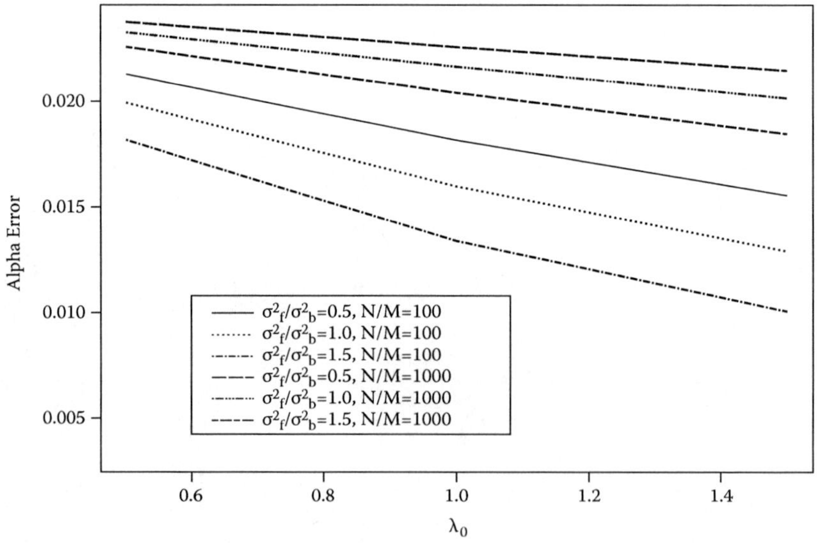

FIGURE 9.2
Type I error probability for the indirect method—the interplay for *N/M* and relative variability between the foreign and the bridging trial, and the level of strength borrowing from the foreign trial.

of the relative sample sizes, the closer the α level is to the planned level. When the variability in the foreign trial is larger than the bridging trial, the α error would be more conservative. As λ_0 increases, α error decreases. Of note, when $\lambda_0 > 1$ the bridging effect is larger than the foreign effect.

9.4.1.3 Direct Evaluation

In the direct method, the point estimate of the treatment effect in the foreign trial is directly used to test the strength of effect borrowing null hypothesis H_0 versus H_1 in Equation 9.1. The test statistic Z is

$$Z = \frac{\hat{\theta}_b - \lambda_0 \tilde{\theta}_f}{\sqrt{\sigma_b^2 / M + \lambda_0^2 \, \sigma_f^2 / N}}$$

For any M, $pr\{Z > z_\alpha \mid \partial H_0\} = \alpha$.

Thus, with the direct method, the type I error probability for testing H_0 is always maintained at the planned level, irrespective of the bridging study sample size, the strength of effect borrowing parameter level, or the assumed bridging study variance value.

9.4.1.4 Comparisons of Methods

Let Δ_f be the true standardized effect size in the foreign trial. The power functions $\theta_b = \lambda\theta_f$ for the indirect method and the direct method are

$$\Phi\left(\frac{\sqrt{M}(\lambda - \lambda_0)\Delta_f - Z_\alpha(\lambda_0 \, h\sqrt{v} + \sigma_b / \sigma_f)}{\sqrt{\lambda_0^2 \, v + (\sigma_b / \sigma_d)^2}}\right) \text{ and } \Phi\left(\frac{\sqrt{M}(\lambda - \lambda_0)\Delta_f}{\sqrt{\lambda_0^2 v + (\sigma_b / \sigma_f)^2}} - Z_\alpha\right)$$

We compare the power performance of the two approaches in Figure 9.3. Consider $\Delta_f = 0.4$. The power increases as the sample size in the bridging trial, the sample size ratio ($N/M > 1$), and the variance ratio ($\sigma_f^2 / \sigma_b^2 > 1$) of the foreign trial over the bridging trial increase and if the true strength of effect borrowing of the foreign trial is larger than the postulated strength borrowing. Of the scenarios considered, the bridging trial is underpowered for $M = 40$. The direct method performs consistently more powerfully than the indirect method. Suppose the bridging effect is smaller than the foreign effect, that is, $\lambda_0 < 1$, for example, $\lambda_0 = 0.9$. Consider the bridging sample size of $M = 100$. The direct method gains about 10% more in power than the indirect method for $N/M = 10$ when $\sigma_f^2 / \sigma_b^2 = 2$. However, the direct method is relatively insensitive to power improvement when N/M increases from 10 to 100 (results not shown).

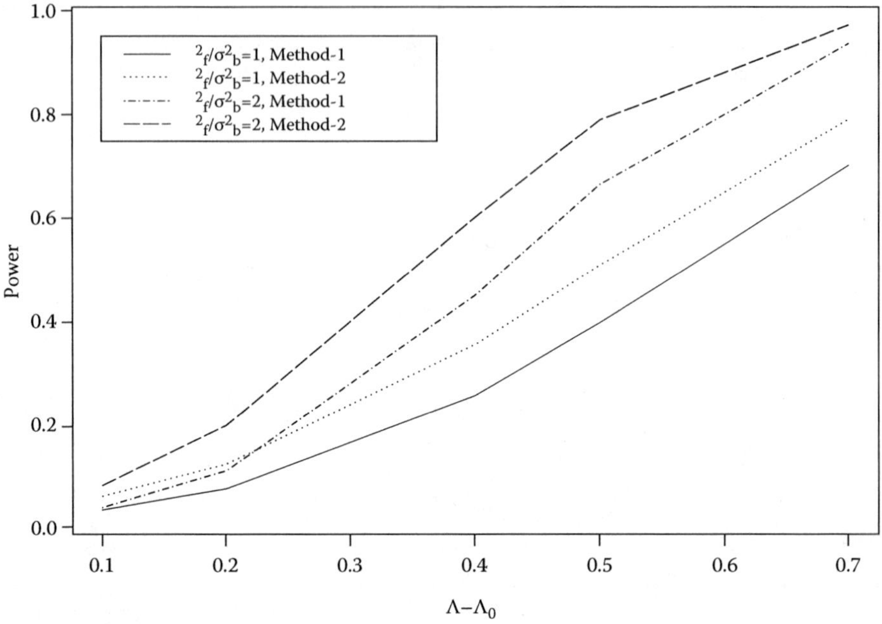

FIGURE 9.3
Power performance, *Effsize* = 0.4, $M = 100$, $N/M = 10$.

9.4.2 Treatment Effect Not Demonstrated in Original Region

The major utility of external bridging strategy stems from the spirit of extrapolation (Hung et al., 2012). With pharmacogenomics development, the formulation of a genomic predictor might be predominately ethnicity driven due to, for example, difference in allele frequency and in prevalence of a genomic biomarker classifier that can include multiple genes. The example cited in the development of gefitinib therapy as first-line treatment in advanced NSCLC patients may belong to this category. First, gefitinib was not shown effective in the two large foreign trials (INTACT1 and INTACT 2) in which at least 90% were Caucasians from the U.S. or European regions. However, it is yet to be demonstrated if gefitinib would be effective in patients of East Asian ethnicity overall or only in East Asian patients who have a EGFR mutation.

In such cases bridging trials should be designed with sufficient statistical power and analyzed as a stand-alone trial, which can be considered adequate and well controlled. These bridging trials do not directly use the original trial results of foreign regions for planning. Conceptually, this type of bridging trial is the same as a statistically sized original trial in the foreign region in terms of parameters needed to consider for designing the trial. The original trial results in the foreign region can be useful for the purpose of understanding the intrinsic and extrinsic ethnic differences when the bridging trial conducted in a new region is completed and compared.

Without loss of generality, such a bridging trial can be a multicenter trial consisting of one country with several sites located in different cities (e.g., NEJ002, WJTOG3405), a multinational clinical trial consisting of one region that includes multiple countries (e.g., IPASS), or a multiregional clinical trial consisting of patients from five continents (e.g., TRITON TIMI 38). In this spirit, in the following section we introduce two different adaptive design approaches to an MRCT for internal bridging strategy.

9.4.3 Internal Bridging Strategy in Multiregional Clinical Trial

In contrast to the external bridging strategy, the statistical inference of an MRCT trial is entirely based on within-trial comparison, and for the purpose of internal bridging there is one common protocol for all regions participating. The common protocol harmonizes the design and analysis of an MRCT for assessing an overall treatment effect across all regions and to bridge the treatment effect to regions evaluated in the same MRCT. In principle, the overall sample size for the MRCT is planned based on the overall effect size, which at the design stage is often assumed to be the same for all regions under the common protocol. Alternatively, if potential heterogeneity of the treatment effect, for example, due to intrinsic or extrinsic ethnic factors, is anticipated, a random-effect model can be used to explore the impact of regional heterogeneity and variability on the efficiency of a trial design (Hung et al., 2011).

9.4.3.1 Blinded Two-Stage Adaptive Test

At the design stage, an internal bridging strategy can be useful if a common treatment effect with a typical level of variability is anticipated. Countries that belong to regions of interest should be prespecified; for instance, the United States and Canada belong to North America. The regions in an MRCT act as mutually exclusive subgroups or subsets within the same trial. The prespecified region factor can easily be incorporated for a stratified randomization to ensure in probability the homogeneous characteristics of patients between the treated group and the control group within each region stratum.

A blinded two-stage adaptive design aims at a consistent treatment effect across regions (Wang, 2009). As such at the end of stage 1, preferably late in the information time where the majority of patients has been accrued, the region-specific pooled variances are estimated using the blinded interim accumulated data. If the estimated pooled variance of the specific region is obviously much larger than that based on all trial data or the data from the remaining regions obtained in the unblinded interim analyses, the prespecified region-specific null hypothesis for that region would not be pursued further. Otherwise, the study would proceed to the end. For the final analyses, the null hypothesis of the overall treatment effect is tested first followed

TABLE 9.4

Final Sample Statistics of Primary Endpoint Including the Prespecified Region

	Asia	Non-Asia	Multiregional Trial
Sample size per arm	105	155	260
Mean difference ($T - P$)	1.76	0.81	1.19
Pooled standard deviation	4.742	3.936	4.247
Nominal p-value	0.0071	0.070	0.0014

by the region-specific null hypothesis if not removed at the end of stage 1 analysis. It is possible to increase the sample size of the prespecified region to achieve both the type I error level and the statistical power level required by the regional health authority.

For illustration, suppose it is of interest to achieve the bridging goal to Asia. Assume the randomization was stratified by region and the sample size was equal between the treated and the placebo within each region. Table 9.4 shows an example MRCT where the bridging efficacy hypothesis for Asia region is prespecified. Suppose the stage 1 blinded analysis was performed at 90% information time and the pooled variance estimate between the Asia region and the MRCT was very similar. This would result in keeping the Asia-specific hypothesis for a final analysis. In other words, the Asia-specific treatment effect hypothesis test would be performed after the overall null hypothesis from the MRCT is rejected at the final analysis. In this example, the final analysis of the ITT patients in the MRCT resulted in a significant treatment effect (p = 0.0014), and the treatment effect appeared to be more profound in the prespecified region, Asia (p = 0.0071).

9.4.3.2 Unblinded Two-Stage Adaptive Test

The two-stage adaptive designs considered in Wang et al. (2007) and Wang et al. (2009) are unblinded two-stage adaptive tests. Following Wang et al. (2007), let the null hypothesis of the overall treatment effect in the MRCT be H_{0M}:$\Delta = 0$, and the null hypothesis of the treatment effect in the prespecified region be H_{01}:$\Delta_1 = 0$. We extend from Wang et al. (2007) to allow futility analysis of the two complementary subset hypotheses, H_{01}:$\Delta_1 = 0$ of the prespecified region and H_{0_1}:$\Delta_{\_1} = 0$ of the remaining regions. If the futility of the treatment effects in both the prespecified region and the remaining regions cannot be concluded, the trial proceeds with recruitment of all patients in stage 2. Otherwise, the accrual continues with only those regions not early terminated for futility. The approach does not entertain an interim efficacy conclusion. The final analysis for testing the overall treatment effect uses patients from both stages if there is no futility stopping for the entire trial at the end of stage 1. If the result of the final test is statistically significant at a prespecified alpha level, the treatment effect in the prespecified region can be further evaluated if the prespecified region was not early terminated for futility.

What follows is a more elaborate approach that generalizes the approach by Wang et al. (2009). Suppose an MRCT includes four mutually exclusive regions. In addition to $H_{0M}{:}\Delta = 0$, let the prespecified null hypothesis of treatment effect in, say, regions 1, 2, and 3 be $H_{0123}{:}\Delta_{123} = 0$, which includes three mutually exclusive subset null hypotheses: $H_{01}{:}\Delta_1 = 0$, $H_{02}{:}\Delta_2 = 0$, and $H_{03}{:}\Delta_3 = 0$; each is nested in the combined region (regions 1, 2 and 3), which is nested in the MRCT. Let the null hypothesis in the remaining region be $H_{04}{:}\Delta_4 = 0$.

Conceptually, the unblinded adaptation proceeds as follows. First, ad hoc but prespecified interim futility analyses will be performed using an unblinded Z-test statistic at the end of stage 1 that should not be early in the information time. These unblinded interim analyses may include the global null hypothesis H_{0M}, H_{0123}, and the lower-level subset null hypotheses H_{0123}, viz., H_{012}, H_{013}, and H_{023}, and the elementary region-specific null hypotheses H_{01}, H_{02}, H_{03}, and H_{04}. The prespecified adaptation rules will govern exclusion of a region, if any, at the interim futility analyses. These futility analyses are nonbinding in terms of alpha spending.

If some regions are excluded, the available sample size can be redistributed to those regions remaining for further accrual. If no real heterogeneity among regions is anticipated, then the final analyses will be performed in a hierarchical manner and the treatment effect in individual regions should be tested only after an overall treatment effect can be conclusively shown in those regions that remain. The MRCT could be designed anticipating the heterogeneity among regions, similar to what we experienced with the development of gefitinib first-line treatment. In such cases, the nested adaptive approach does not require the assumption of homogeneity of the treatment effects across the regions and allows the final analyses to be performed to test the MRCT null hypothesis and the prespecified region null hypotheses with appropriate alpha allocations.

In addition to not considering a potential efficacy conclusion at the interim time, the premise of the proposed unblinded two-stage adaptive trial lies in a few key design considerations. First, the number of regions should be kept to a minimum. Second, the sample size of each region should not be too disproportionate. For sample size planning in an MRCT, see, for example, Quan, Zhao, Zhang, Roessner, and Aizawa (2009), Kawai, Chuang-Stein, Komiyama, and Li (2008), and Hung et al. (2011). Third, the interim futility analysis should be performed with sufficient information time so that the interim estimates will unlikely be random high or random low results. Fourth, the adaptation rules for futility need to be well thought out. For instance, the ideas of the futility analyses may include penalizing those regions with low data quality or poor trial conduct if they exist or anticipating futile treatment effect may be observed if data quality is not an issue. Fifth, the design allows early termination of the entire trial due to futility.

Sixth, if there is no early termination due to futility, the number of regions not to be considered for further accrual should be kept to a minimum.

The objective of such a two-stage adaptation is to maximize the power for either the overall treatment effect or the region-specific treatment effect, if not early terminated for further accrual, while maintaining the type I error rate control with respect to the originally prespecified null hypotheses. There are several variations to the adaptation previously described, depending on the number of regions and how the nested pattern is prespecified. For instance, the four nonoverlapping elementary null hypotheses in a pharmacogenomics MRCT with a prespecified region could represent the true treatment effects in the $g+$ subset of the region of interest, the $g-$ subset of the region of interest, the $g+$ subset of the remaining regions, and the $g-$ subset of the remaining regions.

9.5 Challenges of Bridging Strategy in Pharmacogenomics

Pharmacogenomics trials aim at determining if a treatment effect as observed can be explained by genomic factors that may be associated with disease pathophysiology or the drug's mechanism of action (Wang, 2006). The genomic factors are also known as genomic biomarkers. The following sections point out several challenges facing the pharmacogenomics community.

9.5.1 Prospective–Retrospective Design and Analysis

In a pharmacogenomics study, the genomic samples collected may be genotyped only later in the clinical trial or even after trial completion when a hypothesis of genomic relevance becomes more compelling, introducing into the trial design a new hypothesis of treatment efficacy in a genomic subgroup or a genotype association within the drug treatment arm. Such a trial design is often referred to as prospective–retrospective study design (Wang, 2007, 2008; Wang, Cohen, Katz, Ruano, Shaw, and Spear, 2006; Wang, O'Neill, and Hung, 2010).

A prospective–retrospective study design we discussed is in a conventional adequate and well-controlled clinical trial setting designed to demonstrate a treatment effect in the ITT patient population but where a genomic substudy with genomic convenience samples is embedded in the trial's ITT cohort. We interpret a prospective–retrospective design and analysis to have the following properties. First, the genomic samples are collected in a clinical study, either prior to, during, or after trial completion. Second, specification of the genomic hypothesis may arguably be prospective because it is stated prior to genomic diagnostic assay testing; thus, the genomic biomarker status (positive versus negative) of each subject has not been classified or is unknown at that time. Third, the clinical outcome data have already been (partially) collected and analyzed without the presence of genomic information. In brief, the retrospective aspects are those considered after the trial has been initiated, although defining the genomic hypothesis might be considered "prospective" (Wang, O'Neill et al., 2010). It is important to judiciously collect genomic samples when acquiring specimens for genomic analysis in prospective–retrospective studies.

As a general statistical principle for biomarker analysis, a prospective–retrospective design and analysis may yield interpretable study results if the genomic samples with sufficient amount of genomic materials in an ITT patient population can be fully ascertained. The remaining issues include the availability of an acceptable genomic diagnostic assay that has a high probability of correctly classifying patients into biomarker positive versus biomarker negative status. The genomic biomarker indicator serves as a stratification factor for assessing the treatment effect, which can be incorporated for a stratified randomization requiring the genomic biomarker classification to be completed prior to trial initiation. The stratified randomization would be important if the sample size were small. With an MRCT without preplanning how to incorporate the genomic stratification factor into the design and the analysis, the potential differences in minor allele frequency, the Hardy-Weinberg equilibrium, and the genomic biomarker prevalence can exist due to different allele frequencies among races unevenly distributed among different regions.

9.5.1.1 Probability of Observed Imbalance with Small Sample Size

Cui et al. (2002) explored the impact of small sample sizes on the probability of observed imbalance between two treatment groups with a binary indicator. We apply the binary indicator to a binary genomic biomarker. Cui et al. defined the imbalance as a 20% observed difference in clinical outcomes between the (biomarker) positive and (biomarker) negative patient subsets. As shown in Table 9.5, the probability of observed imbalance decreases as

TABLE 9.5

Probability of Observed Imbalance between Two Treatment Groups: A Binary Genomic Biomarker

True Prevalence	N = 20/arm	N = 50/arm	N = 100/arm
10%	0.0631	0.0017	0.0000
20%	0.1636	0.0173	0.0006
30%	0.2258	0.0377	0.0026
40%	0.2582	0.0519	0.0048
50%	0.2682	0.0569	0.0057

Note: Imbalance is defined as a 20% observed difference.

Source: From Cui, L., H. M. J. Hung, S. J. Wang, and Y. Tsong, *Journal of Biopharmaceutical Statistics*, 12, 347–358, 2002, Table 1.

TABLE 9.6

Probability of Imbalance with Given Sample Size and Percent Imbalance

Prevalence	N = 1350/arm d = 5%	N = 350/arm d = 10%	N = 150/arm d = 15%
10%	0.0000	0.0000	0.0000
20%	0.0012	0.0011	0.0012
30%	0.0046	0.0044	0.0045
40%	0.0080	0.0077	0.0079
50%	0.0094	0.0091	0.0093

Note: d is % observed imbalance between the treated group and the comparator group.

Source: Wang, S. J., R. T. O'Neill, and H. M. J. Hung, *Clinical Trials*, 7, 525–536, 2010, Table 5.2.

the sample size per arm increases for a given prevalence. However, the probability of observed imbalance increases as the true prevalence approaches 50%. This is especially the case when the sample size per arm is not large, say, less than 50 per arm. The genomic biomarker positive or negative patient subset, if not carefully considered at the design stage of a pharmacogenomics clinical trial, can easily fall into small sample sizes similar to those seen in Table 9.5 in a prespecified region of an MRCT.

The sample size needed for narrower imbalance, say, 15%, 10% and 5% observed difference between the treatment group and the control group. As shown in Table 9.6 (extracted from Table 5.2 of Wang, O'Neill et al. 2010a), the sample size needed can be as large as 150/arm, 350/arm to 1350/arm if it is of interest to minimize the probability of imbalance down to less than 0.01 where the imbalance is at a level of 15%, 10% and 5%, respectively, and the important stratification factors including a genomic biomarker classifier are not used to stratify patients at study randomization.

9.5.1.2 Close to Full Ascertainment of Genomic Samples in Pharmacogenomics Trials

When there is an urgent need of sound scientific principles to evaluate the evidence as observed in controlled pharmacogenomics trials, it appears that it is possible to achieve close to full ascertainment through complete genomic consent. Next, we briefly summarize the development of panitumumab belonging to such an example. Panitumumab is a monoclonal antibody selective for EGFR (Amgen, 2006). During the development of panitumumab, several studies have identified that the presence of mutant kRAS in metastatic colorectal cancer (mCRC) tumors correlates with poor prognosis (see, e.g., Andreyev, Norman, and Cunningham, 2001). In addition, others have also showed that mutant EGFR (EGFR+) is associated with lack of response to

EGFR inhibitors such as panitumumab (see, e.g., Benvenuti et al., 2007). The emerging science prompted pharmaceutical sponsors' interests to amend their protocols of ongoing studies to limit the accrual of mCRC patients who are wild-type kRAS. There were differences between the U.S. and Europe regions in their regulatory actions. Panitumumab was approved for monotherapy of relapsed/refractory mCRC by the U.S. Food and Drug Administration (FDA, 2006). But it was approved conditionally in patients with tumors harboring wild-type kRAS by the European Medicines Agency (EMA, 2007).

Following the reports of retrospective analyses of several phase 3 trials at the Annual Society of Clinical Oncology (ASCO) in 2008, a study protocol of North Central Cancer Treatment Group (NCCTG) (http://www.multicare.org/files/crp/5302b2d37d6c8ea326723d2cfde7285c.pdf) was modified and stated that "it no longer appears appropriate to use an EGFR inhibitor in patients with tumors expressing mutated kRAS." These reports were only in abstract forms and included 45% genomic convenience sample in Study CRYSTAL using PCR-based technology to classify the kRAS status (Van Cutsem et al., 2008). Regulatory concerns were raised at the 2008 oncologic advisory committee meeting (http://www.fda.gov/ohrms/dockets/ac/08/minutes/2008-4409m1-Final.pdf). Specifically, there was a critical need to also collect mCRC patients who are kRAS mutant to properly assess to which patient population the panitumumab effect (or cetuximab effect) would be responsible.

As a result, the genomic samples were more diligently collected by the pharmaceutical drug sponsor. Eventually the genomic EGFR biomarker data were available in 92% of mCRC patients who were chemorefractory (Amado et al., 2008), in 91% of mCRC patients who failed initial treatment of mCRC (Peeters et al., 2010), and in 93% of mCRC patients for first-line treatment (Douillard et al., 2010). Not only did all three controlled trials report more than 90% patients with available genomic EGFR biomarker data, but also the estimated wild-type kRAS prevalences were 57% (third-line treatment), 55% (second-line treatment), and 60% (first-line treatment), respectively. However, for consideration of a bridging strategy, although these phase 3 trials are of reasonable sample size, the panitumumab effect by region or ethnicity cannot be properly assessed because the percentages of whites were 97% to 100% in Amado et al. (2008), 95% to 97% in Peeters et al. (2010), and 89% to 93% in Douillard et al. (2010).

The next section uses case studies to illustrate the design and analysis issues with a prospective–retrospective approach that reflects more of the current practice with genomic sample collection. It is hoped that the regulatory concerns described in Section 9.5.2 will prompt urgent considerations of full ascertainment and appropriate coverage of regional patient population diversity.

9.5.2 Genomic Convenience Samples

With the current practice of pharmacogenomics clinical trials, collection of genomic samples requires a separate consent form which is on a voluntary basis. There is no control over which a subject's genomic information is collected; hence, the genomic sample collection process essentially creates convenience samples. That is, the genomic convenience sample is not a random sample in the statistical sense but rather a collection of genomic patient samples where the patients are selected in part or wholly at their own convenience so that self-selected patients or whoever volunteered are evaluable for investigating the hypothesis of genomic interest.

Wang, O'Neill et al. (2010) used four typical genomic convenience sample case studies from prospective–retrospective randomized controlled trials seen in regulatory application to highlight the different issues with the design and analysis of genomic convenience samples not fully obtained from all randomized subjects. The sample size in the original clinical trials ranged from as small as 100 per arm to moderate to large trials with 650, 1000, and 5000 per arm. To illustrate, we provide one example of observed baseline imbalance and four examples with inferential dilemmas. These issues can be more complex when region-specific reasons dominate patients' genomic voluntary consent for treatment effect evaluation in pharmacogenomics clinical trials.

9.5.2.1 Baseline Imbalance

Case study 1 was a three-arm placebo-controlled trial investigating treatment effect in a low-dose group and in a high-dose group for a psychiatric treatment. The study size was approximately 100 patients per arm. The genomic convenience samples consented constitutes only 30% of the entire sample. From Table 9.7, dramatically fewer male patients were observed in the placebo arm, about 24%–25% lower compared with the two drug dose groups. In contrast, the maximum difference in percent of males was 14% in the nonconsented sample. The different gender ratios occur both among treatment groups within the convenience sample and between convenience and nonconsented samples (26% in absolute difference).

In addition (not shown here), the observed imbalance in percent of Caucasians was 13% in the convenience sample and 5% in nonconsented sample, and, in general, older patients (with median age of 1 to 3.5 years

TABLE 9.7

Demographics and Baseline Disease Characteristics

Case Study 1 (100 patients/arm) 30% Convenience Sample	Placebo	Low Dose	High Dose
% Male: Convenience (consented) sample	43%	67%	68%
Nonconsented sample	69%	62%	76%
Disease severity (higher is sicker): Convenience	93.0	92.5	92.0
Nonconsented sample	95.0	96.0	98.0

Source: Wang, S. J., R. T. O'Neill, and H. M. J. Hung, *Clinical Trials*, 7, 525–536, 2010, Table 5.2.

difference) who were less severe (lower baseline value of the prognostic factor of which three points or higher can be shown statistically significantly different for this disease) tended to consent for their genomic materials. As such, moderate to large numerical differences on multiple baseline covariates were alarming and seem to, at least, suggest that baseline characteristics between consented and nonconsented patients were different.

Data from the case studies suggested that the numerical baseline imbalances in the convenience samples appear to decrease as the size of the genomic convenience sample increases as a proportion of the ITT population. For more details, the readers are referred to Wang, O'Neill et al. (2010). The observed imbalance can easily occur in regions with small sample sizes.

9.5.2.2 Inferential Problems

A primary intent behind the use of genomic convenience samples in the prospective–retrospective trial design is to inferentially demonstrate a treatment difference in a genomic biomarker subset from the genomic convenience sample. There are two sources of imbalance of concern in making inference based on comparison in the convenience sample: (1) the convenience sample relative to the ITT sample and (2) the biomarker subsets within the genomic convenience sample.

The genomic hypothesis is not usually specified at the design stage because the particular genomic biomarker may not be well defined until midtrial or at trial end. In the next section we show from case studies to highlight the problems of statistical inference with genomic convenience samples.

9.5.2.2.1 Potential Poor Dose Selection

Continuing from Case study 1 and as shown in Table 9.8, only the low dose showed drug effects nominally based on both coprimary efficacy endpoints

TABLE 9.8

Treatment Effect Estimates of Low Dose and High Dose Relative to Placebo

Case Study 1 (100 Patients/Arm)	Coprimary 1		Coprimary 2	
	L vs. P	**H vs. P**	**L vs. P**	**H vs. P**
Convenience sample (30%)	5.0*	3.4	7.9*	6.6
Nonconsented sample (70%)	1.7	4.9**	2.9	8.5**
ITT sample	3.1*	4.5**	5.1*	8.1**

* Nominally significant at $p < 0.05$ without adjusting for the number of hypotheses tested.

** Nominally significant at $p < 0.01$ without adjusting for the number of hypotheses tested.

Source: Wang, S. J., R. T. O'Neill, and H. M. J. Hung, *Clinical Trials*, 7, 525–536, 2010, Table 2.a.

in the 30% convenience sample; that is, the p-value without adjusting for the number of hypotheses tested is significant. However, this result is very inconsistent with that in the nonconsented sample. In fact, the ITT sample demonstrated a positive dose response relationship with greater statistical significance in the high-dose group.

If the truth is that a dose-response relationship exists, as shown in the ITT patient population, the estimates shown in the genomic convenience sample may exaggerate the effect of the low dose and be biased against the high dose. As a strategy that searches for the genomically favorable patient subset, then, a subset receiving low dose is likely to be selected based on the results of the genomic convenience sample. On the contrary, a subset in the high-dose group is likely to be the favorable genomic subset based on the results of the nonconsented or the ITT sample. Thus, if one relies more on the results of the genomic convenience sample, it might lead to poor dose selection.

When patient characteristics among the regions are quite different such that one region resembles the convenience sample and the other region resembles the nonconsented samples, the "effective" dose regimen applicable to each region may differ if one is willing to assume that each sample is representative of its own region.

9.5.2.2.2 Inconsistent Evidence across Endpoints

Case study 2 was a treatment add-on study for a recurrent cancer. The study size was approximately 650 patients per arm. The ITT analysis failed to demonstrate an effect on the primary efficacy endpoint of add-on therapy when compared to the standard of care ($p > 0.7$). The tumor response results were very inconsistent with the overall survival results in the ITT cohort (see Table 9.9).

However, the results of overall survival and tumor response were consistent in the genomic convenient sample (23% of the ITT). Whether one should

TABLE 9.9

Response Rate by Treatment Group and Nominal Significance of Add-on Effect

Case Study 2 (650 Patients/Arm)	Primary Overall Survival		Secondary Tumor Response	
	SOC	Add-on	SOC	Add-on
Convenience sample (23%)	60%	72%	6.5%	11%
Nonconsented sample (77%)	68%	68%	3.4%*	18%*
ITT sample	66%	69%	4.2%*	16%*

Note: SOC, standard of care. Add-on effect, effect of add-on treatment relative to SOC.

* Nominally significant at $p < 0.0001$ without adjusting for the number of hypotheses tested.

Source: Wang, S. J., R. T. O'Neill, and H. M. J. Hung, *Clinical Trials*, 7, 525–536, 2010, Table 2.b.

TABLE 9.10

Response Rate by Treatment Group and Relative Risk of Treatment over Placebo with Interval Estimates

Case Study 3 (1000 Patients/Arm)	Placebo	Treatment	RR (95% CI)
Convenience (38%)	20%	16%	0.82 (0.63, 2.30)
Nonconsented (62%)	40%	38%	0.94 (0.84, 1.06)
ITT sample (100%)	32%	30%	0.92 (0.82, 1.02)

Source: Wang, S. J., R. T. O'Neill, and H. M. J. Hung, *Clinical Trials*, 7, 525–536, 2010, Table 2.c.

try to explain the numerically somewhat favorable finding in the 23% convenience sample as anything more than a chance exploratory finding is the issue. In fact, while the genomic convenience sample showed an improved survival trend, the nonconsented sample showed no benefit on overall survival, which was supported by the ITT sample. Thus, any conclusion based on genomic convenience samples would be more appropriately viewed as hypothesis generating when the overall study result failed.

9.5.2.2.3 Inconsistent Response Rates

Case study 3 was a placebo-controlled two-arm cardiovascular outcome trial. The trial recruited approximately 1000 patients per arm. The overall treatment effect was inconclusive or marginal at best. There appeared to be a twofold difference in treatment response between the convenience sample and the nonconsented sample in both the placebo (20% vs. 40%) and the treated (16% vs. 38%) groups shown in Table 9.10.

There were few blacks in both study groups, or more severe placebo patients consented for the pharmacogenomics substudy. In addition, there was an obvious difference in the timing of genomic sample collection: some consented and were collected as patients consented into the trial after trial initiation, whereas others entered at some specified time point midtrial (results not shown). These factors might have contributed to the inconsistency in response rate between the consented and the nonconsented genomic samples.

9.5.2.2.4 Inconsistent Treatment Effects

Case study 4 was an active controlled cardiovascular outcome trial with approximately 5000 patients per arm. As shown in Table 9.11, the apparent lack of treatment effect in the genomic convenience sample seemed to be inconsistent with a significant overall treatment effect demonstrated in the ITT sample.

The observed risk reduction might be interpreted as though only nonconsented patients could benefit from the drug treatment. Although apparently

TABLE 9.11

Response Rate by Treatment Group and Odds Ratio of Treatment over Control with Interval Estimates

Case Study 4 (5000 Patients/Arm)	Control	Treatment	OR (95% CI)
Convenience (17%)	9.1%	8.6%	0.95 (0.68,1.31)
Nonconsented (83%)	11.7%	9.4%	0.79 (0.68,0.90)*
ITT sample (100%)	11.2%	9.3%	0.81 (0.71,0.92)*

* Nominally significant at $p \leq 0.001$ without adjusting for the number of hypotheses tested.

Source: Wang, S. J., R. T. O'Neill, and H. M. J. Hung, *Clinical Trials*, 7, 525–536, 2010, Table 2.d.

there was no major imbalance of the four baseline covariates explored in this case study, some mild imbalances in other baseline disease characteristics were observed but are not presented here.

What would be the interpretation had the convenience sample status been the region status in an MRCT that was not used to stratify patients at the design stage? The results shown in Table 9.11 can be perceived to imply that overall treatment effect may be mainly driven by the region defined by the nonconsented patient sample.

9.5.3 Genomics *In Vitro* Diagnostics

Application of genomics in clinical trials requires the use of genomic samples and knowledge of genomic biomarkers (see, e.g., Gutman and Kessler, 2006). The genomic characteristics may be presented by a single biomarker or multiple biomarkers, such as multiple gene features defined using microarray technology known as MammaPrint (FDA cleared this first IVD in 2007) or multiple SNPs defined using genome-wide scanning technology known as RocheChip (Jain, 2005), also known as genomic composite biomarkers (Wang, 2005). It is preferable that all patients in an MRCT are consented to be studied for pharmacogenomics. During the exploratory stage, multiple biomarkers could be of interest. To minimize problematic classifications, the genomic samples provided should be of sufficient quantity for biomarker analysis.

There are a number of molecular techniques, such as the microarray and rt-PCR, for detecting presence of a genomic (composite) biomarker. In the simplest setting of a single genomic biomarker, say, EGFR biomarker, multiple techniques can be used to screen NSCLC patients for presence or absence of the EGFR biomarker. In the case of gefitinib development, EGFR protein expression, EGFR gene copy number, and EGFR mutation were used to determine a patient's EGFR biomarker status. The three EGFR biomarkers are correlated. It was not until later that advanced scientific understanding of gefitinib's target biology pinpointed the dependency of EGFR mutation on the EGFR pathway and thus the mechanism of action of gefitinib (Armour and Watkins, 2010).

To prospectively investigate the predictiveness of EGFR mutation (EGFR+) of gefitinib effect as first-line therapy, a genomic diagnostic assay should be readily available. In particular, to improve the accurate assessment of gefitinib efficacy and therefore the statistical power, it is vital to have a genomic IVD assay for classifying the EGFR+ status that determines gefitinib response with use of a consistent definition of positivity via a prespecified cutoff threshold.

In developing an IVD assay to classifying patients based on the genomic biomarker, the prognostic utility of a genomic biomarker is generally not considered a high-risk product (see, e.g., MammaPrint, 2007). For assessing the therapeutics effect, a prognostic genomic biomarker can improve the precision of a treatment effect estimate in a linear model. For instance, MammaPrint, a 70-gene risk score measure derived from microarray biotechnology, was cleared by the FDA as a prognostic genomic biomarker (Glas et al., 2006). It is now incorporated as an IVD test commercially available to classify patients into MP+ versus MP– status prior to study randomization (see, e.g., Baker, Sigman, Kelloff, Hylton, Berry, and Esserman, 2009).

9.5.3.1 Impact of Misclassification of an IVD in Pharmacogenomics Clinical Trial

Unlike the phenotypic characteristics, a genomic diagnostic assay is needed to assess whether a patient truly possesses the genomic characteristics of interest for therapeutic investigation. However, in reality, the diagnostic assay is not perfect without misclassification error. In a targeted or enrichment pharmacogenomics clinical trial, the primary study objective is either a superior treatment (relative to its comparator) or a noninferior treatment (relative to its active comparator) in the preselected patient population who are classified as positive (g+) of a genomic biomarker.

Assume that the probability of response of the misclassified subjects is identical in the treated and control groups because the blinding should yield no preferential misclassification. With a superiority objective, many kinds of problems fatal to a superiority trial, such as nonadherence, misclassification of the primary endpoint, or measurement problems more generally (i.e., "noise"), or many dropouts who must be assessed as part of the treated group, misclassification of a genomic IVD assay can bias the study results toward no treatment difference.

In contrast, with a noninferiority objective, the misclassification works in favor of a noninferiority conclusion. However, the misclassification could also undermine the validity of the trial. Wang, Hung, and O'Neill (2010) showed that the maximum type I error rate associated with falsely concluding noninferiority can be substantially liberal if the accuracy of the genomic IVD assay is much less than perfect. When the genomic IVD assay has moderate to high sensitivity and specificity, a reasonable range of false nondisease prediction rate among test positives can be identified where the maximum type I error rate inflation is much less. To achieve a prescribed level of positive predictive value, the feasibility of a genomic biomarker for enrichment in a noninferiority pharmacogenomics clinical trial is a function of disease prevalence. Given that the evidential standard of much less inflation of type I error rate can be shown, a genomic biomarker, if qualified, may be useful as an adjunct tool for patient selection.

When the external bridging strategy is used, the genomic diagnostics should be cleared or approved or CE marked depending on the health authority region pursued. In addition, the misclassification rate of the genomic diagnostics is likely to be different between, say, the United States and the European Union. The improperness of the type I error probability of concluding a noninferior new treatment when an internal bridging strategy is adopted in an MRCT depends on the difference among regions in disease prevalence, misclassification rate, and effect size. When the differences are obvious and heterogeneous, it may be more practical to conduct regional trials rather than to employ a global strategy.

9.5.4 Region as a Confounder to Ethnic Sensitivity

In a clinical trial comparing a drug treatment with a placebo, a confounding variable is associated with clinical outcome and may significantly affect the outcome of a trial when appropriate randomization has not been employed. A confounder may fully or partially induce a treatment difference, but that difference may not be attributable to the drug treatment. In certain diseases, some indirect translation of intrinsic ethnic factors may impact disease pathophysiology or therapeutic effect, such as a higher somatic mutation rate of EGFR in unselected tumors from Japan (25.9%) than from the United States (1.6%) in NSCLC patients (Paez et al., 2004), a higher response to gefitinib in Japanese patients (27.5%) than in European-derived population (10.4%) (Fukuoka et al., 2003). In such cases, the intrinsic ethnic factor is considered a prognostic indicator. Depending on the patient population included for treatment effect assessment, the intrinsic ethnicity can confound the region in an MRCT (Wang, 2010). The clinical utility of EGFR mutation as a predictor of treatment effect should be studied in a randomized controlled trial whereby the confounding effects potentially caused by region, ethnicity, and EGFR biomarker are adjusted for either at the design stage or in an analysis adjusted for prespecified potential confounding factors.

To evaluate the potential impact of confounding, suppose for simplicity that an MRCT is observed to have very different distributions between the Asia region and the non-Asia region in each of the two treatment groups (Table 9.12). Assume the true disease prevalence is 50% in either the Asia

TABLE 9.12

Observed Percent of Patients by Region, True Response Rate, and Margin Probability of Response under the Null Hypothesis of No Treatment Difference

Treatment Group	Region		True Response Rate		Marginal Probability of Response
	Asia	Non-Asia	Asia	Non-Asia	
T	0.7	0.3	0.3	0.1	(0.7)(0.3) + (0.3)(0.1) = 0.30
P	0.4	0.6	0.3	0.1	(0.4)(0.3) + (0.6)(0.1) = 0.18

or the non-Asia region. Table 9.12 shows what was observed. Suppose that the true response rate is 30% for Asian patients (A+) and 10% for non-Asian patients (A–) regardless of treatment groups. This is the null state that there is no treatment difference in response rate for A+ (30%), for A– (10%), and overall (20%) in both treatment groups. However, the expected probability of response now suggests an apparent treatment effect (30% vs. 18%) solely due to the imbalance among treatment groups in Asia region status. In practice, when sample size is small, the chance of observing an apparent difference, known as statistical bias, in such a frequency distribution may be substantial.

When the genomic factors are confounded with regions in bridging trials for global development, the regions are correlated with ethnic factors and may exhibit ethnic sensitivity affecting the drug response if highly correlated in the study of pharmacogenomics. For common diseases that are not determined purely by genetics, it is generally anticipated that the drug response is more likely to be sensitive to extrinsic ethnic factors than intrinsic ethnic factors. The extrinsic ethnic differences among regions in their environments and medical practices may result in treatment effect differences in an order of magnitude.

9.5.5 Implication of Futility Analysis with an Unblinded Adaptive Test in MRCT

In cases where an adaptive design is of interest seeking a regional claim or a genomic claim of treatment efficacy in an MRCT, two general types of two-stage adaptive tests—blinded and unblinded—are discussed. There is generally no interest to consider early efficacy inference. In the blinded approach, a futility analysis to early terminating a region is not a consideration. The futility analysis with an unblinded two-stage adaptive design including the nested adaptive approaches may terminate further accrual to nonperforming regions. To increase the chance of a successful MRCT, such a futility analysis could serve as a quality control measure and thus penalize regions producing data of poor quality that result in limited contribution to the entire MRCT. The futility analysis in an unblinded two-stage adaptive design of an MRCT is also a way to enrich regions not only collecting data of good quality but also minimizing sources of heterogeneity due to poor data.

The adaptive selection of regions with average to high performance could improve the treatment effect estimate and as such the sampling variability could be much reduced. Appropriate strategies for handling operational bias and design-induced bias due to unblinding should be included in a statistical analysis plan at the design stage. The usual cautions of an unblinded adaptive test including establishment of firewalls and the process to facilitate the communications among the various parties involved in the planning and the conduct would be critical to the success of an unblinded two-stage adaptive designed MRCT. Wang, Hung, and O'Neill (2011) enlisted trial logistics models seen in the regulatory submissions planned as adaptive designs.

It may be arguable on the ethical ground to limit patient participation in regions with poor trial conduct and poor data collection. To raise awareness of the importance of collecting good quality data, especially in an MRCT that includes diverse patient population with ethnic sensitivity, it should be possible to give training on conductance of clinical trials to participating regions prior to trial initiation. After the training, a futility analysis may serve as a way to increase the quality of an MRCT by restricting participation of regions that do not comply with good clinical practice.

On the other hand, if the data quality is not an issue, the futility analysis may exclude regions that may pose different prognostic or predictive factors. Armour and Watkins (2010) reported that overall mutation positive rate in non-Asian patients was 10% based on voluntary consented data collected in seven studies (920 patients total) and was 39% in Asian patients in six studies (140 patients). From a genomics perspective and when it is possible to assume little concern with genomic data quality, in such cases an analysis can result in exclusion of a region with few observed biomarker positive patients or low observed prevalence of serious adverse events under investigation.

9.5.6 Other Complex Issues

Both gefitinib (IRESSA) and erlotinib (Tarceva) are EGFR TKIs. Hidalgo et al. (2001) showed that the approved daily dose of erlotinib (150 mg/day) is equal to the maximum tolerated dose and leads to a steady-state serum concentration of 3 μM. In contrast, Baselga et al. (2000) showed that the approved daily dose leads to a steady-state serum concentration of < 1 μM. The gefitinib dosing information implies that the differences observed in the original trials (INTACT1 and INTACT2) and the regional trial (IPASS) based on all patients studied could be due to suboptimal dose regimens studied in the original trials (INTACT1 and INTACT2) and that there might also be differences in treatment exposure due to ethnicity (IPASS) resulting in a superior gefitinib effect on OTR and PFS not observed in INTACT1 and INTACT2.

When a nested case-control design is used from a completed pharmacogenomics controlled trial to explore drug treatment associated serious adverse events, the apparent association of a genomic biomarker and treatment response can be due to differences in genomic biomarker prevalence or in treatment response rate between the regions, also known as population stratification. Such spurious association can lead to false reports of associated adverse events when there is no association with drug treatment.

Although the bridging trial is generally of much smaller size than the original trial, it is worthwhile to note that the IPASS regional pharmacogenomics clinical trial was two-thirds larger than the original trials in the number of patients per treatment arm. In an MRCT not necessarily focused on pharmacogenomics, the complexity arises when there are regional differences in the regulatory requirements for licensing a test medical product. One difference could be the primary efficacy measure of importance; for example, in a diabetes trial the primary efficacy measure is changed from baseline in HbA1C at 6 months for the FDA following the guidance for industry on diabetes mellitus: developing drugs and therapeutic biologics for treatment and prevention (2008) but is changed from baseline at 12 months for EMA. Another difference could be the number of patients studied in a region. Currently, Japan is probably the only country recommending the number of patients satisfying its country or region requirement (Ministry of Health, Labour and Welfare of Japan, 2007). As for pharmacogenomics bridging, the differences in regulatory requirements include mainly that (1) patient genomic consent may be limited to what laws are applicable in a country and therefore a region, and (2) that the genomic IVD assay that is either a risk-based approach of its intended use of a device in the United States (FDA Guidance on harmacogenetic test and genetic tests for heritable markers issued in 2007) or CE marked in Europe (see also Section 9.2.4).

9.5.7 Replication Issue

The low precision of treatment effect estimate in a genomic subset, say, $g+$, may increase the chance of an apparent heterogeneity occurring in treatment effects observed between the biomarker positive and negative subsets when in fact the treatment effect is homogeneous. Even though the genomic subset is prespecified, when the sample size is not large enough or the outcome measure is highly variable, the uncertainty in the subset effect estimate tends to push the point estimates of both subsets toward the more opposite extreme and thus generates false heterogeneity (Wang, O'Neill et al., 2010). Hypothesis test of treatment by subset interaction is known to have low statistical power to detect an apparent quantitative heterogeneity. A statistically insignificant interaction does not provide evidence for or against the assertion of real heterogeneity.

For illustration, we employ an example of a drug development program for rheumatoid arthritis treatment indication mimicking a real biologic licensing application (Table 9.13). Here, $g+$ represents a subset of patients who are classified as positive based on a molecular biomarker, and $g-$ is its counterpart. In the beginning of the clinical development, an early phase 2a controlled trial was launched only for the $g+$ patients to explore drug activity.

TABLE 9.13

Study Results from Three Placebo-Controlled Trials of a Drug Development Program

Response	P	T	p-value
ph2a n	140	140	< 0.005
g+ only	38%	73%	
ph2b n	131	176	<0.0001
g+ (74%)	28% (n+ = 96)	54% (n+ = 130)	(primary)
g– (26%)	53% (n– = 35)	47% (n– = 46)	ns
ITT	31%	51%	< 0.001
ph3 n	201	298	< 0.0001
g+ (79%)	19% (n+ = 159)	54% (n+ = 235)	
g– (21%)	12% (n– = 42)	41% (n– = 63)	
ITT	18%	51%	

Source: Wang, S. J., R. T. O'Neill, and H. M. J. Hung, *Clinical Trials*, 7, 525–536, 2010, Table 6.

Sample size for each patient set was approximately 140. The results of this phase 2a trial suggested a significant treatment improvement in the response rate with a nominal p-value < 0.005. A phase 2b trial was then conducted to include g+ and g– patients, with g+ being the primary hypothesis followed by the overall hypothesis. Subsequently, a phase 3 trial was sufficiently powered for detecting an overall treatment effect defined by the difference in response rates between T and P. As seen in Table 9.13, both the smaller phase 2b trial and the larger phase 3 trial observed a 75% to 80% prevalence in the biomarker positive subset and showed a significant treatment effect in the ITT patient set.

Given a high prevalence, the overall treatment effect was dominated by the effect seen in the biomarker positive subset. We note that the seemingly inconsistent treatment effect in the biomarker negative subset due to small sample size is likely because of a low precision in this subset regardless of whether randomization was stratified by the genomic biomarker status.

In this case example, there was a clear consensus about an overall treatment effect replicated in the phase 2b and phase 3 trials. However, if a claim in the g+ subgroup is pursued, it is unclear that one can conclusively rule out a lack of benefit in the g– subset. From a public health perspective, a specific subset claim might not be sensible unless there is sufficient evidence that the complementary subset lacks a favorable benefit–risk ratio.

As a general principle, replication of a positive trial finding is important. This is applicable to the original trials and the bridging pharmacogenomics trials and is equally applicable to clinical biomarkers not genomically classified. The usual standard for replication is that two adequate and well-controlled trials should be planned with sufficient power for detecting a treatment effect, and the treatment effect shown in one trial is also shown in the other trial. It would be interesting to see the updated OS results by EGFR mutation status in the regional pharmacogenomics trial (WJTOG3405) per personal communication with the same authors (2011).

9.6 Concluding Remarks

The growing genomic biotechnology for drug development has increased the capability of a randomized controlled pharmacogenomics trial to evaluate the treatment efficacy relative to its comparator in the interested genomic biomarker subset $g+$ or $g-$. The developed genomic (composite) biomarker is characterized by the genomic IVD assay explored from among plausible genomic biomarkers using the sophisticated genomic biotechnology. In late-phase drug development, traditional study designs of multiregional clinical trials for an internal bridging strategy or bridging trials for an external bridging strategy could be improved when incorporating the developed genomic (composite) biomarker as such clinical hypotheses of treatment effects in each of the genomic biomarker subset in the prespecified region in addition to the overall treatment effect of all regions can be formally tested. Both fixed design and adaptive design blinded or unblinded can be devised.

An important question for pharmacogenomics bridging is when will the intrinsic ethnic factor play a large role in treatment efficacy? Common wisdom pointing to how large the heterogeneity among race/ethnic groups that may be predominantly region driven should be expected at the planning stage. If the majority of the genetic polymorphisms selected for analysis are functional polymorphisms, conceivably the heterogeneity of intrinsic difference would be the ethnic variability in allele frequencies. On the other hand, if the majority of the associated genetic polymorphisms is due to linkage disequilibrium with other functional variants, the amount of linkage can differ significantly in populations between regions mainly represented by ethnics with different concentration. In such cases, the region factor and the race/ethnic factor are confounded, and it is possible that a pharmacogenomics biomarker for one ethnically concentrated population may not translate into another ethnically concentrated population.

With pharmacogenomics, it is difficult to replicate single-population results in ethnically mixed and disproportionate patient population. In addition, small but significant differences in allele frequencies in individual ethnic groups may lead to false positive or false negative results. Thus, in planning the sample sizes that appropriately represent different regions in a multiregional clinical trial, an analysis plan should be devised to incorporate the anticipated or expected heterogeneity. Alternatively, the design should include genomic and region subset hypotheses in addition to the single hypothesis of an overall treatment effect when the heterogeneity among regions and ethnicity due to genomics can be expected to be too wide. Prior knowledge of disease epidemiology among regions and prospective partition of the sample sizes into individual regions can help maximize the region-specific study power and the power of the study overall. Whether the genomic factor is the major determinant of the overall treatment effect, we believe the ultimate interest of a pharmacogenomics bridging strategy lies in the balance of risk and benefit to the public health of that particular region or all regions in the genomic biomarker enriched $g+$ patient subset.

References

Amado, R. G., Wolf, M., Peeters, M., Van Cutsem, E., Siena, S., Freeman, D. J. et al. (2008). Wild-type KRAS is required for panitumumab efficacy in patients with metastatic colorectal cancer. *Journal of Clinical Oncology*, 26: 1626–1634.

Amgen. (2006). Package Insert. *Panitumumab (Vectibix)*. Thousand Oaks, CA: Amgen, September.

Andreyev, H. J., Norman, A. R., and Cunningham, D. (2001). Kirsten ras mutations in patients with colorectal cancer: The "RASCAL II" study. *British Journal of Cancer*, 85: 692–696.

Armour, A. A., and Watkins, C. L. (2010). The challenge of targeting EGFR: Experience with gefitinib in nonsmall cell lung cancer. *European Respiratory Review*, 19(117): 186–196.

Baker, A. D., Sigman, C. C., Kelloff, G. J., Hylton, N. M., Berry, D. A., and Esserman, L. J. (2009). I-SPY 2: An adaptive breast cancer trial design in the setting of neoadjuvant chemotherapy. *Clinical Pharmacology & Therapeutics*, 86: 97–100.

Baselga, J. (2001). Herceptin alone or in combination with chemotherapy in the treatment of HER2-positive metastatic breast cancer: Pivotal trials. *Oncology*, 61(suppl. 2): 14–21.

Baselga, J., Rischin, D., Ranson, M., Calvert, H., Raymond, E., Kieback, D. G. et al. (2000). Phase I safety, pharmacokinetic, and pharmacodynamic trial of ZD1839, a selective oral epidermal growth factor receptor tyrosine kinase inhibitor, in patients with five selected solid tumor types. *Journal of Clinical Oncology*, 20: 4292–4302.

Benvenuti, S., Sartore-Bianchi, A., Di Nicolantonio, F., Zanon, C., Moroni, M., Veronese, S. et al. (2007). Oncogenic activation of the RAS/RAF signaling pathway impairs the response of metastatic colorectal cancers to anti-epidermal growth factor receptor antibody therapies. *Cancer Research*, 67: 2643–2648.

Biomarkers Definitions Working Group. (2001). Commentary: Biomarkers and surrogate endpoints: Preferred definitions and conceptual framework. *Clinical Pharmacology and Therapeutics*, 69(3): 89–95.

Brown, T., Boland, A., Bagust, A., Oyee, J., Hockenhull, J., Dundar, Y. et al. (2010). Gefitinib for the first line treatment of locally advanced or metastatic non-small cell lung cancer. *Health Technology Access*, 14(s2): 71–79.

Chan, J. C. N., Wat, N. M. S., So, W. Y., Lam, K. S. L., Chua, C. T., Wong, K. S. et al. (2004) Renin angiotensin aldosterone system blockade and renal disease in patients with type 2 diabetes. *Diabetes Care*, 27(4): 874–879.

Chang, G. C., Tsai, C. M., Chen, K. C., Yu, C. J., Shih, J. Y., Yang, T. Y. et al. (2006). Predictive factors of gefitinib antitumor activity in East Asian advanced non-small cell lung cancer patients. *Journal of Thoracic Oncology*, 1(6): 520–525.

Chang, W. C., Midodzi, W. K., Westerhout, C. M., Boersma, E., Cooper, J., Barnathan, E. S. et al. (2005). Are international differences in the outcome of acute coronary syndromes apparent or real? A multivariate analysis. *Journal of Epidemiology Community Health*, 59: 427–433.

Cui, L., Hung, H. M. J., Wang, S. J., and Tsong, Y. (2002). Issues related to subgroup analysis in clinical trials. *Journal of Biopharmaceutical Statistics*, 12: 347–358.

Dancey, J. E. (2006). Early clinical trials of targeted agents: Issues and designs. Paper presented at the Practical Strategies for Speeding Up Developing and Testing New Treatments Session, 42nd ASCO Annual Meeting, Atlanta, GA, June 4.

Douillard, J. Y., Siena, S., Cassidy, J., Tabernero, J., Burkes, R., Barugel, M. et al. (2010). Randomized phase III trial of panitumumab with infusional fluorouracil, leucovorin, and oxaliplatin (FOLFOX4) versus FOLFOX4 alone as first line treatment in patients with previously untreated metastatic colorectal cancer: The PRIME Study. *Journal of Clinical Oncology*, 28: 4697–4705.

Eiermann, W. (2001). Trastuzumab combined with chemotherapy for the treatment of HER2-positive metastatic breast cancer: Pivotal trial data. *Annals of Oncology*, 12(suppl. 1): S57–S62.

European Medicines Agency. (EMA). (2007). Committee for Medicinal Products for Human Use December 2007 Plenary Meeting Monthly Report. Retrieved February 12, 2011, from: http://www.ema.europa.eu/docs/en_GB/document_library/EPAR_-_Procedural_steps_taken_before_authorisation/human/000741/WC500047708.pdf.

FDA Label—USDA Clearance. (2007). http://www.accessdata.fda.gov/cdrh_docs/reviews/k062694.pdf.

Fukuoka, M., Yano, S., Giaccone, G., Tamura, T., Nakagawa, K., Douillard, J. Y. et al. (2003). Multi-institutional randomized phase II trial of gefitinib for previously treated patients with advanced non-small-cell lung cancer. *Journal of Clinical Oncology*, 21(12): 2297–2246.

Ge, J., Zhu, J., Hong, B. K., Boonbaichaiyapruck, S., Goh, Y. S., Hou, C. J. et al. (2010). Presugrel versus clopidogrel in Asian patients with acute coronary syndromes: Design and rationale of a multi-dose, pharmacodynamic, phase 3 clinical trials. *Current Medical Research Opinion*, 26(9): 2077–2085.

Giaccone, G., Herbst, R. S., Manegold, C., Scagliotti, G., Roselll, R., Miller, V. et al. (2004). Gefitinib in combination with Gemcitabine and Cisplatin in advanced non-small-cell lung cancer: A phase 3 trial—INTACT 1. *Journal of Clinical Oncology*, 22: 777–784.

Glas, A. M., Floore, A., Delahaye, L., Witteveen, A. T., Pover, R., Bakx, N. et al. (2006). Converting a breast cancer microarray signature into a high-throughput diagnostic test. *BMC Genomics*, 7: 278–287.

Gomes, M. F., Faiz, M. A., Gyapong, J. O., Warsame, M., Agbenyega, T., Babiker, A. et al. (2009). Pre-referral rectal artesunate to prevent death and disability in severe malaria: A placebo-controlled trial. *Lancet*, 373(9663): 557–566.

Gutman, S., and Kessler, L. G. (2006). The US Food and Drug Administration perspective on cancer biomarker development. *Nature Reviews: Cancer*, 6: 565–571.

Herbst, R. S., Giaccone, G., Schiller, J. H., Natale, R. B., Miller, V., Manegold, C. et al. (2004). Gefitinib in combination with paclitaxel and carboplatin in advanced non-small-cell lung cancer: A phase 3 trial—INTACT2. *Journal of Clinical Oncology*, 22: 785–794.

Hidalgo, M., Siu, L. L., Nemunaitis, J., Rizzo, J., Hammond, L. A., Takimoto, C. et al. (2001). Phase I and pharmacologic study of OSI-774, an epidermal growth factor receptor tyrosin kinase inhibitor, in patients with advanced solid malignancies. *Journal of Clinical Oncology*, 19(13): 3267–3279.

Hsiao, C. F., Chern, H. D., Chen, L. K., and Lin, M. S. (2003). Algorithm for evaluation of bridging studies in Taiwan. *Drug Information Journal*, 37: 123(s)–128(s).

Hsiao, C. F., Wang, M., Hsu, Y. Y., and Liu, J. P. (2005). An overview of bridging evaluations in Taiwan. *International Chinese Statistical Association Bulletin, Special Feature Article*, 29–36.

International Conference on Harmonisation. (ICH). (1998). *Ethnic Factors in the Acceptability of Foreign Clinical Data (ICH E-5)*. CPMP/ICH/289/95. London: European Agency for the Evaluation of Medicinal Products.

International Conference on Harmonisation. (ICH). (2006). ICH E-5 ethnic factors in the acceptability of foreign clinical data. Questions & Answers. CPMP/ICH/5746/03. Available at: http://www.ich.org/cache/compo/276-254-1.html

International Conference on Harmonisation. (ICH). (2007). ICH E15. Definitions for genomic biomarkers, pharmacogenomics, genomic data, and sample coding categories. U.S. Food and Drug Administration, DHHS, Current Step 4 version, November.

International HapMap Consortium. (2005). A haplotype map of the human genome. *Nature*, 437(7063): 1299–1320.

Jain, K. K. (2005). Applications of AmpliChip CYP450. *Molecular Diagnostics*, 9: 119–127.

Kalow, W. (1962). *Pharmacogenetics: Heredity and the response to drugs*. Philadelphia: W.B. Saunders.

Kawai, N., Chuang-Stein, C., Komiyama, O., and Li, Y. (2007). An approach to rationalize partitioning sample size into individual regions in a multiregional trial. *Drug Information Journal*, 42: 139–147.

Kosaka, T., Yatabe, Y., Endoh, H., Kuwano, H., Takahashi, T., and Mitsudomi, T. (2004). Mutations of the epidermal growth factor receptor gene in lung cancer: biological and clinical implications. *Cancer Research*, 64: 8919–8923.

Lynch, T. J., Bell, D. W., Sordella, R., Gurubhagavatula, S., Okimoto, R. A., Brannigan, B. W. et al. (2004). Activating mutations in the epidermal growth factor receptor underlying responsiveness of non-small-cell lung cancer to gefitinib. *New England Journal of Medicine*, 350: 2129–2139.

Maemondo, M., Knoue, A., Kobayashi, K., Sugawara, S., Oizumi, S., Isobe, H. et al. (2010). Gefitinib or chemotherapy for non-small-cell lung cancer with mutated EGFR. *New England Journal of Medicine*, 362(25): 2380–2388.

Mahbub ul Haq, Amartya Sen. (1990). History of the Human Development Report. United Nations Development Programme. Retrieved January 30, 2011, from: http:hdr.undp.org/en/humandev/reports/ and http://en.wikipedia.org/wiki/Human_Development_Index

Mega, J., Close, S. L., Wiviott, S. D., Shen, L., Walker, J. R., Simon, T. et al. (2010). Genetic variants in ABCB1 and CYP2C19 and cardiovascular outcomes after treatment with clopidogrel and prasugrel in the TRITON-TIMI 38 trial: A pharmacogenetic analysis. *Lancet*, 376: 1312–1319.

Ministry of Health, Labour and Welfare of Japan. (2007). Basic principles on global clinical trials. Available at: http://www.pmda.go.jp/english/service/pdf/notifications/0928010-e.pdf

Mitsudomi, T., Morita, S., Yatabe, Y., Negoro, S., Okamoto, I., Tsurutani, J. et al. (2010). *Lancet Oncology*, 11: 121–128.

Mok, T. S., Wu, Y. L., Thongprasert, S., Tang, C. H., Chu, D. T., Saijo, N. et al. (2009). Gefitinib or carboplatin-paclitaxel in pulmonary adenocarcinoma. *New England Journal of Medicine*, 361: 947–957.

Molina-Vila, M. A., Bertran-Alamillo, J., Reguart, N., Taron, M., Castella, E., Llatjos, M. et al. (2008). A sensitive method for detecting EGFR mutations in non-small cell lung cancer samples with few tumor cells. *Journal of Thoracic Oncology*, 3: 1224–1235.

Nagai, Y., Miyazawa, H., Huqun, Tanaka, T., Udagawa, K., Kato, M. et al. (2005). Genetic heterogeneity of the epidermal growth factor receptor in non-small cell lung cancer cell lines revealed by a rapid and sensitive detection system, the peptdie nucleic acid-locked nucleic acid PCR clamp. *Cancer Research*, 65: 7276–7282.

Newton, C. R., Graham, A., Heptinstall, L. E., Powell, S. J., Summers, C., Kalsheker, N. et al. (1989). Analysis of any point mutation in DNA: The Amplification Refractory Mutation System (ARMS). *Nucleic Acids Research*, 17: 2503–2516.

O'Donogue, M., Antman, E. M., Braunwald, E., Murphy, S. A., Steg, G., Finkelstein, A. et al. (2009). A TRITON-TIMI 38 (Trial to Access Improvement in Therapeutic Outcomes by Optimizing Platelet Inhibition with Prasugrel-Thrombolysis in Myocardial Infarction 38) Analysis. *Journal of American College of Cardiology*, 54: 678–685.

O'Shea, J. C., and Califf, R. M. (2000). Inter-regional differences in acute coronary syndrome trials. *European Heart Journal*, 21: 1397–1399.

Paez, J. G., Janne, P. A., Lee, J. C., Tracy, S., Greulich, H., Gabriel, S. et al. (2004). EGFR mutations in lung cancer: Correlation with clinical response to gefitinib therapy. *Science*, 304(5676): 1497–1500.

Paik, S., Shak, S., Tang, G., Kim, C., Baker, J., Cronin, M. et al. (2004). A multigene assay to predict recurrence of tamoxifen-treated, node-negative breast cancer. *New England Journal of Medicine*, 351: 2817–2826.

Pao, W., Miller, V., Zakowski, M., Doherty, J., Politi, K., Sarkaria, I. et al. (2004). EGF receptor gene mutations are common in lung cancers from "never smokers" and are associated with sensitivity of tumors to gefitinib and erlotinib. *Proceedings of National Academy Science U.S.A.*, 101(36): 13306–13311.

Peeters, M., Price, T. J., Cervantes, A., Sobrero, A. F., Ducreux, M., Hotko, Y. et al. (2010). Randomized phase III study of panitumumab with fluorouracil, leucovorin, and irinotecan (FOLFIRI) compared with FOLFIRI alone as second-line treatment in patients with metastatic colorectal cancer. *Journal of Clinical Oncology*, 28: 4706–4713.

Polanczyk, G., Faraone, S. V., Bau, C. H. D., Victor, M. M., Becker, K., Pelz, R. et al. (2008). The impact of individual and methodological factors in the variability of response to methylphenidate in ADHD pharmacogenetic studies from four different continenets. *American Journal of Medical Genetics B Neuropsychiatric Genetic*, 147B(8): 1419–1424.

Quan, H., Zhao, P. L., Zhang, J., Roessner, M., and Aizawa, K. (2009). Sample size considerations for Japanese patients in a multi-regional trial based on MHLW guidance. *Pharmaceutical Statistics*, 9: 1–14.

Reck, M. (2010). A major step towards individualized therapy of lung cancer with gefitinib: The IPASS trial and beyond. *Expert Review Anticancer Therapy,* 10(6): 955–965.

Rosell, R., Moran, T., Queralt, C., Porta, R., Cardenal, F., Camps, C. et al. (2009). Screening for epidermal growth factor receptor mutations in lung cancer. *New England Journal of Medicine,* 361: 958–967.

Ruff, C. T., Giugliano, R. P., Antman, E. M., Murphy, S. A., Lotan, C., Heuer, H. et al. (2010). Safety and efficacy of prasugrel compared with clopidogrel in different regions of the world. *International Journal of Cardiology,* 155(3): 424–429.

Simon, R., and Wang, S. J. (2006). Use of genomic signatures in therapeutics development in oncology and other diseases. *Pharmacogenomics Journal,* 6: 166–173.

Simon, R. M., Korn, E. L., McShane, L. M., Radmacher, M. D., Wright, G. W., and Zhao, Y. (2003). *Design and analysis of DNA microarray investigations.* New York: Springer.

Simon, R. M., Paik, S., and Hayes, D. F. (2009). Use of archived specimens in evaluation of prognostic and predictive biomarkers. *Journal of National Cancer Institute,* 101: 1446–1452.

Shepherd, P. A., Pereira, J. R., and Ciuleanu, T. (2005). Erlotinib in previously treated non-small-cell lung cancer. *New England Journal of Medicine,* 353: 123–132.

Sullivan, P. M., Etzioni, R., Feng, Z., Potter, J. D., Thompson, M. L., Thornquist, M. et al. (2001). Phases of biomarker development for early detection of cancer. *Journal of National Cancer Institute,* 93: 1054–1061.

Tanaka, T., Matsuoka, M., Sutani, A., Gemma, A., Maemondo, M., Inoue, A. et al. (2010). Frequency of any variables associated with the EGFR mutation and its subtypes. *International Journal of Cancer,* 126: 651–655.

Taron, M., Ichinose, Y., Rosell, R., Mok, T., Massuti, B., Zamora, L. et al. (2005). Activating mutations in the tyrosine kinase domain of the epidermal growth factor receptor are associated with improved survival in gefitinib-treated chemorefractory lung adenocarcimona. *Clinical Cancer Research,* 11: 5878–5885.

Temple, R. J. (2005). Enrichment designs: Efficiency in development of cancer treatments. *Journal of Clinical Oncology,* 23(22): 4838–4839.

U.S. Food and Drug Administration. (FDA). (2006). FDA approves a new drug for colorectal cancer. Vectibix. September 27. Retrieved February 12, 2011, from: http://www.fda.gov/NewsEvents/Newsroom/PressAnnouncements/2006/ucm108745.htm

U.S. Food and Drug Administration. (FDA). (2007). FDA Guidance for Industry and FDA Staff: Pharmacogenetic tests and genetic tests for heritable markers. June 19. Retrieved February 12, 2011, from: http://www.fda.gov/MedicalDevices/DeviceRegulationandGuidance/GuidanceDocuments/ucm077862.htm

U.S. Food and Drug Administration. (FDA). (n.d.). FDA Guidance for Industry: Diabetes Mellitus: Developing drugs and therapeutic biologics for treatment and prevention. Retrieved March 16, 2012 from: http://www.fda.gov/downloads/Drugs/GuidanceComplianceRegulatoryInformation/Guidances/ucm071624.pdf

Van Cutsem, E., Lang, I., D'haens, G., Moiseyenko, V., Zaluski, J., Folprecht, G. et al. (2008). KRAS status and efficacy in the first-line treatment of patients with metastatic colorectal cancer (mCRC) treated with FOLFIRI with or without cetuximab: The CRYSTAL experience. Annual Society of Clinical Oncology 2008, Abstract #4001. *Journal of Clinical Oncology* 26: (May 20 suppl.; abstr. 2).

van'tVeer, L. J., Dai, H., Vijver, MJvd et al. (2002). Gene expression profiling predicts clinical outcome of breast cancer. *Nature*, 415: 530–536.

Vogel, F. (1959). Moderne probleme der humangenetic. *Ergeb Inn Med Kinderheilkd*, 165: 835–837.

Wallentin, L., Becker, R. C., Budaj, A., Cannon, C. P., Emanuelsson, H., Held, C. et al. (2009). Ticagrelor versus clopidogrel in patients with acute coronary syndromes. *New England Journal of Medicine*, 361: 1045–1057.

Wang, S. J. (2005). Utility of high dimensional genomic biomarkers in therapeutic and/or diagnostic development. The IEEE Conference Proceedings of the Fifth International Emerging Information Technology Conference. doi:10.1109/EITC.2005.1544330, 13–16.

Wang, S. J. (2006). Genomic biomarker derived therapeutic effect in pharmacogenomics clinical trials: A biostatistics view of personalized medicine. *Taiwan Clinical Trials*, 4: 57–66.

Wang, S. J. (2007). Biomarker as a classifier in pharmacugenomics clinical trials: A tribute to 30th anniversary of Pharmaceutical Statistician Institute (PSI). *Pharmaceutical Statistics*, 6: 283–296.

Wang, S. J. (2008). Utility of adaptive strategy and adaptive design for biomarker facilitated patient selection in pharmacogenomics or pharmacogenetics clinical development program. *Clinical Formosan Medical Association*, 107(12): S18–26.

Wang, S. J. (2009). Bridging study versus pre-specified regions nested in global trials. *Drug Information Journal*, 43: 27–34.

Wang, S. J. (2010). Editorials: Multi-regional clinical trials—What are the challenges. *Pharmaceutical Statistics*, 9: 171–172.

Wang, S. J., Cohen, N., Katz, D. A., Ruano, G., Shaw, P., and Spear, B. (2006). Retrospective validation of genomic biomarkers—what are the questions, challenges and strategies for developing useful relationships to clinical outcomes—Workshop Summary. *Pharmacogenomics Journal*, 6: 82–88.

Wang, S. J., Hung, H. M. J., and O'Neill, R. T. (2009). Adaptive patient enrichment designs in therapeutic trials. *Biometrical Journal*, 51: 358–374.

Wang, S. J., Hung, H. M. J., and O'Neill, T. (2011). Genomic classifier for patient enrichment: Misclassification and type I error issues in pharmacogenomics noninferiority trial. *Statistics in Biopharmaceutical Research*, 3: 310–319.

Wang, S. J., Hung, H. M. J., and O'Neill, T. (2011). Adaptive design clinical trials and logistics models in CNS drug development. *European Neuropsychopharmacology Journal*, 21: 159–166.

Wang, S. J., O'Neill, R. T., and Hung, H. M. J. (2007). Approaches to evaluation of treatment effect in randomized clinical trials with genomic subset. *Pharmaceutical Statistics*, 6: 227–244.

Wang, S. J., O'Neill, R. T., and Hung, H. M. J. (2010). Some statistical considerations in evaluating pharmacogenomics confirmatory clinical trials. *Clinical Trials*, 7: 525–536.

Wellcome Trust Case Control Consortium. (2007). Genome-wide association study of 14,000 cases of seven common diseases and 3,000 shared controls. *Nature*, 447: 661–683.

Wellkang Tech Consulting. (1996–2012). What is CE Marking (CE Mark)? Accessed February 12, 2011 from: http://www.ce-marking.org/what-is-ce-marking.html

Whitcombe, D., Theaker, J., Guy, S. P., Brown, T., and Little, S. (2000). Detection of PCR products using self-probing amplicons and fluorescence. *Nature Biotechnology*, 17: 804–807.

Wiviott, S. D., Braunwald, E., McCabe, C. H., Montalescot, G., Ruzyllo, W., Gottlieb, S. et al. (2007). Prosugrel versus clopidogrel in patients with acute coronary syndromes. *New England Journal of Medicine*, 357: 2001–2015.

World Health Organization. (WHO). (2000). *The World Health Report 2000 health systems: improving performance*. Geneva: WHO, pp. 21–46.

Yang, C. H., Shih, J. Y., Chen, K. C., Yu, C. J., Yang, T. Y., Lin, C. P. et al. (2006). Survival outcome and predictors of gefitinib antitumor activity in East Asian chemonaive patients with advanced nonsmall cell lung cancer. *Cancer*, 107: 1873–1882.

10

Interaction Effects in Bridging Studies[*]

Eric Tsung-Cheng Hsieh
Buddhist Tzu-Chi University and Hospital

Jen-pei Liu
National Taiwan University

10.1 Introduction

Although a drug has been approved by regulatory authorities to treat a certain disease or illness due to its overall effectiveness and safety, there may still exist a considerable variability of responses to the drug among different ethnic, geographic, genetic, and demographic factors of the patients. In particular, the International Conference on Harmonisation (ICH) E5 guideline "Ethnic Factors in the Acceptability of Foreign Clinical Data" addresses the issue of extensive duplication of clinical evaluation to address the geographic variation of efficacy and safety of a drug product (ICH, 1998). Therefore, according to the ICH E5 guideline, the supplementary pharmacodynamic and clinical data on efficacy, safety, dosage, and dose regimen from bridging studies conducted in the new region makes it possible for us to extrapolate the foreign clinical data to the population of the new region. In addition, the ICH E5 guideline suggests the use of the concept of similarity for evaluation of extrapolation of the foreign clinical data. Currently, different statistical procedures or methods are proposed to evaluate the similarity of the treatment effects obtained from the bridging studies in the new region and those from the original regions for the assessment of extrapolation of foreign clinical data (Chow, Shao, and Hu, 2002; Hsiao, Hsu, Tsou, and Liu, 2007; Hsiao,

* Part of this chapter was published in *Drug Information Journal* (Liv, J. P., J. R. Lin, and E. Hsieh, A Noninferiority Test for Treatment-by-Factor Interaction with Application to Bridging Studies and Global Trials, *Drug Information Journal*, 43(1), 11–16, 2009). The views expressed in this article are personal opinions of the authors and may not necessarily represent the position of National Taiwan University, the National Health Research Institutes, or Buddhist Tzu-Chi University and Hospital. This research is partially supported by the Taiwan National Science Council Grant NSC 95 2118-M-002-007-MY2 to Jen-pei Liu.

Xu, and Liu, 2003, 2005; Ko, 2010; Liu and Chow, 2002; Liu, Hsiao, and Hsueh, 2002; Liu, Hsueh, and Hsiao, 2004; Shih, 2001).

However, assessment of treatment similarity is not limited to only the geographic variation. Other variability such as ethic or demographic variations of treatment effects is equally important. For example, reduction in blood pressures of an antihypertensive drug may be different among Caucasians, Hispanics, and African Americans. Other examples include whether the treatment effect of a drug treating chronic hepatitis B observed in the adult population above 18 years old can be extrapolated to the pediatric subpopulation under 11 years old or whether the treatment effect of a cancer drug is consistent across different cancer stages.

The evaluation of consistency of treatment effects is, however, not confined just to the framework of between-study comparisons. As indicated in the E5 "Implementation Working Group Questions and Answers" (ICH, 2006), it would be more efficient to assess potential regional differences as part of a global development program, that is, for development of data to occur simultaneously in various regions rather than sequentially. For example, multiregional trials can be conducted to collect the clinical information from each region concurrently within the same studies. As a result, the impact of ethnic differences can be investigated for determining whether the entire database is pertinent to the new region by evaluating the consistency of treatment effect across regions concurrently within the study. As a result, similarity of the treatment effects of a drug product among different intrinsic and extrinsic ethnic, demographic, or geographic factors is vital not only to regulatory agencies for the approval of the drug but also to the public health in the postapproval applications.

Evaluation of similarity of treatment effects among different levels of ethnic, geographic, or demographic factors is to assess treatment-by-factor interaction. Most current approaches are for detection of the existence of treatment-by-factor interaction. As pointed out by Liu, Lin, and Hsieh (2009), a well-designed and carefully conducted clinical trial will provide estimated treatment effects with high precision so that it can detect a very small and inconsequential treatment-by-factor interaction with a magnitude of no clinical importance. On the other hand, a poorly executed clinical trial generating an estimated treatment effect with large variability may fail to detect an important treatment-by-factor interaction even though such an interaction in fact exists. Therefore, good clinical trials are penalized for their small variability. The main reason for this paradox is the incorrect formulation of hypotheses for evaluation of the similarity of the treatment effects between different levels of ethnic, geographic, or demographic factors. Assessment of the similarity of treatment effects among ethnical or demographic factors is not to detect the existence of treatment-by-factor interaction but rather to evaluate whether the magnitude of treatment-by-factor interaction is within a clinically allowable margin. It follows that evaluation of similarity of treatment effects between different levels of a factor should be formulated as the noninferiority hypothesis.

As a result, Liu et al. (2009) proposed the sum of squares of deviations from the overall (SSDO) mean treatment difference as a measure for the treatment-by-factor interaction. In addition, they employed the methods of generalized pivotal quantities (GPQ) and bootstrap technique to derive testing procedures for the noninferiority inference of evaluation of the similarity of treatment effects among different ethnical or demographic factors (Efron and Tibshirani, 1993; Weerahandi, 1993). In the next section, SSDO is introduced, and a noninferiority hypothesis for evaluating the similarity of treatment effects between different levels of a factor is proposed. In Section 10.3, testing procedures based on the GPQ method and the bootstrap approach are suggested. Simulation results are reported in Section 10.4. In Section 10.5, numerical examples illustrate the proposed methods under different scenarios and therapeutic areas. Discussion and final remarks are provided in the final section.

10.2 Noninferiority Hypothesis for Treatment Similarity

Following Liu et al. (2009), suppose that there is a factor that divides the targeted patient population into L mutually exclusive subpopulations. Therefore, we use subpopulation as a generic term for different levels of ethnic, geographic, or demographic factor. For simplicity, we consider a randomized control clinical trial for comparing a test drug, T, with its concurrent control, C, conducted in the L subpopulations. The problem considered here is to evaluate the similarity of treatment effect among L subpopulations. Let and be some efficacy endpoint for patients i and j receiving test product and control product, respectively, in subpopulation k for $i = 1,\ldots,n_{Tk}$, $j = 1,\ldots,n_{Ck}$, and $k = 1,\ldots,L$. Assume that X_{Tki} and Y_{Ckj} are normally distributed with population means μ_{Tk} and μ_{Ck}, variances σ^2_{Tk} and σ^2_{Ck}, respectively. Denote $\Delta k = \mu_{Tk} - \mu$ the mean treatment difference between test product and control product in subpopulation k, $k = 1,\ldots,L$. The overall mean treatment difference is then defined as

$$\overline{\Delta} = \sum_{k=1}^{L} \Delta_k / L$$

It follows that $\theta_k = \Delta - \Delta_k$ represents the deviation of the mean treatment difference of subpopulation k from the overall mean treatment difference, $k = 1,\ldots,L$. As a result, an aggregate metric for assessing the similarity of treatment differences among L subpopulations is the treatment-by-factor interaction expressed as the sum of squares of deviations from overall (SSDO) mean treatment difference as follows:

$$\theta = \frac{\sum_{k=1}^{L} \theta_k^2}{L} = \frac{1}{L}\sum_{k=1}^{L} (\Delta_k - \bar{\Delta})^2 \tag{10.1}$$

As mentioned previously, the evaluation of similarity of treatment effects among k subpopulations is to test whether the magnitude of the treatment-by-factor interaction is less than an allowable clinical margin. It follows that the hypothesis for proving the similarity treatment difference among k subpopulations should be formulated as a noninferiority hypothesis based on SSDO:

$$H_0: \theta \geq \delta^2 \text{ vs. } H_a: < \delta^2 \tag{10.2}$$

where δ is the some clinically allowable upper margin.

Moreover, let $\Delta = (\Delta_1, \Delta_2, \ldots, \Delta_L)$ and $\theta = (\theta_1, \theta_2, \ldots, \theta_L)$. Denote as an L × L symmetric and idempotent matrix with the diagonal elements $1 - 1/L$ and off-diagonal elements $-1/L$. It follows that

$$\sum_{k=1}^{L} \theta_k^2$$

can be expressed as $\theta'\theta = \Delta' A \Delta$ and the noninferiority hypothesis in Equation 10.2 can be then represented as

$$H_0: \delta \frac{1}{L} \Delta' A \Delta \geq \delta^2 \text{ vs. } H_a: \frac{1}{L} \Delta' A \Delta < \delta^2 \tag{10.3}$$

10.3 Statistical Testing Procedures

Liu et al. (2009) applied the GPQ method and bootstrap approach to derive statistical testing procedures for the noninferiority hypothesis in Equation 10.3. First, the procedure based on the GPQ method is derived. Suppose that W is a random variable whose distribution depends on a vector of unknown parameters $\zeta = (\theta, \eta)$, where θ is a parameter of interest, and η is a vector of nuisance parameter. Let **V** be a random sample from *V*, and **v** be the observed value of **V**. Also let **R** = **R**(**V**; **v**, ζ) be a function of **V**, **v**, and ζ. The random quantity **R** is said to be a GPQ if satisfies the following two conditions:

(a) The distribution of **R** does not depend on any unknown parameter.
(b) The observed value of **R**, say, **r** = **R**(**V**; **v**, θ, η), is free of the vector of nuisance parameters η. Namely, **r** is only a function of (**v**, θ).

Furthermore, let r_1 and r_2 be such that

$$P\{ r_1 \le \mathbf{R}(\mathbf{V}; \mathbf{v}, \theta, \eta) \le r_2 \} = 1 - \alpha$$

Then $\{\theta: r_1 \le \mathbf{R}(\mathbf{V}; \mathbf{v}, \theta, \eta) \le r_2 \}$ is a 100(1 – α)100% generalized confidence interval (GCI) for θ.

Specifically, if the observed quantity $r = \theta$, then the GPQ is called the fiducial generalized pivotal quantity (FGPQ), and the GCIs based on the FGPQ are proven to have asymptotically correct frequent coverage probability (Hanning, Iyer, and Patterson, 2006). Consequently, an upper 100(1 – α)-th percentile GCI for θ is given by $(0, R_{1-\alpha})$, where $R_{1-\alpha}$ are the 100(1 – α)-th percentile of the distribution of **R**. The percentile of **R** can be analytically estimated using Monte-Carlo algorithms.

Let $\mathbf{M} = \hat{\Delta} = (\hat{\Delta}_1,\ldots,\hat{\Delta}_L)'$, and the variance–covariance matrix of **M** is given as

$$\Sigma_{\widehat{\Delta L}} = \text{diag}(\sigma^2_{\hat{\Delta}_1},\ldots,\sigma^2_{\hat{\Delta}L}) = \text{diag}(\sigma^2_{T1}/n_{T1} + \sigma^2_{C1}/n_{C1},\ldots,\sigma^2_{TL}/n_{TL} + \sigma^2_{CL}/n_{CL})$$

where $\hat{\Delta}_k = \overline{X}_{Tk} - \overline{Y}_{Ck}$.

It follows that $\hat{\Delta}$ is distributed as a multivariate normal distribution with mean and variance–covariance matrix $\Sigma_{\bar{\Delta}}$. Unbiased and sufficient estimators for $\sigma^2_{Tk}, \sigma^2_{Ck}$, and the variance of the estimator of are given, respectively, as

$$\hat{\sigma}^2_{Tk} = S^2_{TK} = \sum_{i=1}^{n_{Tk}} \left(X_i - \overline{X}_{Tk}\right)^2 / \left(n_{Tk} - 1\right)$$

$$\hat{\sigma}^2_{Ck} = S^2_{CK} = \sum_{i=1}^{n_{Ck}} \left(Y_{Cki} - \overline{Y}_{Ck}\right)^2 / \left(n_{Ck} - 1\right) \tag{10.4}$$

$$\hat{\sigma}^2_{\hat{\Delta}_k} = \frac{\hat{\sigma}^2_{Tk}}{n_{Tk}} + \frac{\hat{\sigma}^2_{Ck}}{n_{Ck}} = \frac{S^2_{TK}}{n_{Tk}} + \frac{S^2_{CK}}{n_{Ck}}$$

where S^2_{Tk}, and S^2_{Ck} are the sample variances of test drug and control observed from subpopulation k; $k = 1,\ldots,L$.

Then the unbiased and sufficient estimator for and its estimated variance–covariance matrix $\Sigma_{\hat{\Delta}}$ are given, respectively, as

$$\hat{\Delta} = M = (\hat{\Delta}_1, \ldots, \hat{\Delta}_L)'$$

$$\hat{\Sigma}_{\hat{\Delta}} = diag(\hat{\sigma}^2_{\hat{\Delta}_1}, \ldots, \hat{\sigma}^2_{\hat{\Delta}_L})$$

$$= diag(\hat{\sigma}^2_{T1}/n_{T1} + \hat{\sigma}^2_{C1}/n_{C1}, \ \ldots, \ \hat{\sigma}^2_{TL}/n_{TL} + \hat{\sigma}^2_{CL}/n_{CL}) \tag{10.5}$$

$$= diag(S^2_{T1}/n_{T1} + S^2_{C1}/n_{C1}, \ \ldots, \ S^2_{TL}/n_{TL} + S^2_{CL}/n_{CL})$$

In addition, since k subpopulations are mutually disjoint, it follows that $\hat{\Delta}_k$ and $S^2_{Tk}/n_{Tk} + S^2_{Ck}/n_{Ck}$ are mutually independent, $k = 1,\ldots,L$.

It is easy to verify that the estimators **M** and S^2_{TK} and S^2_{CK} are associated with the pivotal quantities **Z** and U_{Tk} and U_{Ck} for $k = 1,..,L$, which are mutually independent with the following known distributions:

$$Z = \Sigma_{\hat{\Delta}}^{-1/2}\left[\mathbf{M} - \Delta\right] \sim N_L(\mathbf{0}, \mathbf{I})$$

$$U_{Tk} = \frac{(n_{Tk} - 1)S^2_{Tk}}{\sigma^2_{Tk}} \sim \chi^2_{n_{Tk}-1}, \text{ and} \tag{10.6}$$

$$U_{Ck} = \frac{(n_{Ck} - 1)S^2_{Ck}}{\sigma^2_{Ck}} \sim \chi^2_{n_{Ck}-1}$$

where $\chi^2_{n_{Tk}-1}$ and $\chi^2_{n_{Ck}-1}$ denote the central chi-square distribution with $n_{Tk} - 1$, and $n_{Ck} - 1$ degrees of freedom, respectively, and $N_L(\mathbf{0},\mathbf{I})$ is the standard multivariate normal distribution with mean vector **0** and variance–covariance matrix **I**. In addition, matrix $\Lambda^{1/1}$ denotes the positive definite square root of a positive definite matrix Λ and $\Lambda^{-1/2} = (\Lambda^{1/2})^{-1}$. Then the GPQs for $\sigma^2_{\hat{\Delta}k}$ and Σ_{Λ} are given, respectively,

$$R_{\sigma^2_{\hat{\Delta}k}} = \frac{s^2_{Tk}\sigma^2_{Tk}}{S^2_{Tk}n_{Tk}} + \frac{s^2_{Ck}\sigma^2_{Ck}}{S^2_{Ck}n_{Ck}} = \frac{(n_{Tk}-1)s^2_{Tk}}{U_{Tk}n_{Tk}} + \frac{(n_{Ck}-1)s^2_{Ck}}{U_{Ck}n_{Ck}} \quad \text{for k=1,...,L}$$

$$\mathbf{R}_{\Sigma_{\hat{\Lambda}}} = \text{diag}\left(R_{\sigma^2_{\hat{\Delta}1}}, \ldots, R_{\sigma^2_{\hat{\Delta}L}}\right) \tag{10.7}$$

It follows from Equation 10.6 that SSDO can be expressed as

$$\begin{aligned}
\text{SSDO} &= \frac{1}{L}\Delta'\mathbf{A}\Delta \\
&= \frac{1}{L}\left(\mathbf{M}-\Sigma_{\hat{\Delta}}^{1/2}\mathbf{Z}\right)'\mathbf{A}\left(\mathbf{M}-\Sigma_{\hat{\Delta}}^{1/2}\mathbf{Z}\right) \\
&= \frac{1}{L}\left(\mathbf{M}-diag(\sqrt{d_1},\ldots,\sqrt{d_L})\mathbf{Z}\right)'\mathbf{A}\left(\mathbf{M}-diag(\sqrt{d_1},\ldots,\sqrt{d_L})\mathbf{Z}\right)
\end{aligned} \tag{10.8}$$

where

$$d_k = \frac{(n_{Tk}-1)S_{Tk}^2}{U_{Tk}n_{Tk}} + \frac{(n_{Ck}-1)S_{Ck}^2}{U_{Ck}n_{Ck}} \quad \text{for } k = 1,\ldots,L$$

Let m, and be the observed values of **M**, and S_{Tk}^2, and S_{Ck}^2, respectively. From Equation 10.8, a GPQ for SSDO is given by

$$\begin{aligned}
UR_{SSDO} &= \frac{1}{L}\left(\mathbf{m}-R_{\Sigma_{\hat{\Delta}}}^{1/2}\mathbf{Z}\right)'\mathbf{A}\left(\mathbf{m} - R_{\Sigma_{\hat{\Delta}}}^{1/2}\mathbf{Z}\right) \\
&= \frac{1}{L}\left(\mathbf{m}-\text{diag}(\sqrt{R_{\sigma^2_{\hat{\Delta}_1}}},\ldots,\sqrt{R_{\sigma^2_{\hat{\Delta}_L}}})\mathbf{Z}\right)'\mathbf{A}\left(\mathbf{m}-\text{diag}(\sqrt{R_{\sigma^2_{\hat{\Delta}_1}}},\ldots,\sqrt{R_{\sigma^2_{\hat{\Delta}_L}}})\mathbf{Z}\right)
\end{aligned} \tag{10.9}$$

It is easy to verify that the observed values of $(R_{\sigma^2_{\hat{\Delta}_1}},\ldots,R_{\sigma^2_{\hat{\Delta}_L}})$ have distributions that are free of parameters $(\sigma^2_{\hat{\Delta}_1},\ldots,\sigma^2_{\hat{\Delta}_L})$. For the second expression of $R_{\sigma^2_{\hat{\Delta}_k}}$ in Equation 10.7, the observed value of $(R_{\sigma^2_{\hat{\Delta}_1}},\ldots,R_{\sigma^2_{\hat{\Delta}_L}})$ has the distribution that is free of parameters $(\sigma^2_{\hat{\Delta}_1},\ldots,\sigma^2_{\hat{\Delta}_L})$. Since the expression of UR_{SSDO} in Equation 10.9 involves only the observed values of **M** and S_{TK}^2 and S_{CK}^2 ; the pivotal quantities of U_{Tk} and U_{Ck}, and **Z**; and the constant matrix **A**, it has the distribution that is free of parameters. For the first expression of $R_{\sigma^2_{\hat{\Delta}_k}}$ in Equation 10.7, when **M**, S_{TK}^2 and S_{CK}^2, are substituted by their observed values **m**, s_{Tk}^2 and s_{Ck}^2 in Equation 10.9, the observed value of UR_{SSDO} turns out to be SSDO, which is free of the nuisance parameters . Hence, it fulfills the requirements of (a) and (b) for a GPQ previously mentioned.

Furthermore, since $\hat{\Delta}$ follows a multivariate normal distribution with mean and variance–covariance matrix $\Sigma_{\bar{\Delta}}$, it follows that may overestimate SSDO with a magnitude of

$$\frac{L-1}{L^2}\sum_{k=1}^{L}\left(\frac{\sigma_{Tk}^2}{n_{Tk}}+\frac{\sigma_{Ck}^2}{n_{Ck}}\right)$$

To correct this possible bias, we propose the following GPQ for SSDO:

$$R_{SSDO} = UR_{SSDO} - \frac{L-1}{L^2}\sum_{k=1}^{L} R_{\sigma^2_{\hat{\Delta}k}} \tag{10.10}$$

where UR_{SSDO} and $R_{\sigma^2_{\hat{\Delta}k}}$ are defined as same as Equation 10.9 and Equation 10.7, respectively.

An upper 100(1 – α)-th percentile generalized confidence interval for SSDO based on R_{SSDO} can be then obtained from the following Monte-Carlo algorithm:

Step 1: Choose a large simulation sample size, say, G = 10,000. For t equal to 1 through G, carry out the following two steps.

Step 2: Generate the $L \times 1$ standard normal random vector and the central chi-square random variables U_{Tk} and U_{Ck} with degree of freedom $n_{Tk} - 1$ and $n_{Ck} - 1$, respectively, for $k = 1,\ldots,L$.

Step 3: For the realized values of **M**, S_{Tk}^2, and S_{Ck}^2, compute R_{SSDO} as defined in Equation 10.10.

The required upper 100(1 – α)-th percentiles of the distribution of R_{SSDO} for SSDO then are estimated by the 100(1 – α)-th sample percentiles of the collection of G = 10,000 realizations $R_{SSDO},\ldots\ldots, R_{SSDO,1000}$.

The upper 100(1 – α)-th percentile GCI for SSDO based on R_{SSDO} can be used to test the noninferiority hypothesis in Equation 10.3 for the similarity of treatment effects among L subpopulations. The null hypothesis in Equation 10.3 is rejected and the treatment effects can be concluded to be similar among L subpopulations at the α significance level if the upper 100(1 – α)% generalized confidence limit for SSDO is less than δ^2.

Next, the testing procedure for the noninferiority hypothesis using the bootstrap approach is described. Since $\hat{\Delta}$ is distributed as a multivariate normal distribution with mean and variance Δ and $\Sigma_{\hat{\Delta}}$, the following parametric bootstrap algorithm is proposed to obtain an upper 100(1 – α)% confidence interval for SSDO:

Step 1: Use the observed response $\overline{X}_{Tk}$, $\overline{Y}_{Ck}$, S_{Tk}^2, and S_{Ck}^2, for k = 1,..,L, to estimate the parameters of the parametric distribution, Δ, and $\Sigma_{\hat{\Delta}}$, by **m** and $\text{diag}(s_{T1}^2/n_{T1}+s_{C1}^2/n_{C1},\ldots,s_{TL}^2/n_{TL}+s_{CL}^2/n_{CL})$ respectively.

Step 2: Select a large number of bootstrap samples, say, $B = 3000$, from the multivariate normal distribution

$$N_L\left(\mathbf{m}, diag\left(s_{T1}^2 / n_{T1} + s_{C1}^2 / n_{C1}, \ldots, s_{TL}^2 / n_{TL} + s_{CL}^2 / n_{CL}\right)\right)$$

Step 3: For each bootstrap sample compute $\hat{\Delta}^{*g}$ and $\widehat{SSDO}_g^{*} = \hat{\Delta}^{*g\prime}\mathbf{A}\hat{\Delta}^{*g} / L$, $g = 1, 2, \ldots, B$.

Step 4: The upper $100(1 - \alpha)\%$ confidence limit is given as $\widehat{SSDO}_{du} = \widehat{SSDO}^{*}_{(1+(1-\alpha)B)}$, where $\widehat{SSDO}^{*}_{(1)} < \ldots < \widehat{SSDO}^{*}_{(B)}$ are the order statistics of $\widehat{SSDO}^{*}_1, \ldots, \widehat{SSDO}^{*}_B$.

Similarly, the null hypothesis in Equation 10.3 is rejected, and the treatment effects can be concluded similar among L subpopulations at the α significance level if the bootstrap upper $100(1 - \alpha)\%$ confidence limit for SSDO, $\widehat{SSDO}_{du}$ is less than δ^2.

10.4 Simulation Studies

Simulation studies were conducted to investigate and compare performance of the empirical sizes and powers based on the GPQ approach and parameter bootstrap method for two major types of applications. The first type is under the framework of between-study comparisons where a bridging study is conducted in a new region to investigate the similarity of treatment effects for comparing the test drug with placebo control between the new and original regions. For the simulation study, the scenario of Hsiao et al. (2007) for one bridging study in the new region and three trials in the original region is considered. In addition, a mean difference in reduction of 10 for the change from baseline of the primary endpoint between test drug and placebo is considered efficacious. Various combinations of treatment means for test drug and placebo with an overall treatment mean difference of –10 for the four studies are specified. In addition, the efficacy result of the bridging study of the new region is assumed to be noninferior to that from the original region if it can retain half of the magnitude of the overall mean treatment difference. As a result, the clinically allowable upper margins of 3, 4, of 5 were selected in the simulation to represent the stringent, moderate, and liberal margins. It follows that the true values of SSDO are 9, 16, and 25, respectively. To investigate the impact of sample sizes and standard deviations of treatment on the empirical size, four sets of sample sizes per group—(100, 100, 100, 20), (150, 150, 150, 30), (300, 300, 300, 60), (450, 450, 450,

90)—were chosen, where the first three sample sizes per group in parentheses are those for three studies in the original region and the last sample size per group is the sample size of the bridging study in the new region. To follow the spirit of avoiding unnecessary duplication of clinical evaluation of the ICH E5 guideline, the sample size for the bridging study in the new region was set as 20% of the trials conducted in original region. In addition, the standard deviation of 4, 6, 10, 12, and 16 were also chosen to study its impact on the empirical size.. For the 5% nominal significance level, a simulation study with 10,000 random samples implies that 95% of the empirical type I error rates evaluated at the allowable margins will be within 0.0457 and 0.0543 if the proposed methods can adequately control the type I error rate at the nominal level of 0.05.

Table 10.1 presents the results of the empirical sizes for simulation of the bridging study. In general, the empirical size increases when sample size increases and decreases when standard deviation increases. In addition, the empirical size also increases when the clinically allowable upper margin relaxes. Overall, 80.5% (58/72) of the empirical type I error rates of all combinations for the GPQ methods are within the interval of (0.0457, 0.0543). A total of 10 of 14 empirical type I error rates of the GPQ method is below the lower limit of 0.0457 when the sample size is small (< 60 for the bridging study), the standard deviation is large (> 8), and clinically allowable upper margin is stringent (= 3). This indicates that the GPQ method is conservative under the situations mentioned above. Furthermore, 92% (44/48) of the empirical type I error rates of the GPQ method are within the interval of (0.0457, 0.0543) when $\delta \geq 4$. However, only 43.6% of the empirical type I error rates of the bootstrap approach are within the interval of (0.0457, 0.0543). Similar conservatism is observed for the bootstrap approach for the combinations with a large standard deviation, a stringent margin, and a smaller sample size. On the other hand, 60.4% (29/48) of the empirical type I error rates of the bootstrap approach are above the upper limit of 0.543 when the clinically allowable upper margin is greater than 3. This shows that the bootstrap approach seems a little liberal with relaxation of the clinically allowable upper margin. On the other hand, the GPQ method can adequately control the type I error rates at the nominal level when the standard deviation is small (< 8), the sample size is moderate (≥ 60 for the bridging study), or the clinically allowable upper margin is not too stringent (≥ 4).

Figure 10.1 presents the empirical power curves for simulation of the bridging study for the combination when the upper allowable limit δ is 4, standard deviation is 10, and the sample sizes are 150, 150, 150, and 30 for three trials in the original regions and one bridging study in the new region, respectively. Figure 10.1 demonstrates that although the bootstrap approach seems more powerful than the GPQ method the difference is negligible. In addition, the empirical type I error rate of the bootstrap method is 0.0568, which is greater than the upper limit of 0.0543. Therefore, the power advantage of

TABLE 10.1

Empirical Type I Error Rate for Simulation of the Bridging Study

Sample Sizes		$\delta = 3$		$\delta = 4$		$\delta = 5$	
(O1,O2,O3,N)	**SD**	**GPQ**	**Bootstrap**	**GPQ**	**Bootstrap**	**GPQ**	**Bootstrap**
(100,100,100,20)	4	0.0468	0.0517	0.0506	***0.0581***	0.0457	***0.0544***
	6	0.0472	0.0522	0.0517	***0.0576***	0.0475	***0.0545***
	8	***0.0337***	***0.0401***	0.0504	***0.0582***	0.0479	***0.0547***
	10	***0.0147***	***0.0206***	0.0495	***0.0554***	0.0497	***0.0544***
	12	***0.0023***	***0.0047***	***0.0442***	0.0513	0.0498	***0.0561***
	16	***0.0000***	***0.0000***	***0.0056***	***0.0115***	***0.0330***	***0.0402***
(150,150,150,30)	4	0.0471	0.0509	0.0499	***0.0548***	0.0506	***0.0549***
	6	0.0483	0.0520	0.0511	***0.0555***	0.0519	***0.0553***
	8	***0.0453***	0.0485	0.0536	***0.0576***	0.0505	***0.0552***
	10	***0.0323***	***0.0366***	0.0532	***0.0572***	0.0492	0.0541
	12	***0.0173***	***0.0222***	0.0513	***0.0555***	0.0541	***0.0578***
	16	***0.0002***	***0.0010***	***0.0367***	***0.0416***	0.0514	***0.0555***
(300,300,300,60)	4	0.0498	0.0520	0.0522	***0.0543***	0.0504	0.0528
	6	0.0498	0.0519	0.0502	0.0523	0.0507	0.0524
	8	0.0492	0.0519	0.0517	0.0530	0.0504	0.0520
	10	0.0489	0.0511	0.0542	***0.0563***	0.0516	0.0539
	12	0.0465	0.0468	0.0540	***0.0577***	0.0540	***0.0574***
	16	***0.0255***	***0.0277***	0.0527	***0.0552***	0.0543	***0.0571***
(450,450,450,90)	4	0.0527	0.0536	0.0473	0.0497	0.0476	0.0497
	6	0.0512	0.0523	0.0529	***0.0550***	0.0497	0.0521
	8	0.0513	0.0532	0.0527	***0.0553***	0.0513	0.0529
	10	0.0508	0.0506	0.0539	***0.0555***	0.0498	0.0520
	12	0.0485	0.0491	0.0535	0.0541	0.0488	0.0507
	16	***0.0415***	***0.0422***	0.0532	0.0534	0.0526	***0.0549***

Note: O1, clinical trial I in the original region. O2, clinical trial II in the original region. O3, clinical trial III in the original region. N, bridging study in new region I. Values in bold italic are the empirical sizes outside the range of (0.0457, 0.0543).

the bootstrap approach comes at the expense of an inflated size. As a result, the GPQ method not only can control the type I error rates at the nominal level but also can provide the sufficient power. Although this type of the simulation study was conducted under the framework of the bridging study, the results can also be applied to the situation where there is a subpopulation with a smaller sample size compared with other subpopulations.

The simulation study for the second type of applications is for the within-study comparisons where a multiregion study is currently being conducted in three geographic or ethnic regions with approximately the same sample sizes. Although we consider only one multiregion trial, the same specifications of the overall treatment mean difference, standard deviation, and

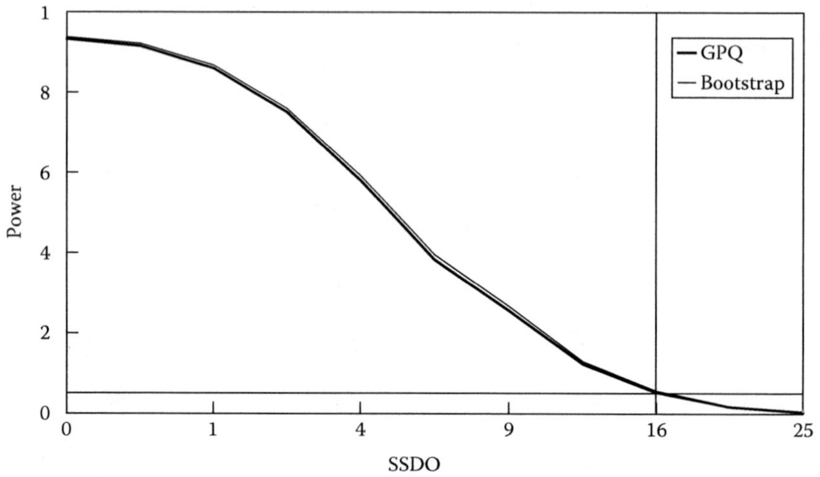

FIGURE 10.1
The empirical power curve when the upper limit of δ is 4 (SSDO of 16), sample sizes (O1,O2,O3,N) are (150,150,150,30) and standard deviation is 10.

clinically allowable upper margins employed in the first type of applications are also used here. The same sample size of 100, 150, 300, and 450 is assumed for each of the three regions. Table 10.2 presents the results of the type I error rates for simulation under the framework of a multiregion study. Empirical type I error rates increase when sample size increases or δ relaxes and decreases when standard deviation increases. The results of the GPQ method are very similar to those obtained under the situation of the bridging study. A total of 81.9% of empirical sizes (59 out of 72) of all combinations for the GPQ method is within the interval (0.0457, 0.0543). However, the results of the bootstrap approach under the multiregion studies are different. Unlike the results obtained under the bridging studies, the liberal performance of the bootstrap approach improves when the clinically allowable upper margin is relaxed. Therefore, 83.3 (60/72) of all combinations for the bootstrap approach are within the interval (0.0457, 0.0543). In summary, both the GPQ and bootstrap testing procedures can adequately control the type I error rates at the nominal level when the clinically allowable upper margin is not too stringent (≥ 4).

Figure 10.2 presents the empirical power curves under the situation of the multiregion study for the combination when the upper allowable limit δ is 4, standard deviation is 12, and the sample size is 150 for each of the three regions. Figure 10.2 shows that the power curves of the two methods are indistinguishable. Therefore, for the multiregion studies with approximately the same sample size for each region, the GPQ and bootstrap procedures yield almost identical performances on empirical sizes and powers.

TABLE 10.2

Empirical Type I Error Rate for Simulation of Multicenter Study

Sample Sizes (R1,R2,R3)	SD	δ = 3 GPQ	δ = 3 Bootstrap	δ = 5 GPQ	δ = 5 Bootstrap	δ = 4 GPQ	δ = 4 Bootstrap
(100,100,100)	4	0.0474	0.0490	0.0470	0.0479	0.0505	0.0520
	6	0.0473	0.0494	0.0480	0.0503	0.0457	0.0476
	8	0.0457	0.0466	0.0478	0.0499	0.0484	0.0494
	10	***0.0407***	***0.0422***	0.0460	0.0473	0.0474	0.0482
	12	***0.0380***	***0.0382***	***0.0443***	***0.0446***	***0.0426***	***0.0432***
	16	***0.0162***	***0.0184***	***0.0349***	***0.0360***	***0.0427***	***0.0435***
(150,150,150)	4	0.0469	0.0485	0.0495	0.0506	0.0477	0.0469
	6	0.0464	0.0474	0.0472	0.0484	0.0492	0.0496
	8	0.0490	0.0495	0.0473	0.0472	0.0479	0.0499
	10	***0.0441***	***0.0445***	0.0465	0.0486	0.0462	0.0465
	12	***0.0353***	***0.0365***	0.0467	0.0476	0.0468	0.0482
	16	***0.0324***	***0.0335***	***0.0427***	***0.0431***	***0.0445***	***0.0447***
(300,300,300)	4	0.0462	0.0479	0.0513	0.0516	0.0521	0.0527
	6	0.0462	0.0463	0.0491	0.0490	0.0499	0.0507
	8	0.0498	0.0514	0.0484	0.0480	0.0491	0.0488
	10	0.0491	0.0499	0.0491	0.0497	0.0539	0.0538
	12	0.0468	0.0473	0.0474	0.0479	0.0501	0.0507
	16	***0.0449***	0.0458	0.0514	0.0513	0.0518	0.0522
(450,450,450)	4	0.0506	0.0506	0.0508	0.0515	0.0514	0.0509
	6	0.0497	0.0498	0.0512	0.0503	0.0502	0.0506
	8	0.0505	0.0495	0.0505	0.0498	0.0509	0.0517
	10	0.0518	0.0513	0.0482	0.0482	0.0481	0.0484
	12	0.0489	0.0480	0.0466	0.0470	0.0473	0.0480
	16	0.0463	0.0472	0.0503	0.0504	0.0503	0.0496

Note: R1, region I. R2, region II. R3, region III. Values in bold italic are the empirical sizes outside the range of (0.0457, 0.0543).

10.5 Numerical Examples

Two examples for illustration of the proposed testing procedures to the between-study comparisons and within-study comparisons that are provided in Liu et al. (2009) are also given in this section.

10.5.1 Applications to Evaluation of Bridging Studies

The data sets of Hsiao et al. (2007) are modified to illustrate applications of the proposed testing procedures for evaluation of bridging studies. In short, the foreign clinical data contained in the complete clinical data package

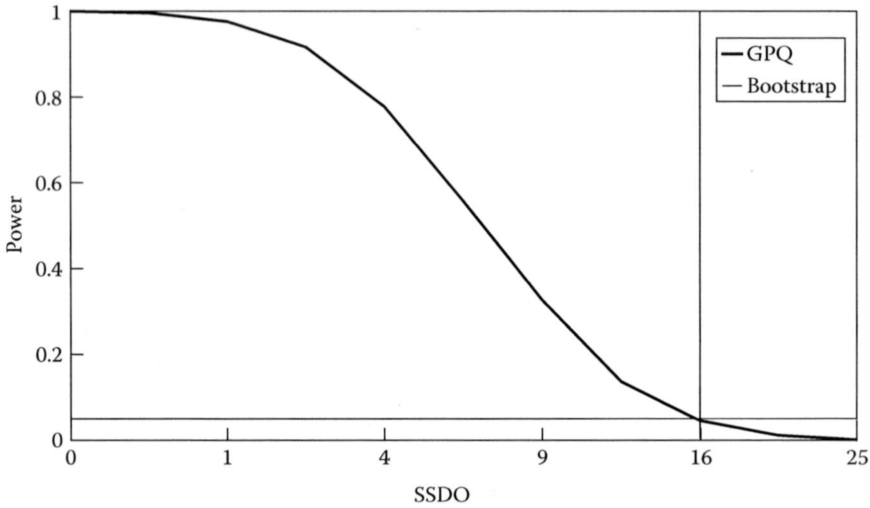

FIGURE 10.2
The empirical power curve when the upper limit of δ is 4 (SSDO of 16), sample sizes (C1,C2,C3) are (150,150,150) and standard deviation is 12.

(CCDP) include the results of three randomized, placebo-controlled pivotal trials conducted in the original region for comparing a new antihypertensive drug with a concurrent placebo. The primary endpoint is the change from baseline of sitting diastolic blood pressure (SDBP, mmHg) at week 12. A bridging study was conducted in the new region with the similar design for evaluation of extrapolation of the foreign clinical data to the new regions. Similar to Hsiao et al., three scenarios of the results of the bridging study were considered. The first scenario presents the situation where the new antihypertensive drug fails to demonstrate its efficacy over the placebo in the population of the new region. The second scenario presents the situation where the efficacy of the new antihypertensive drug is statistically superior to the placebo with a magnitude of mean reduction of SDBP at week 12 quite close to those observed in three pivotal trials in the original region. The last scenario is that the difference in mean reduction of SDBP at week 12 between the new antihypertensive drug and placebo observed in the bridging study is approximately half of those from the three pivotal trials in the original region. Table 10.3 provides the descriptive statistics for the data sets. Figure 10.3 presents the 95% confidence intervals of the difference in mean reduction of SDBP at week 12 between the new antihypertensive drug and placebo for the three scenarios.

The overall mean treatment difference in reduction of SDBP at week 12 computed from the three pivotal trials in the original region is –14.3 mmHg. Since there are currently numerous different types of drugs available in the new region for treatment of high blood pressure, the regulatory agency

TABLE 10.3

Descriptive Statistics of Reduction from Baseline in Sitting Diastolic Blood Pressure (mmHg)

Clinical Trials in Original Region	Treatment Group	Mean	SD	*N*	Bridging Study in New Region	Treatment group	Mean	SD	*N*	Test for Difference (*p*-value)
I	Drug	–18	11	138	Example I	Drug	–5	11	64	0.607
	Placebo	–3	12	132		Placebo	–4	11	65	
II	Drug	–17	10	185	Example II	Drug	–15	11	64	<0.0001
	Placebo	–2	11	179		Placebo	–2	11	65	
III	Drug	–15	13	141	Example III	Drug	–10.4	13	64	0.006
	Placebo	–2	14	143		Placebo	–4	13	65	

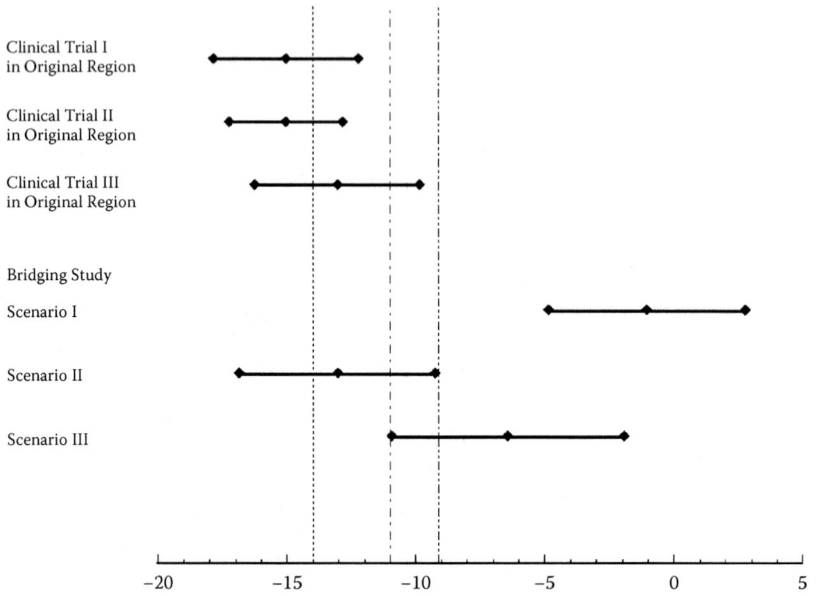

FIGURE 10.3
The 95% confidence intervals of treatment difference of reduction from baseline in sitting diastolic blood pressure for each of original regions and scenarios in the new region.

chooses a rather stringent clinically allowable upper limit of 4 mmHg, which retains approximately 72% of the efficacy of the new antihypertensive drug provided by the three pivotal trials in the original region.

Table 10.4 provides the results of each statistical test procedure as well as the *p*-values for detecting the existence of the treatment-by-region interaction by one-way analysis of variance (ANOVA). For the first scenario, the 95% upper confidence limits of SSDO by the GPQ and bootstrap methods are 39.3235 and 39.3513, respectively, which both are larger than the allowable upper limit for SSDO of 16. Hence, both GPQ and bootstrap methods show that at the 5% significance level not enough evidence supports the similarity of the treatment effects between the bridging study in new region and the three clinical trials in the original region. The result is consistent with the ANOVA results, which show that the treatment-by-study interaction effect is very statistically significantly different from 0 with a p-value < 0.0001. The nonoverlapping 95% confidence intervals of treatment effects of the bridging studies and original regions also confirm this conclusion.

For the second scenario, the estimated mean difference between the new antihypertensive drug and the placebo is –13 mmHg, which is very close to the overall mean treatment difference of –14.3 mmHg. In addition, the 95% confidence interval for the mean difference of the bridging study is almost overlapped with those from the original study. As a result, the 95% upper confidence limits of SSDO by the GPQ and bootstrap methods are,

TABLE 10.4

Results of Evaluation of the Similarity of Treatment Effect of Reduction from Baseline in Sitting Diastolic Blood Pressure across Regions by Proposed Test Procedures

	Test for Similarity Across Regions (SSDO = 16)			Test for Interaction
New Region	**Result**	**GPQ**	**Bootstrap**	**ANOVA (p-value)**
Scenario I	Upper Limit of 95% CI	39.3345	39.3567	< 0.0001
	Conclusion	Not Reject	Not Reject	**Reject**
Scenario II	Upper Limit of 95% CI	1.8589	1.8803	0.8755
	Conclusion	**Reject**	**Reject**	Not Reject
Scenario III	Upper Limit of 95% CI	15.9665	15.9019	0.0055
	Conclusion	**Reject**	**Reject**	**Reject**

Note: ANOVA, one-way analysis of variance; CI, confidence interval.
Source: Liu, J. P., J. R. Lin, and E. Hsieh, *Drug Information Journal*, 43(1), 11–16, 2009. With permission.

respectively, 1.8848 and 2.0183, which are smaller than 16. Both GPQ and bootstrap methods conclude at the 5% significance level the similarity of the treatment effect between the bridging study in new region and the three clinical trials in the original region. The conclusion is also consistent with the ANOVA result, which fails to show the existence of the treatment-by-region interaction (p-value − 0.8755).

For the third scenario, only a small portion of the 95% confidence interval for the mean difference of the bridging study is overlapped with those from the original study. As a result, the ANOVA shows a statistically significant treatment-by-region interaction with a p-value 0.0055. However, the 95% upper confidence limits of SSDO by the GPQ and bootstrap methods are, respectively, 15.9665 and 15.9019 which are smaller than 16. The last scenario demonstrates the situation of a statistically significant treatment-by-region interaction with a magnitude of treatment effect of no clinical consequence. As mentioned previously, the clinically allowable upper margin is chosen as 4 mmHg, which can retain 72% of the overall treatment mean difference of –14.3 mmHg observed from the clinical trials in the original region. It should also be noted that a treatment mean difference of –6.4 mmHg observed in the bridging study with a total sample size of 129 patients for the third scenario is also statistically significant at the 0.05 significance level.

10.5.2 Application to Evaluation of Age Groups within the Same Study

The change from baseline in HBV DNA at week 48 in the "Statistical Review and Evaluation, Clinical Studies" (FDA, 2007, Table 4) is one of the key secondary endpoints of a clinical trial for assessment of Hepsera (Adefovir Dipivoxil) in treating chronic hepatitis B in patients less than 18 years old. These data are used to illustrate the similarity between different age groups

TABLE 10.5

Change from Baseline in HBV DNA (log10 copies/mL)

Age Group	Treatment Group	Mean	SD	*N*
2–6 years	Adefovir	–3.19	1.71	21
	Placebo	–0.93	1.23	12
7–11 years	Adefovir	–3.38	1.68	36
	Placebo	–0.51	0.95	18
12–17 years	Adefovir	–3.72	1.45	51
	Placebo	–0.66	1.04	27

Source: FDA, Statistical Review and Evaluation, Clinical Studies, NDA/Serial Number: 21449/SE5-011.

within the same study. Table 10.5 provides the mean change from baseline in HBV DNA (log10 copies/mL) with standard deviation of adefovir and placebo for age groups of 1–6 years, 7–11 years, and 12–17 years. The 95% confidence intervals for treatment difference for each age group are also presented in Figure 10.4. The figure shows the confidence intervals of three age groups are overlapped. The overall mean treatment difference between adefovir and placebo of three age groups is –2.83. The allowable upper limit of δ is set as 1 to reflect retention of 65% of efficacy. This implies that the allowable upper limit of SSDO is also 1. The results presented in Table 10.6 shows that the 95% upper confidence limit of SSDO by the GPQ and bootstrap methods are 0.4743 and 0.4516, respectively. Because both 95% upper confidence limits are smaller than 1, the null hypothesis in Equation 10.3 is rejected at the 5% significance level by either the GPQ method or bootstrap approach. It follows that the treatment effects of adefovir are similar among the three age groups. In addition, the ANOVA also fails to reject the null hypothesis of no treatment-by-age interaction (p-value = 0.5667)

10.6 Discussion and Final Remarks

Evaluation of similarity of treatment effects among different subpopulations for an investigational drug not only is one of major interests for pharmaceutical industries and regulatory agencies but also is extremely important to public health of a country. Several statistical procedures for assessing the similarity of the treatment effect for an investigational product by conducting a bridging study in a new region have already been proposed based on Bayesian and other statistical theories. The statistical hypothesis with the corresponding exact test procedures proposed based on SSDO for evaluation

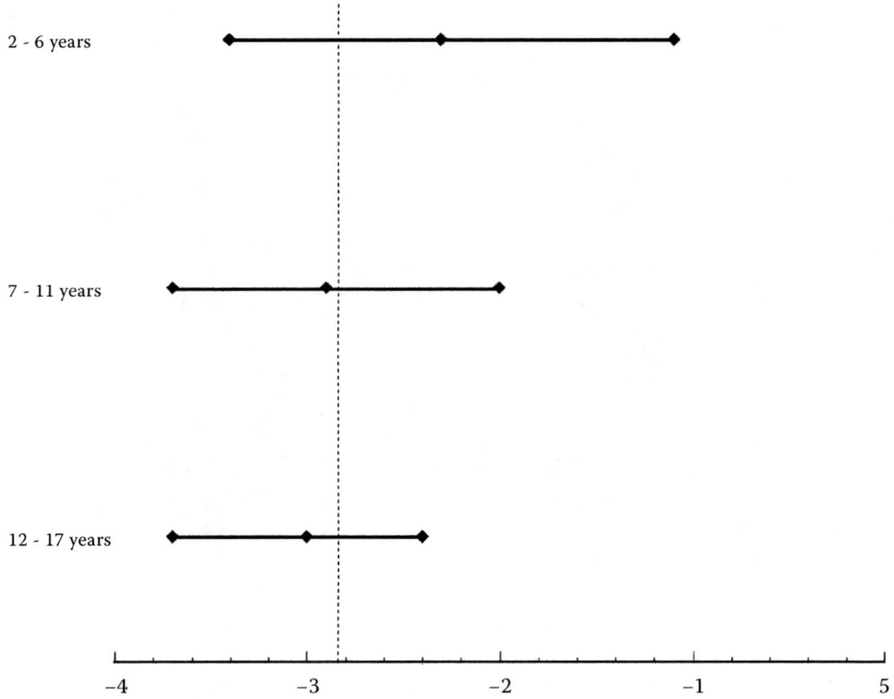

FIGURE 10.4
The 95% confidence intervals of treatment differences in changes from baseline of HBV DNA for age groups. (From Liu, J. P., Lin, J. R., and Hsieh, E., *Drug Information Journal*, 43(1), 11–16, 2009. With permission.)

TABLE 10.6

Results of Evaluation of the Similarity of Treatment Effect of Change from Baseline in HBV DNA across Age Groups by Proposed Test Procedures

Test for Similarity Across Age Groups			Test for Interaction
Result	**GPQ**	**Bootstrap**	**ANOVA (*p*-value)**
Upper limit of 95% CI	0.4743	0.4516	0.5667
Conclusion	**Reject**	**Reject**	Not Reject

Note: ANOVA, one-way analysis of variance; CI, confidence interval.
Source: Liu, J. P., J. R. Lin, and E. Hsieh, *Drug Information Journal*, 43(1), 11–16, 2009. With permission.

of the similarity considers the differences of the treatment effect across populations as the effect of treatment-by-population interaction. However, unlike the traditional approach for detecting the existence of the treatment-by-population interaction, the aim is to evaluate if the treatment-by-population interaction is less than some allowable upper limit where the allowable limit is decided from the clinical point of view. The simulation study described herein demonstrates the proposed GPQ method not only can adequately control the type I error at the nominal level but also can keep the good performance of the power, whereas the bootstrap method cannot. Besides, the numerical examples also show the proposed GPQ method can reach the conclusion consistent with the data.

Although the proposed statistical test procedures in Section 10.2 are derived by considering a two-arm study for comparing the treatment difference of a continuous endpoint for a test product with its control product, it is easy to extend the proposed methods to the applications for the study design which only investigational product is compared without control product. For example, the vaccine development company is willing to evaluate if a similar anti-HPV response for the investigational vaccine in adult women can also be observed in female adolescents. Therefore, a single-arm, noncontrolled study is conducted for comparing the geometric mean titers of female patients in age groups 9–15 years and 16–26 years after receiving the test treatment. For this type of applications, the proposed GPQ method can be applied by redefining in Equation 10.2 the proposed hypothesis as the difference between the treatment mean of k-th population and the average of treatment means, and is the allowable upper bound of θ_k, for each $k = 1,\ldots,L$. The corresponding GPQ is then the same form as Equation 10.13 by replacing the definition of **m** and $R_{\sigma^2_{\hat{\Delta}k}}$ in Equation 10.8 as

$$\mathbf{m} = (\bar{x}_1, \bar{x}_2, \ldots, \bar{x}_L)$$

$$R_{\sigma^2_{\hat{\Delta}k}} = \frac{(n_k - 1)s_k^2}{U_k n_k} \qquad \text{for } k = 1, \ldots, L$$

where $n_k, \bar{X}_k,$ and s_k^2 denote the sample size, sample mean, and sample variance for k-th population of the investigational product, respectively, and $\chi^2_{n_k-1}$ denotes the central chi-square distribution with $n_k - 1$. The 95% confidence limit of the corresponding SSDO and the assessment for the similarity for the single-arm study can be obtained and conducted by the same procedures previously described.

In addition to the application for the single-arm study, the study is often designed by considering the multiple, categorical, or survival endpoints based on the requirements for different indications. Further research is needed for these considerations and applications.

References

Chow, S. C., Shao, J., and Hu, O. Y. P. (2002). Assessing sensitivity and similarity in bridging studies. *Journal of Biopharmaceutical Statistics*, 12: 385–400.

Efron, B. and Tibshirani, R. J. (1993). *An introduction to the bootstrap, monographs on statistics, and applied probability*. New York, NY: Chapman & Hall.

Hanning, J., Iyer, H. K., and Patterson, P. (2006). Fiducial generalized confidence intervals. *Journal of the American Statistical Association*, 101: 254–269.

Hsiao, C. F., Hsu, Y. Y., Tsou, H. H., and Liu, J. P. (2007). Use of prior information for Bayesian evaluation of bridging studies. *Journal of Biopharmaceutical Statistics*, 17: 109–131.

Hsiao, C. F., Xu, J. Z., and Liu, J. P. (2003). A group sequential approach to evaluation of bridging studies. *Journal of Biopharmaceutical Statistics*, 13: 793–801.

Hsiao, C. F., Xu, J. Z., and Liu, J. P. (2005). A two-stage design for bridging studies. *Journal of Biopharmaceutical Statistics*, 15: 75–83.

International Conference on Harmonisation. (ICH). (1998). Tripartite guidance E5 ethnic factors in the acceptability of foreign data. *U.S. Federal Register*, 83: 31790–31796.

Ko, F. S., Tsou, H. H., Liu, J. P., and Hsiao, C. F. (2010). Sample size determination for a specific region in a multiregional trial. *Journal of Biopharmaceutical Statistics*, 20: 870–885.

Lawrence, J., and Belisle, P. (1997). Bayesian sample size determination for normal means and differences between normal means. *Statistician*, 46: 209–226.

Liu, J. P., and Chow, S. C. (2002). Bridging studies for clinical development. *Journal of Biopharmaceutical Statistics*, 12: 357–369.

Liu, J. P., Hsiao, C. F., and Hsueh, H. M. (2002). Bayesian approach to evaluation of bridging studies. *J. Biopharm. Stat*, 12: 401–408.

Liu, J. P., Hsueh, H. M., and Hsiao, C. F. (2004). Bayesian non-inferior approach to evaluation of bridging studies. *Journal of Biopharmaceutical Statistics*, 14: 291–300.

Liu, J. P., Lin, J. R., and Hsieh, E. (2009). A noninferiority test for treatment-by-factor interaction with application to bridging studies and global trials. *Drug Information Journal*, 43(1): 11–16.

Shih, W. J. (2001). Clinical trials for drug registration in Asian-Pacific countries: Proposal for a new paradigm from a statistical perspective. *Controlled Clinical Trials*, 22: 357–366.

U.S. Food and Drug Administration. (FDA). (2007). U.S. Department of Health and Human Services. Statistical review and evaluation, clinical studies. NDA/Serial Number: 21449/SE5-011.

Weerahandi, S. (1993). Generalized confidence intervals. *Journal of the American Statistical Association*, 88: 899–905.

11

Multiregional Clinical Trials[*]

Yi Tsong
U.S. Food and Drug Administration

Hsiao-Hui Tsou
National Health Research Institutes

11.1 Introduction

With increasing globalization in the development of medicines, developing strategies for when and how to address geographic variations of efficacy and safety for product development has become essential. To shorten the time for drug development and regulatory approval, it would be desirable to conduct a trial for simultaneous drug development, submission, and approval around the world. Recently, the number of clinical trials simultaneously conducted in Asian countries, Europe, and the United States has increased significantly. In particular, the Japanese government has the initiative to participate in global development and international clinical studies. The 11th Q&A for the ICH E5 (ICH, 2006) guideline described points to consider for evaluating the possibility of bridging among regions in a multiregional trial and stated that "it may be desirable in certain situations to achieve the goal of bridging by conducting a multi-regional trial under a common protocol that includes sufficient numbers of patients from each of multiple regions to reach a conclusion about the effect of the drug in all regions." Basically, a multiregional clinical trial is designed for two objectives. The first objective is to assess the efficacy of the test treatment over all regions in the trial. The second objective is to bridge the overall effect of the test treatment to each of the regions in the trial.

Differences in the regulatory requirements among regions complicate the assessment of effect of the test treatment over all regions (Girman et al., 2011; Hsiao, Tsong, Wang, Dong, and Tsou, 2012; Peterson et al., 2011; Tsong, Chang, Dong, and Tsou, 2012). The issues of designing and analyzing

[*] This chapter represents the professional opinions of the authors. They do not necessarily reflect the official positions of the FDA or NHRI.

a multiregional clinical trial when there are differences in the regulatory requirement among the regions have been well documented in articles published in statistical journals and have been discussed at length at professional conferences. From a statistical point of view, these differences are typically related to endpoints, noninferiority or superiority testing, noninferiority margin, study length, and trial design. Most of the differences lead to complications in trial design, analysis, and sample size requirements. In some situations, these differences may even lead to unsolvable design complications. In Section 11.2, we discuss in detail the issues and impacts of designing a multiregional trial to assess the overall effect of a test treatment when there are differences in requirements between the regional authorities.

To assess region-specific treatment effects after establishing the overall treatment effect in a multiregional trial, it is important to realize that there will never be a sufficiently large sample to establish the treatment effect of the region or consistency between regional and overall effects. Therefore, with the sample size and power planned to access the overall effect, one has to modify the type I error rate for hypothesis testing or the significance level of estimation of regional effect (MHLW, 2007; Tsong, Chang et al., 2012). In Section 11.3, we discuss the issues of assessing the regional treatment effect in detail after establishing the overall treatment effect in a multiregional trial.

11.2 Different Regional Requirements

PhRMA organized a statistical workshop October 29–30, 2007, to facilitate discussions between industrial sponsors and regulatory agencies on issues regarding multiregional clinical trials. Following these discussions, the Drug Information Association (DIA) organized a workshop titled "Ensuring Quality and Balancing Risks for Multiregional Clinical Trials: Clinical, Regulatory, and Ethnic Factors" on October 26–27, 2010. One of the issues discussed, "Conducting MRCTs When Regulatory Guidances Differ between Regions," generated great interest within both the industrial and regulatory segments of the drug development community. Different medical endpoint requirements by regional regulatory agencies have a significant impact on the study design, hypothesis setting, sample size determination, and implementation of multiregional clinical trials (MRCTs) in global drug-development programs. The resulting impacts of these differences on implementing MRCTs are both logistical and operational. Medical endpoint requirements may vary in terms of which endpoints are considered primary, coprimary, or secondary. They are sometimes even viewed by the regulatory authorities with the acceptability of prespecified endpoints differently. In addition, differences across regions in required endpoints may involve differences in clinical or patient-reported outcomes (PROs), or in how the endpoints are implemented in trials, differences in time points, differences in noninferiority margins, differences in experimental designs, or differences in patient populations studied or analyzed (Girman et al., 2011; Hung, Wang, and O'Neill, 2010). Such differences may have a substantial impact on power and sample size requirements.

Girman et al. (2011) classified the scenarios involving different regional requirements among the EMA and the U.S. Food and Drug Administration (FDA) into five categories. We will briefly describe those categories and the impact on multiplicity adjustment and sample size requirement.

11.2.1 Different Noninferiority Margins

A key issue when designing a noninferiority clinical trial is to prespecify the noninferiority margin. How to define this margin has been discussed extensively (Tsong, Wang, Hung, and Cui, 2003). The basis of such margin may also be different across therapeutic areas. In some therapeutic areas, the recommendations on the noninferiority margin are consistent among all the regions. However, in other therapeutic areas, there still is a need for broad consensus regarding the noninferiority margin. For example, Girman et al. (2011) pointed out that a wide range of 10–15% margin has been used in noninferiority clinical trials with treatment-naive HIV-infected patients. However, in the FDA guidance document, a noninferiority margin of 10–12 percentage points for the response rate in treatment-naive HIV-infected patients is considered appropriate, while the CHMP guidance document has suggested a 10 percentage point margin during consultation. Girman et al. stated that the inconsistency in the recommendations by different regulatory agencies may cause confusion and sometimes leads to different development strategies for different regions. Collaboration across regions is helpful to reach a consistent recommendation. When there is no common fixed margin, the study sample size needs to be determined with the narrower margin to satisfy the different requirements. It has been well established that no multiple comparison adjustment is needed to test for both margins in a single sample size testing setting (Hung and Wang, 2004; Tsong and Zhang, 2007; Wang, Hung, Tsong, Cui, and Nuri, 2001). However, it requires type I error rate adjustment when it is designed with a multiple testing stages group sequential approach (Tsong, Dong, Hsiao, Wang, and Tsou, 2012).

11.2.2 Different Time Points Requirements

As Girman et al. (2011) pointed out, the expected treatment duration or time point for assessment of treatment response in a clinical trial to support efficacy or duration of response may be different between the EMA and the FDA. Girman et al. listed two examples. In pretreated HIV-infected patients, the FDA requires HIV-RNA levels at week 24 to support efficacy while the EMA accepts HIV-RNA levels at week 16. On the other hand, for Fondaparinux

Sodium (Arixtra), trials were conducted in patients with acute coronary syndrome, with a primary endpoint of major adverse cardiac events (MACE). The FDA requests the events 14 or more days after exposure, while the EMA accepts the MACE events in the first 9 days.

In planning an MRCT for the two regions, the sponsors need to negotiate a common time point or to measure the endpoints at both time points to satisfy the different requirements. An MRCT designed with two regional different endpoints presents many statistical challenges (Tsong, Dong et al., 2012). First, if efficacy is being evaluated at two different time points, one for the EMA and the other one for the FDA, there may be a need to correct for inflation of the type I error rate. When the outcome is binary, such as cumulative response, or survival, the group sequential adjustment may be applicable with the information time defined by the cumulative number of events for interim analysis using a Pocock or other sequential boundary. However, it poses a complication when the response is continuous. The conventional information time (defined by the cumulated number of subjects exposed to the treatments) will not work in this situation. Since the trial would not be terminated due to a significant testing result at the earlier time point, the type I error rate adjustment may be further complicated unless the interim testing performed at the early time point is blinded. Furthermore, when the results at the two time points are inconsistent, this complicates the interpretation of the data (Tsong, Dong et al.).

11.2.3 Different Experimental Designs

The difficulties of modifying standard experimental designs for different regions within a single MRCT trial depend on the magnitude and impact of the different design features. Adding an earlier time point for a safety assessment in specific regions or using a different rescue therapy within specific regions may be easy to implement without complicating the analysis of data or interpretation of the results. It becomes more complicated when the treatment effect assessment requirements are different among regions. Taking a multiregional trial with three treatment arms (placebo, positive control, and test), for example, some regions require that it be shown that the test treatment is better than a placebo for treatment efficacy and that the positive control is better than a placebo for validation. Other regions may simply require that the mean of (test – placebo) be greater than λ% of the mean of (positive control – placebo). In some applications, some regions may require that the test treatment be compared with the positive control in a noninferiority setting. Other regions may require that the test treatment be more effective than a placebo in a superiority setting. Testing the two sets of hypotheses may lead to multiple comparison issues. On the other hand, changing a simple single-stage design to a two-stage design to incorporate different requirements may often lead to more complications in design and analysis. For example, the sponsor may plan a two-stage trial to accommodate the different requirements. With such a two-stage trial, the sponsor may plan the first stage with a two-arm (test and placebo) designed trial. At the end of the first stage, when it is shown that the test treatment is more effective than a placebo (to satisfy the requirement of some regions), the sponsor may randomize the placebo arm into two arms (test and active control arms) to show that the test treatment is noninferior to the active control treatment. This leads to the complication that the superiority test at the end of the first stage and the noninferiority test at the end of the second stage are correlated. A complicated type I error rate adjustment is needed for such two-stage trials. Furthermore, it leads to an issue about how to interpret the study result if the results at the end of the two stages are inconsistent.

11.2.4 Different Endpoints Required by Two Regions

The regulatory authorities in the two regions may have different requirements on the clinical endpoints or other endpoints such as patient-reported outcome measures. In some cases, the authorities may require completely different efficacy endpoints, which can cause significant complexity in the design, implementation, analysis, and interpretation of data related to a development program. Sponsors interested in getting simultaneous approval in multiple regions in a global drug development program may be interested in handling this issue by using multiple primary or key secondary endpoints in a single MRCT protocol. There are many examples of the differences. Girman et al. (2011) listed the following four examples. For virology products, the EMA requires a combined composite of virological, histological, and biochemical responses for HBV phase III trials, while the FDA requires a complete virological response at 52 weeks in MITT population. For bronchodilators in chronic obstructive pulmonary disease, the EMA recommends using St. Georges' Respiratory Questionnaire (SGRQ) as a primary endpoint for assessing improvement in lung function and symptomatic benefit. On the other hand, the FDA does not include SGRQ-based primary endpoint in its draft guidance. For overactive bladder, the EMA recommends a subjective measure of treatment benefit as a coprimary endpoint along with incontinence episodes, micturitions, or urgency episodes based on a voiding diary. The FDA does not accept the subject measurement as coprimary endpoint. For atrial fibrillation (AF), the EMA guidance clearly specifies that prevention of any recurrence is the primary endpoint in patients with AF. The FDA recommends "delay in symptomatic recurrence of AF" instead.

Although in most applications, when the regions cannot reach a consensus on a common endpoint, the regulatory agencies allow the sponsors to use different hypotheses (prespecified) for the two different regions within the same MRCT protocol. The handling of testing multiple hypotheses may lead to complications in data analysis and sample size determinations as discussed in Hsiao et al. (2012). For example, considering the situation of two different regional endpoints, assuming X_{ij} and Y_{ij} with $i = T$ for test, C

for control treatment, $j = 1, 2$ for the two regions, represent the response of the endpoints in the study population of the two regions. Furthermore, we assume that $X_{ij} \sim N(\mu_{Xi}, \sigma_X)$, $Y_{ij} \sim N(\mu_{Xi}, \sigma_Y)$, and correlation of X_i and Y_i is ρ. Let

$$\Delta_X = \mu_{XT} - \mu_{XC}, \Delta_Y = \mu_{YT} - \mu_{YC}, \Delta_{Xj} = \mu_{XTj} - \mu_{XCj}, \Delta_{Yj} = \mu_{YTj} - \mu_{YCj}$$

The study may be designed to test for any of the four hypothesis sets.

11.2.4.1 Two Subset Testing

Test endpoint 1 with region 1 data for the hypothesis

$$H_{10} : \Delta_{X1} \leq -\delta_X$$

vs.

$$H_{1A} : \Delta_{X1} > -\delta_X$$

and test endpoint 2 with region 2 data for the following hypothesis:

$$H_{20} : \Delta_{Y2} \leq -\delta_Y$$

vs.

$$H_{2A} : \Delta_{Y2} > -\delta_Y$$

It is to be tested with no type I error rate adjustment. This would require different sample sizes for each region. To target for approval at both regions, sample size needs to be determined with power adjusted by either using $\beta^* = 1 - \sqrt{(1-\beta)}$ or incorporating the correlation of the two endpoints.

11.2.4.2 Testing Two Sequential Overall Hypotheses Using All Sample Size

Tests

$$H_{10} : \Delta_X \leq -\delta_X \text{ vs. } H_{1A} : \Delta_X > -\delta_X$$

If H_{10} is rejected, then we proceed to test

$$H_{20} : \Delta_Y \leq -\delta_Y \text{ vs. } H_{2A} : \Delta_Y > -\delta_Y$$

With this setting, H_{10} is tested with data of both regions. However, H_{20} is tested only if H_{10} is rejected. The type I error rate is under control with no adjustment required. Sample size determination needs to take into consideration approval in two regions.

11.2.4.3 Testing Two Parallel Overall Hypotheses with No Adjustment

Tests

$$H_{10} : \Delta_X \leq -\delta_X \text{ vs. } H_{1A} : \Delta_X > -\delta_X$$

$$\text{and } H_{20} : \Delta_Y \leq -\delta_X \text{ vs. } H_{2A} : \Delta_Y > -\delta_Y \text{ simultaneously}$$

There are four potential results: "Reject both H_{10} and H_{20}", "Reject H_{10} only", "Reject H_{20} only" and "Cannot reject either null." Without type I error rate adjustment, one may control regional type I error rate but not family-wise type I error rate. It would be considered statistically naive. Sample size determination needs to take into consideration for approval in two regions.

11.2.4.4 Testing Two Parallel Overall Hypotheses with Type I Error Rate Adjustment

Tests

$$H_{10} : \Delta_X \leq -\delta_X \text{ vs. } H_{1A} : \Delta_X > -\delta_X$$

$$\text{and } H_{20} : \Delta_Y \leq -\delta_X \text{ vs. } H_{2A} : \Delta_Y > -\delta_Y \text{ simultaneously}$$

To control the family wise type I error rate, one may use Bonferoni adjustment or Hochberg testing scheme. In sample size determination, one needs to adjust the type I error rate as well as the power.

11.3 Bridging the Overall Treatment Effect to Regions

On September 28, 2007, the Japanese Ministry of Health, Labour and Welfare (MHLW) published the "Basic Principles on Global Clinical Trials" guidance about the planning and implementation of global clinical studies. By this guidance, "global clinical studies refer to studies planned with the objective of world-scale development and approval of new drugs in which study sites of a multiple number of countries and regions participate in a single study based on a common protocol and conducted at the same time in parallel." The MHLW guideline focused on how to assess the efficacy of a drug in all participating regions and how to evaluate the possibility of applying the overall trial results to each region by conducting a multiregional trial. To be more specific, MHLW recommended two methods to address the issues on establishing efficacy in a specific region and consistency in efficacy among regions. Method 1 described consistency between the results of the Japanese region and all regions combined. The guidance described consistency by showing the ratio of the treatment effect estimate of the Japanese region to that of the overall multiregion to be greater than 50%. Method 2 described consistency in the sense that in addition to overall treatment in all regions combined, estimate of treatment effect needs to exceed zero in the Japanese region. To be more specific, let D and D_i be the estimated treatment effect of all participants and of the i-th region, $I = 1,2,\ldots,K$.

Method 1 (Consistency)

$D_i/D>\pi$ (with $\pi \geq 0.50$) occurs with a probability 80% or higher

Method 2 (Efficacy)

$D > 0$ and $D_i > 0$ occurs with a probability 80% or higher.

When it is a noninferiority test, we us $D > -\delta$ and $D_i > -\delta$ (where $\delta \geq 0$ is the fixed margin) instead. Each of the two methods is established if there is more than 80% chance of success.

The sample size requirement for the Japanese population or any specific region based on the two MHLW methods became the topics of many clinical trial researches. For example, Uyama et al. (2005) and Uesaka (2009) described the two methods focusing on the requirement of 80% or greater power for the Japanese region conditioning on the effect of overall global trial. Quan, Zhao, Zhang, Roessner, and Aizawa (2009) and Uesaka discussed the sample size requirements based on method 1. Quan et al. further extend the results to trials with various endpoints. Kawai, Stein, Komiyama, and Li (2008) employed an approach to rationalize partitioning the total sample size among the regions to reach a high probability for a consistent trend (method 2) under the assumption that the treatment effect is positive and homogeneous among the regions in a confirmatory multiregional trial. Due to the limited sample sizes allocated to the region, the regular interaction test for treatment by region is not practical. Ko, Tsou, Liu, and Hsiao (2010) proposed a statistical criteria for consistency between the region of interest and overall results. However, in all the articles, the authors discussed the sample size needs without the proper framework in terms of hypothesis and type I error rate to be used.

Tsong, Chang et al. (2012) lay out the scenarios of assessing regional efficacy when the MRCT was designed with proper power to test for the overall efficacy with the conventional type I error rate of 2.5%. They discussed that with the prespecified sample size for a targeted treatment effect size, the power to show efficacy for any region is restricted by the given sample size. Therefore, proper assessment of treatment efficacy in the region needs to accommodate the adjusted type I error rate for the same target size of efficacy under the assumption of uniform effect across the regions. As an example, if a three-region clinical trial is designed for noninferiority testing of the following hypothesis:

$$H_{0,All} : \Delta \le -0.5 \text{ vs. } H_{a,All} : \Delta > -0.5$$

with the assumption that the standard deviation σ, a total sample size of 566 subjects is needed for each treatment group given an expected treatment difference Δ' = 0, α = 0.025, β = 0.20. At the completion of the trial, the results show that the average overall treatment effect is −0.001 with the lower 95% confidence limit of −0.350. Given three regions consisting of 50%, 30%, and 20% of the overall sample size, the average regional treatment differences are 0.005, 0.025, and −0.056, respectively. The corresponding lower 95% confidence limits of the mean treatment difference are −0.490, −0.614, and −0.842 for the three regions, respectively (see Table 11.1). Accordingly, the treatment difference is not significant for regions 2 and 3. Such statistics are constrained by the 2.5% type I error rate and unfitted sample sizes. If the three regions have the same treatment effect as the overall effect to have the same power of 80% to show the difference in all three regions, the type I error rate needs to be adjusted with

$$\alpha_i = 1 - \Phi\left(\sqrt{\frac{N_i}{2}}\frac{\Delta^* + \delta}{\sigma} + z_{\beta^*}\right)$$

where δ = 0.5, σ = 3, $\beta^* = 1 - (1-\beta)^{1/3}$. The adjusted type I error rates for the three regions are therefore 0.302, 0.471, and 0.583, respectively. The adjusted lower confidence limits for the three regions are −0.126, 0.002, and 0.027, respectively. They are all consistent with the overall results. Note that the analysis procedure satisfies the testing requirement stated as method 2 in MHLW (2007).

For the sample size requirement derivation, we need to introduce a few notations. Let *X* and *Y* be the efficacy responses for patients taking the test drug and the control, respectively. For simplicity, we assume both *X* and *Y* are normally distributed with a common variance σ^2. Let μ_T and μ_C denote the population means for the test-drug group and control group, respectively. Let $\Delta = \mu_T - \mu_C$ denote the population mean difference, assuming the effect size (Δ/σ) is uniform across regions. The hypothesis of testing for the overall treatment effect is

$$H_0 : \Delta \le -\delta \text{ vs. } H_A : \Delta > -\delta \tag{11.1}$$

with a prespecified noninferiority margin δ. When testing a superiority hypothesis, we define margin δ = 0.

Let N denote the total sample size for each group planned for detecting an expected treatment difference Δ^* at the desired significance level α and with power $1 - \beta$. Thus,

$$N = 2\left[\left(z_{1-\alpha} + z_{1-\beta}\right)\sigma / \left(\Delta^* + \delta\right)\right]^2$$

where $z_{1-\alpha}$ is the $(1-\alpha)$-th percentile of the standard normal distribution. Suppose that we are interested in assessing whether the treatment is effective in an individual region of the trial, $\Delta = \mu_{Ti} - \mu_{Pi}$ say, the i-th region, where $1 \le i \le K$. We assume further that the mean difference Δ is uniform across regions, that is, $\Delta_i = \Delta$. The hypothesis of testing the treatment effect for the i-th region is

$$H_{0i} : \Delta_i \le -\delta \text{ vs. } H_{Ai} : \Delta_i > -\delta \tag{11.2}$$

Let X_{ij} and Y_{ij}' be efficacy responses for patients j and j' receiving the test product and the control respectively in the i-th region. Let K be the number of regions, and p_i denote the proportion of patients out of $2N$ in the i-th region, $i = 1,\ldots,K$, where

$$\sum_{i=1}^{K} p_i = 1$$

Also let N_i be the number of patients per group in the i-th region. That is, $N_i - p_i N$. Let D_i be the observed mean difference in the i-th region, and D the observed mean difference from all regions. That is,

$$D_i = \bar{X}_{i.} - \bar{Y}_{i.} \text{ and } D = \sum_{i=1}^{K} N_i(\bar{X}_{i.} - \bar{Y}_{i.}) / N$$

where

$$\bar{X}_{i.} = \sum_{j=1}^{N_i} X_{ij} / N_i \quad \text{and} \quad \bar{Y}_{i.} = \sum_{j=1}^{N_i} Y_{ij} / N_i$$

Also, let Z_i be the test statistic in the i-th region, and Z the test statistic for the overall results. In other words,

$$Z_i = \frac{\bar{X}_{i.} - \bar{Y}_{i.} + \delta}{\sigma\sqrt{\frac{2}{N_i}}} \quad \text{and} \quad Z = \frac{\sum_{i=1}^{K} N_i(\bar{X}_{i.} - \bar{Y}_{i.})/N + \delta}{\sigma\sqrt{\frac{2}{N}}}$$

When the treatment effect in the regions is tested only if the overall null hypothesis H_0 is rejected, we need to consider a conditional test whose power is represented as conditional power in the following form:

$$P_{\Delta^*}(Z_i > z_{1-\alpha_i} \mid H_{A_i}, \text{ reject } H_0)$$

where $P_{\Delta^*}(x)$ is the probability measure with respect to $\Delta = \Delta^*$ and is the significant level required in the i-th region. It can be derived that

$$P_{\Delta^*}(Z_i > z_{1-\alpha_i} \mid H_{A_i}, \text{ reject } H_0) = \frac{\int_{z_{1-\alpha_i} - \sqrt{p_i}(z_{1-\alpha} + z_{1-\beta})}^{\infty} \Phi\left(\frac{z_{1-\beta} + \sqrt{p_i}\,u}{\sqrt{1-p_i}}\right)\varphi(u)du}{1-\beta} \tag{11.3}$$

where Φ denotes the cumulative probability function of the standard normal distribution and ϕ denotes the probability density function of the standard normal distribution. The details of the derivations of Equation 11.3 are given in Tsong, Chang et al. (2012).

We assume that the conditional power (Equation 11.3) for the i-th region has to achieve the same level as the power of the global trial. That is,

$$P_{\Delta^*}(Z_i > z_{1-\alpha_i} \mid H_{A_i}, \text{ reject } H_0) = 1-\beta \tag{11.4}$$

By Equation 11.3 and Equation 11.4, we have

$$(1-\beta)^2 = \int_{z_{1-\alpha_i} - \sqrt{p_i}(z_{1-\alpha} + z_{1-\beta})}^{\infty} \Phi\left(\frac{z_{1-\beta} + \sqrt{p_i}\,u}{\sqrt{1-p_i}}\right)\varphi(u)du \tag{11.5}$$

When α, β, and the proportion p_i are given, we can obtain the significance level for α_i the region by Equation 11.5 with numerical analysis technique.

For assessing a consistent trend of efficacy across the specific region and the overall region, we use the confidence interval to be the assessable criterion to ensure whether the efficacy is consistent between the overall region and the i-th region. The confidence interval of the mean treatment difference, the overall region, and the i-th region are

$$\left(D \pm z_{1-\alpha}\sqrt{\frac{2}{N}}\sigma\right) \quad \text{and} \quad \left(D_i \pm z_{1-\alpha_i}\sqrt{\frac{2}{N_i}}\sigma\right)$$

respectively. If the level α confidence interval for the overall region and the level α_i confidence interval for the i-th region both exclude $-\delta$, we say that the efficacy is qualitative consistency between the overall region and the i-th region in the way consistent with method 2 of MHLW (2007) with $\delta = 0$.

When we consider the power of the regional efficacy testing in terms of the joint probability of rejection at all regions, the joint power is expressed as

$$\begin{aligned} &P_{\Delta}(Z_1 > z_{1-\alpha_1},\ Z_2 > z_{1-\alpha_2},\ Z_3 > z_{1-\alpha_3},\ Z_4 > z_{1-\alpha_4} \mid Z > z_{1-\alpha}) \\ &= P_0(Z_1 > z_{1-\alpha_1} - \sqrt{p_1}\left(z_{1-\alpha} + z_{1-\beta}\right),\ Z_2 > z_{1-\alpha_2} - \sqrt{p_2}\left(z_{1-\alpha} + z_{1-\beta}\right) \\ &\quad Z_3 > z_{1-\alpha_3} - \sqrt{p_3}\left(z_{1-\alpha} + z_{1-\beta}\right), Z_4 > z_{1-\alpha_4} - \sqrt{p_4}\left(z_{1-\alpha} + z_{1-\beta}\right) \\ &\quad \mid \sqrt{p_1}Z_1 + \sqrt{p_2}Z_2 + \sqrt{p_3}Z_3 + \sqrt{p_4}Z_4 > -z_{1-\beta}) \end{aligned} \tag{11.6}$$

where α_i is the significant level for the i-th region, which is prespecified, and α is a function of the total sample size N. For sample size determination, for $\Delta = \Delta^*$, Equation 11.6 can further be derived as

$$\begin{aligned} &P_{\Delta^*}(Z_1 > z_{1-\alpha_1},\ Z_2 > z_{1-\alpha_2},\ Z_3 > z_{1-\alpha_3},\ Z_4 > z_{1-\alpha_4} \mid Z > z_{1-\alpha}) \\ &= \frac{P_0(Z_1 > c_1,\ Z_2 > c_2,\ Z_3 > c_3,\ Z_4 > c_4, c_5Z_1 + c_6Z_2 + c_7Z_3 + c_8Z_4 > c_9)}{P_0(Z > c_9)} \\ &= \frac{\int_{c_4}^{\infty}\int_{c_3}^{\infty}\int_{c_2}^{\infty}\int_{\max\left\{c_1,\ \frac{c_9 - c_6u_2 - c_7u_3 - c_8u_4}{c_5}\right\}}^{\infty} \varphi(u_1)du_1\varphi(u_2)du_2\varphi(u_3)du_3\varphi(u_4)du_4}{\int_{c_9}^{\infty}\varphi(u)du} \\ &\geq (1-\beta) \end{aligned} \tag{11.7}$$

where

$$c_1 = z_{1-\alpha_1} - \sqrt{p_1}\frac{\Delta^* + \delta}{\sigma\sqrt{\frac{2}{N}}}, c_2 = z_{1-\alpha_2} - \sqrt{p_2}\frac{\Delta^* + \delta}{\sigma\sqrt{\frac{2}{N}}}, c_3 = z_{1-\alpha_3} - \sqrt{p_3}\frac{\Delta^* + \delta}{\sigma\sqrt{\frac{2}{N}}}$$

$$c_4 = z_{1-\alpha_4} - \sqrt{p_4}\frac{\Delta^* + \delta}{\sigma\sqrt{\frac{2}{N}}}, c_5 = \sqrt{p_1}, c_6 = \sqrt{p_2}, c_7 = \sqrt{p_3}, c_8 = \sqrt{p_4} \text{ and } c_9 = z_{1-\alpha} - \frac{\Delta^* + \delta}{\sigma\sqrt{\frac{2}{N}}}$$

The derivation details of Equations 11.7 are given in Tsong, Chang et al. (2012). To solve N for Equation 11.7, we need to specify p_i for each of the regions. This can be done by using p_i derived from the unconditional sample size formula. As a comparison, we recalculate the regional and overall sample size with the same configurations of Table 11.1. The results of simultaneous power approach with various configurations of α_i are given in Table 11.2. As expected, the sample sizes are much larger than that determined without accommodating regional efficacy in sample size consideration.

TABLE 11.1

Assessing the Regional Treatment Effect for a Multi-Regional Trial of Three Regions Using 0.025 Type I Error Rate, 0.20 Type II Error Rate (0.5, 0.3, 0.2) as the Weight for the Three Regions

Region	N_i	$\hat{\Delta}_i$	Lower $CL^{0.95}$	α_i^*	Lower $CL^{1-\alpha_i^*}$
1	283	0.005	−0.490	0.302	−0.126
2	170	0.025	−0.614	0.471	0.002
3	113	−0.056	−0.842	0.583	0.027

TABLE 11.2

Sample Size Requirements for a Multiregional Trial of Three Regions Using Conditional Simultaneous Test Formula (Equation 11.7)

Region	α_i	Sample Size	p_i	Overall Sample Size	Overall α
1	0.10	425	0.3835	1109	0.0010
2	0.10	425	0.3835		
3	0.25	259	0.2231		
1	0.10	422	0.4104	1029	0.0016
2	0.15	350	0.3401		
3	0.25	257	0.2494		
1	0.20	292	0.3333	876	0.0041
2	0.20	292	0.3333		
3	0.20	292	0.3333		
1	0.25	245	0.3333	735	0.0093
2	0.25	245	0.3333		
3	0.25	245	0.3333		

11.4 Summary

From a statistical point of view, a multiregional clinical trial has two objectives. The first is to assess the treatment effect of the test treatment over all regions. The second objective is to bridge the overall effect of the test treatment to the member regions in the trial. Due to the differences in the regulatory requirements of individual regions, study design and analysis become much more complicated for multiregional clinical trials than for clinical trials conducted in a single region, even for the assessment of overall treatment effect. If a single multiregional trial can be designed for assessing the overall treatment effect, the sample size of the multiregional trial can be increased significantly from that of a single-region trial. Furthermore, we described various strategies for hypothesis testing with two different regional endpoints. We discussed the risk and sample size requirement of each strategy. On the other hand, when the regional authorities of the multiregional trial interest in assessing regional treatment effect in a multiregional clinical trial, it impacts on the sample size requirement of a multiregional clinical trial. A reasonable approach is to reach an agreement between the sponsor and the regional authorities on the compromised type I error rate used in each of the regions. This leads to sample size recalculation based on such agreements.

References

Chen, C.-T., Hung, H. M. J., and Hsiao, C.-F. (2012). Design and evaluation of multiregional trials with heterogeneous treatment effect across regions. *Journal of Biopharmaceutical Statistics* (in press).

Chen, J., Quan, H., Binkowitz, B., Ouyang, S. P., Tanaka, Y., Li, G. et al. (2010). Assessing consistent treatment effect in a multi-regional clinical trial: A systematic review. *Pharmaceutical Statistics*, 9: 242–253.

Chen, Y.-H., and Wang, M. (2012). Assessing dose-region profile of drug efficacy: A multiregional trial strategy. *Journal of Biopharmaceutical Statistics* (in press).

Chung-Stein, C., Anderson, K., Gallo, P., and Collins, S. (2006). Sample size reestimation: A review and recommendations. *Drug Information Journal*, 40: 475–484.

Church, J. D., and Harris, B. (1970). The estimation of reliability from stress-strength relationships. *Technometrics*, 12: 49–54.

Eis, P., and Geisser, S. (1971). Estimation of the probability that Y<X. *Journal of American Statistical Association*, 66: 162–168.

European Medicines Agency. (EMA). (2009). Reflection paper on the extrapolation of results from clinical studies conducted outside the EU to the EU-population.

Girman, C. J., Ibia, E., Menjoge, S., Mak, C., Chen, J., Agarwal, A. et al. (2011). Impact of different regulatory requirements for trial endpoints in multiregional clinical trials. *Drug Information Journal* 45: 587–594.

Hsiao, C.-F., Tsong, Y., Wang, W.-J., Dong, X., and Tsou, H.-H. (2012). Designing multi-regional clinical trials with difference regional endpoints. *Journal of Biopharmaceutical Statistics* (in review).

Hung, H. M. J., and Wang, S. J. (2004). Multiple testing of noninferiority hypotheses in active controlled trials. *Journal of Biopharmaceutical Statistics* 14: 327–335.

Hung, H. M. J., Wang, S.-J., and O'Neill, R. T. (2010). Consideration of regional difference in design and analysis of multi-regional trials. *Pharmaceutical Statistics* 9: 173–178.

International Conference on Harmonisation. (ICH). (1998). Tripartite guidance E5 ethnic factors in the acceptability of foreign data. *U.S. Federal Register* 83: 31790–31796.

International Conference on Harmonisation. ICH). (2006). Technical Requirements for Registration of Pharmaceuticals for Human Use. *Q&A for the ICH E5 Guldeline on Ethnic Factors in the Acceptability of Foreign Data*. Available at: http://www.ich.org/LOB/media/MEDIA 1194.pdf.

Kawai, N., Stein, C., Komiyama, O., and Li, Y. (2008). An approach to rationalize partitioning sample size into individual regions in a multiregional trial. *Drug Information Journal*, 42: 139–147.

Ko, F. S., Tsou, H. H., Liu, J. P., and Hsiao, C. F. (2010). Sample size determination for a specific region in a multi-regional trial. *Journal of Biopharmaceutical Statistics* 20: 4, 870–885.

Lu, N., Chen, X., Nair, N., Xu, Y., Kang, C., and Li, N. (2012). Decision rules and associated sample size planning for regional approval utilizing multi-regional clinical trials. *Journal of Biopharmaceutical Statistics* (in press).

Ministry of Health, Labour and Welfare of Japan. (MHLW). (2007). Basic principles on global clinical trials, Notification No. 092810, Evaluation and Licensing Division, Pharmaceutical and Food Safety Bureau, Ministry of Health, Labor, and Welfare: Tokyo, MHLW.

Peterson, P., Carroll, K., Chuang-Stein, C., Ho, Y., Jiang, Q., Li, G. et al. (2010). *PISC* expert team white paper: Toward a consistent standard of evidence when evaluating the efficacy of an experimental treatment from a randomized, active controlled trial. *Statistics in Biopharmaceutical Research* 2: 4, 522–531.

Posch, M. and Bauer, P. (1999). Adaptive two-stage designs and the conditional error function. *Biometrical Journal*, 41: 689–696.

Proschan, M. A. (2005). Two-stage sample size re-estimation based on a nuisance parameter: A review. *Journal of Biopharmaceutical Statistics* 15: 539–574.

Proschan, M. A., and Hunsberger, S. A. (1995). Designed extension of studies based on conditional power. *Biometrics*, 51: 1315–1324.

Quan, H., Zhao, P. L., Zhang, J., Roessner, M., and Aizawa, K. (2009). Sample size considerations for Japanese patients in a multi-regional trial based on MHLW guidance. *Pharmaceutical Statistics*, 9: 100–112.

Tanaka, Y. (2008). Design and inference in multi-regional clinical trials. International Society of Biopharmaceutical Statistics Conference, Shanghai, China.

Tanaka, Y. (2009). Illustration of consistency assessment across tudies using real data. ICSA Applied Statistics Symposium, San Francisco, CA.

Tsong, Y. (2007). The utility of active-controlled noninferiority/equivalence trials in drug development. *International Journal of Pharmaceutical Medicine*, 21(3): 226–233.

Tsong, Y., Chang, W.-J., Dong, X., and Tsou, H.-H. (2012). Assessment of regional treatment effect in a multiregional clinical trial. *Journal of Biopharmaceutical Statistics* (in press).

Tsong, Y., Wang, S.-J., Hung, H.-M., and Cui, L. (2003). Statistical issues on objective, design and analysis of noninferiority active-controlled clinical trial. *Journal of Biopharmaceutical Statistics* 13: 29–41.

Tsong, Y. and Zhang, J. (2007). Simultaneous test for superiority and non-inferiority hypotheses in active controlled clinical trials. *Journal of Biopharmaceutical Statistics,* 17: 247–257.

Uesaka, H. (2009). Sample size allocation to regions in a multiregional trial. *Journal of Biopharmaceutical Statistics,* 19: 580–594.

Uyema, Y., Shibata, T., Nagai, N., Hanaoka, H., Toyoshima, S., and Mori, K. (2005). Successful bridging strategy based on ICH E5 guidance for drug approval in Japan. *Clinical Pharmacology and Therapeutics* 78: 102–113.

Wang, S.-J., Hung, H.-M. J., Tsong, Y., Cui, L., and Nuri, W. A. (2001). Group sequential test strategies for superiority and non-inferiority hypotheses in active controlled clinical trials. *Statistics in Medicine,* 20: 1903–1912.

12

Multiregional Clinical Trials for Global Simultaneous Drug Development in Japan

Kihito Takahashi
GlaxoSmithKline, Japanese Association of Pharmaceutical Medicine, and Japanese Center of Pharmaceutical Medicine

Mari Ikuta and Hiromu Nakajima
GlaxoSmithKline

12.1 Introduction

Recently, many multiregional clinical trials (MRCTs) involving Japanese subjects have been conducted, and it has become a standard approach for pharmaceutical companies in Japan to build clinical development strategy positioning MRCTs as a crucial step. At the time of this writing, 19 drugs have been approved in Japan based on MRCTs that included Japanese patients (Uyama, 2011).

The historical background and the status of MRCTs at the beginning of the 21st century in Japan have been described recently (Takahashi, 2007). In that article, many hurdles preventing pharmaceutical companies from participating in MRCTs involving Japanese trial sites were analyzed from strategic and operational points of view, and the efforts to overcome these hurdles were described. Further, two cases of drug development were reported as successful clinical development projects using MRCTs, leading to regulatory approvals as a new drug and a new indication, namely, tolterodine tartrate for overactive bladder and losartan potassium for diabetic nephropathy, respectively. Finally, expectations for more collaborative efforts between the Japanese government and the pharmaceutical industry in Japan were stated.

In this chapter, the progress and the current status of MRCTs in Japan will be reviewed, with recent updates on some details in two contrasted therapeutic areas: oncology and the cardiovascular/metabolic (CVM) fields.

12.2 Drug Lag

Japan has been the world's second largest national drug market, next to the United States, for the last several years. The Japanese public, however, has been suffering from a lag in terms of access to the newest drugs available in other parts of the world, because new drugs have often been approved and marketed in Japan several years after being available in the United States, the European Union, and even other Asian countries. This situation is called *drug lag* and has been identified as a major or critical issue in Japan.

Among factors leading to the drug lag, delays in new drug application (NDA) submissions for approval of new drugs contribute a large portion. Further, these delays in NDA submissions have been suggested to be due to setbacks in the initiation of drug development in Japan. Earlier access to new drugs without a time lag with respect to the United States or European Union has been an urgent and imperative matter for Japan.

To eliminate the drug lag, the Japanese government, academia, and pharmaceutical companies have been implementing a series of actions, as described in the following sections.

12.3 MRCTs as a Solution to Drug Lag

Until recently, companies as well as physicians tended to attribute the drug lag to the rigid and bureaucratic judgments observed in local regulatory processes of Japan. In response to criticism of the rather inflexible regulatory process, the Japanese regulatory body has made considerable efforts to minimize the lag, one of which is represented by a government action plan called the "New Five Year Plan for Clinical Trial Activation (2007–2012)" (MEXT, MHLW, and METI, 2007). Based on this plan, the Pharmaceuticals and Medical Devices Agency (PMDA) in Japan has increased the number of review officers to shorten the review term, and efforts have been made to improve efficiency in the review process.

On September 28, 2007, the PMDA released a new guideline, titled "Basic Concept for International Joint Clinical Trials," in response to the growing interest in global simultaneous drug development in Japan (MHLW, 2007). Now that the PMDA apparently encourages pharmaceutical companies to join MRCTs to bridge the relevant trial data for NDA submission in Japan, part of the remaining drug lag is attributable to the operating pharmaceutical companies themselves. Under these circumstances, local companies could choose either global simultaneous drug development or domestic stand-alone clinical trial plans, depending on their assessment of their cost–benefit comparisons. However, now that participation in MRCTs has become a crucial step for local companies to introduce the pipelines to Japan consistently with the U.S. and E.U. markets, many local companies, especially subsidiaries of foreign-based multinational pharmaceutical companies, seem to have chosen global simultaneous drug development as a part of their core development strategy.

12.4 Improvements in Clinical Trial Environment in Japan

In the mid-2000s, slow patient recruitment to clinical trials and quality assurance of the data from Japanese trial sites were major issues in Japan (Takahashi, 2007). Pharmaceutical companies in Japan have exerted significant efforts to improve their internal processes to increase productivity to meet the global timelines and to improve the data quality to meet global standards.

Significant changes in the regulatory environment originating from a series of International Conference on Harmonisation (ICH) activities have also dramatically influenced the status of clinical trials in Japan. In the late 1990s, implementation of new rules based on ICH activities was initiated and continued over several years. At that time, many clinical trial sites in Japan were not well aligned with rapid changes in the regulatory environment, and therefore the introduction of new rules was associated with significant turmoil in clinical trial activities in Japan. Particularly, the introduction of the New GCP in 1997 has resulted in significant reduction of the number of clinical trials in Japan. The number of CTNs in 1996 was 722, which decreased to 500 in 1997, and then to 406 in 1998, according to a report from the Ministry of Health, Labour and Welfare (Miyata, 2011).

Under these critical circumstances, the Japanese government has taken the lead in several initiatives to improve the infrastructure and environment for clinical development. In the New Five-Year Strategy for Clinical Trial Activation, 11 core institutions and 35 key institutions were selected to enhance clinical trials and clinical research, and this initiative has evoked the response from major hospitals that include academic sites to build the infrastructure for clinical trials at their sites.

Some improvements, apparently facilitated by the New Strategy, were observed in the infrastructure of clinical trial sites including the core and key institutions mentioned already. For example, clinical research coordinators have been placed and clinical trial centers have been formed in many academic sites, leading to better management of clinical trials at their sites.

The introduction of the New GCP, once regarded as a major inhibitory factor in Japanese drug development, has resulted in various "modernizations" in clinical trial sites and also turned out to be a significant contributor in transforming the quality of clinical trials in Japan. These improvements, coupled with increased productivities in pharmaceutical companies in

Japan, have resulted in improvement in the speed of patient enrollment and the quality of clinical trials, enabling Japan to participate in MRCTs.

12.5 Growing Trends of MRCTs in Japan

12.5.1 Trends in CTN and PMDA Clinical Trial Consultations on MRCTs

For the past five years, the Japan domestic CTN count has consistently been about 200 per fiscal year (FY). As described already, the PMDA released a guideline for MRCTs on September 28, 2007. Since then, the opportunities for participation in MRCTs have increased dramatically. The percentage of CTNs for MRCTs increased from approximately 5% of all CTNs in FY 2007 to 15.6% in FY 2008 and to 20.2% in FY 2009 and was 19.7% in FY 2010 (April to December) (Moriyama, 2011). In early FY 2007, the main target disease was cancer, but the range of target diseases has since rapidly expanded to include other diseases. Clear expansion of clinical trials to metabolic and cardiovascular diseases was achieved in late FY 2008 and early FY 2009 (Ichimaru, Toyoshiima, and Uyama, 2009).

A similar trend has been observed in the number of clinical trial consultations on MRCTs at the PMDA. In FY 2006, the percentage of consultations on MRCTs among all consultations was 13.9%, which increased to 27% in FY 2007, 32.1% in FY 2008, 29.5% in FY 2009, and 30.6% in FY 2010 (April to December) (Ichimaru et al. 2009). These data apparently support the notion that an increasing amount of drug development projects are being conducted as global simultaneous development.

12.5.2 Industry Surveys

Some pharmaceutical industry organizations in Japan, including the Japan Pharmaceutical Manufacturers Association (JPMA) and the European Federation of Pharmaceutical Industries and Associations, Japan (EFPIA, 2010), have recently conducted surveys regarding MRCTs among their member companies.

In the survey conducted by JPMA in June 2011, 65 companies participated, including 47 Japan-based companies and 15 foreign-based companies (Nishida, 2011). The total number of projects in this survey was 573, and 246 projects (42.9%) were planned as global simultaneous development. Oncology-related drug development projects accounted for 25%, and more than half of those projects were intended for global simultaneous development. In nononcology areas, global simultaneous development projects accounted for less than 50%, indicating that oncology is the most advanced therapeutic area in terms of global simultaneous drug development using

MRCTs in Japan. Of note, in both oncology and nononcology therapeutic areas, foreign-based companies used global simultaneous development strategies more often than did Japan-based companies, indicating that foreign-based multinational companies are taking advantage of MRCTs more actively than Japan-based companies. Some of the large Japan-based companies have been expanding their research and development (R&D) activities globally, and therefore the difference observed in this survey between foreign-based and Japan-based companies is expected to become much smaller in the future.

In the survey conducted by EFPIA Japan in June 2010, phase II and III clinical trials that were ongoing or completed in 2009 were analyzed (EFPIA, 2010). In 2009, MRCTs accounted for 74% (49 global studies in a total of 66 CTNs), which is significantly higher than the 29% (18/63) found in a similar survey conducted by the same group in 2007. In terms of specific therapeutic area, oncology accounted for 30.6%, followed by cardiovascular and metabolic (CVM) areas (14.3%) and respiratory areas (14.3%), indicating that MRCTs are most commonly conducted in oncology, which is consistent with the trend observed in the JPMA survey. Obviously, EFPIA Japan is composed only of multinational companies having central operations located in Europe, and therefore it is natural that this result is consistent with that observed in foreign-based companies in the JPMA survey.

In both surveys, it is apparent that MRCTs are most commonly conducted in oncology areas and are expanding in other therapeutic areas such as CVM. In the following sections, specific situations in oncology and CVM will be discussed, areas for which experience with MRCTs is most abundant in Japan.

12.6 MRCTs in the Field of Oncology

12.6.1 Necessity of MRCTs in the Field of Oncology

The necessity of MRCTs in oncology to create scientific evidence for proper use of anticancer drugs has grown. In the development of anticancer drugs, confirmatory clinical trials, which are intended to provide new evidence, need to statistically show clinical benefits of the drugs, including the improvement in overall survival (OS) and quality of life (QOL), besides tumor response. The scale of the clinical trials needs to be large in many cases to demonstrate clinical benefits statistically. Recently, molecular targeted drugs have become the mainstream of anticancer drug development (Gutierrez, Kummar, and Giaccone, 2009).

For such drugs, the mechanism of action, such as harboring specific genetic mutations, restricts the patient population anticipated to respond to the treatment. Therefore, clinical trials covering areas with larger populations are indispensable for enrolling the required numbers of patients.

As discussed in the previous sections, the drug lag has been a significant issue in Japan and has been especially serious in the area of anticancer drugs because of the life-threatening nature of the disease. To eliminate the drug lag, Japanese participation in phase III MRCTs has become a strategic approach to reduce the delay in the initiation of drug development in Japan (Hashimoto, Ueda, and Narukawa, 2009).

This strategy is supported by the Japan Oncology Guideline, which states that phase III confirmatory studies could be conducted globally for the submission of NDAs to seek approval of drugs in Japan (MHLW, 2006). The most feasible strategy to compensate for the delay has been to jump into global Phase III trials after confirming pharmacokinetics (PK) and safety in Japanese patients through reasonably streamlined Japanese phase I studies, as in other therapeutic areas.

12.6.2 PMDA Consultation on MRCTs in the Field of Anticancer Drugs

Recently, Japanese participation in global phase III trials has become common, particularly in oncology, allowing almost simultaneous submission of the approval applications in Japan and in other countries. This is evidenced by the data of PMDA consultations on MRCTs in the field of anticancer drugs.

The PMDA data show that the percentage of consultations on MRCTs relative to the total number of consultations in oncology was 4.3% in 2004, and this number increased to 5.4% in 2005, 10.9% in 2006, 28.0% in 2007, and 40.9% in 2008 and was 35.2% in 2009 (Iguchi, 2011).

The data also showed that, among clinical trial consultations on global studies on anticancer drugs, consultations on the development of molecular targeted drugs have increased. This indicates the current trend of new drug development is moving from cytotoxic drugs to molecular-targeted drugs.

12.6.3 Ethnic or Regional Differences

Ethnic or regional differences may impact on responses to drugs, including the efficacy and safety. For example, in the IRESSA Survival Evaluation in Lung cancer (ISEL) study, conducted as an MRCT, the overall data showed no significant survival prolongation in the active treatment group with gefitinib compared with the placebo group (Thatcher, Chang, Parikh, Rodrigues Pereira, Ciuleanu, von Pawel et al., 2005). However, a subgroup analysis on Asian patients showed prolonged survival of 9.5 months with gefitinib treatment compared with 5.5 months with placebo (Chang, Parikh, Thongprasert, Tan, Perng, Ganzor et al., 2006). As a reason for this difference, gefitinib was later revealed to have a high response rate among patients with EGFR mutation (Paez, Jänne, Lee, Tracy, Greulich, Gabriel et al., 2004). The prevalence of this gene mutation appeared to be 20–30% among Asian patients (including Japanese) with non-small cell lung cancer (NSCLC) and significantly higher than that among Western populations with NSCLC (Mitsudomi and Yatabe, 2007). In fact, the subsequent IRESSA Pan-Asia Study (IPASS), which was conducted in eight Asian countries including Japan, showed the superiority of gefitinib in terms of PFS as the primary endpoint (Mok et al., 2008).

Under the existence of such ethnic difference, justification should be provided as to why the entire study population, across the different study regions, can be treated as one population in MRCTs, so that the MRCT should be accepted as a meaningful MRCT including Japanese patients.

In the case of some cancers, such as liver cancer and gastric cancer, which show high incidences in Asian countries, conducting MRCTs in areas of Asia including China, Korea, and Taiwan is considered to be an effective way for developing anticancer drugs from practical, scientific, and regulatory points of view (Iwasaki, Hinotsu, and Katsura, 2010).

For this strategic scheme to be scientifically supported, it is also particularly important to adequately characterize PK and dose-response relationship in the Japanese population through Japanese phase I studies in advance.

12.6.4 Differences in Clinical Staging and Medical Environment

MRCTs need to employ clinical staging systems that are common to all countries participating in the trials. Use of any Japanese original staging system would be a hindrance to good planning of an MRCT. Also, treatment practices for malignant tumors may differ among different geographic regions or countries, and this factor needs to be taken into consideration when planning MRCTs.

In MRCTs, molecularly targeted drugs are often used in combination with chemotherapy. However, recommended doses of some chemotherapy drugs differ between Japan and Western countries, which can be an issue in the preparation of the common clinical trial protocol. Some drugs intended for use in an MRCT may not be approved in Japan, and differences in medical environment such as standard treatment and available medical devices should also be considered when planning MRCTs. In such instances, discussion with the regulatory agency is required to clarify regulatory requirements for the conduct of MRCTs in Japan.

12.6.5 New Paradigm

As discussed previously, the main stream of anti-cancer drugs has been shifting from cytotoxic chemotherapeutic drugs to the new generation of molecularly targeted drugs. This shift, coupled with the recent emergence of immunotherapeutic biologics including cancer vaccines, requires a new paradigm of drug development in the field of oncology, providing new challenges for Japan to participate in MRCTs in this field (Gutierrez et al., 2009).

For example, some of the drugs with new mechanisms of action might require longer observation period to see the efficacy, and there might be a need to choose endpoints such as progression-free survival or time to progression as opposed to objective response rate even in earlier phases than phase III confirmatory trials. Further, there is a need to identify the appropriate target population for the treatment effects and safety of molecularly targeted drugs to be improved. For those purposes, efforts have been made to establish biomarkers to be used in clinical trials, and interest in companion drug development has recently increased (Hayashi, 2011).

12.7 MRCTs in the Field of CVM

12.7.1 Necessity of MRCTs in the Field of Oncology

Recent medical practice is conducted under significant influence of the relevant clinical guidelines, which claim scientific evidence for each recommended treatment. Therefore, during the drug development, pharmaceutical companies are required to clarify the merit of the medication as well as to provide a sufficient amount of safety data.

In the CVM area, the benefit should be proven by the risk reduction of cardiovascular events, which directly affect the patients' quality and expectancy of life. Such evidence is also required by the FDA during the regulatory review process for new CVM medications. Therefore, a large-scale, multicentered, and multinational outcome trial—namely, a global clinical trial (GCT) or MRCT—should be conducted, in which thousands of subjects are recruited to obtain considerable statistical power.

12.7.2 Ethnic Factors

In Japan, we have experienced a dramatic Westernization of lifestyle during the last decade (Matsuzawa, 2006). We have also accumulated genetic research results on ethnic differences in drug sensitivity and reactions in the CVM area. Thus, the problem of ethnic differences is a matter of new discussion as a major element of drug lag, since the similarity of PK and pharmacodynamics (PD) of the investigational product is required as rationale in an MRCT. Indeed, Japanese were believed to be genetically specific and environmentally isolated in various aspects from the other ethnicities, and thus there was once an established belief that definite ethnic differences should exist in PK and PD between Japanese and Caucasians (Wood and Zhou, 1991). Historically, this belief tended to confine the common dose of approved drugs applied to Japanese patients in CVM areas frequently to almost half of the international dose in treating diabetes, dyslipidemia, and hypertension. Top approved doses were also limited, which resulted in several restrictions for academia to incorporate overseas treatment guidelines into the Japanese guidelines.

If we aim to minimize the lag and gap, it will be necessary to reassess correctly how and where ethnic difference intervenes during the drug development process.

The following is the consideration of the so-called ethnic factors often discussed by the regulatory officers during PMDA consultations. Each element for the lag has been scientifically clarified, and the accumulation of new evidence will guide us to discriminate the true and apparent ethnic differences.

12.7.3 Intrinsic Factors

It has long been believed that ethnic differences reflecting racial genetic background inevitably should be taken into account in dose determination for Japanese subjects. There are several typical examples, such as oral hypoglycemic, lipid-lowering, and hypotensive agents. These have been approved in Japan with lower common doses than those in the United States and the European Union. To note, other Asian countries, such as China and Korea, do not differentiate their dosing from the global doses, for the reason that the clinical trials are conducted as a part of a global development program, and the dosing is forced to follow the global dosing (Kim and Johnston, 2011; Malinowski, Westelinck, Sato, and Ong, 2008). A typical example of a Japan-specific drug lag has been seen in the case of metformin (Ohmura, Tanaka, Mitsuhashi, Atsum, Matsuoka, Onuma et al., 1998). It is only recently that the Japan regulatory body has approved revision of the dose of metformin following the Western countries (i.e., 1,500 mg or more per day).

The neighboring countries of China and Korea have introduced globally compatible doses without creating a lag. Previously, the Japanese government, as well as Japanese experts, was very sensitive about cohering Japanese dosing to global doses, unless sufficient similarity had been obtained in PK and PD data. Therefore, conducting Japan stand-alone clinical trials, rather than bridging strategy for dosing, was a more comfortable solution than to join global MRCTs without dose determination. Academia and the regulatory authorities shared the notion that the Japanese population is more sensitive to beta-blockers, aldosterone converting enzyme inhibitors, sulfonylureas, metformin, thiazolidinediones, statins, and so on, and the common medical practice was established based on this belief.

However, recent genetic research has revealed that ethnic genetic variation of Japanese subjects in the sensitivity to drugs is, at least in part, of little significance, and thus there would not always be such severe genetic variation in drug-tolerability and sensitivity. In addition, safety and efficacy profiles do not significantly differ in Japanese subjects compared with those in Caucasians, even with the considerably high doses, when tested in the early phase clinical trials (Seino, Nakajima, Miyahara, Kurita, Bus, Yang et al., 2009).

12.7.4 Extrinsic Factors

It is a common academic and medical notion that Japanese patients with diabetes mellitus have less insulin resistance and more severe insulin deficiency than Caucasians. These are strong intrinsic factors that define the type of diabetes mellitus in a pathophysiological sense. Indeed, this was true 20 years ago. However, dramatic Westernization of lifestyle has brought about a considerably higher incidence of obesity and metabolic syndrome in the young to middle-aged Japanese population (Matsuzawa, 2006). This phenomenon is now filling the ethnic gaps in the pathophysiology of diabetes and hence the incidence and phenotypes of CVM diseases. This interpretation has been very well validated through the investigation of generational changes of glucose tolerance among emigrants in the same Japanese ethnic group. Several reports demonstrated that even in genetically unique Japanese, emigrants to Hawaii and the U.S. mainland exhibit increasing frequency of insulin resistance and diabetes mellitus according to age, and this tendency is strengthened in the next generation (Fujimoto, Leonetti, Kinyoun, Schuman, Stolov, and Wahl, 1987). From such evidence, even genetically determined intrinsic factors can be affected and overwhelmed by the extrinsic factors postnatal.

In contrast, there can be definitive genetic variations that cannot be affected by lifestyle and environmental factors, and thus strict ethnicity would appear as a racial difference of the response to medications. As an example, the ABCG2/BCRP gene polymorphism, the most influential risk of gout and hyperuricemia, conferring an odds ratio of 5.97, presents a clear ethnic problem (Matsuo, Takada, Ichida, Nakamura, Ikebuchi et al., 2009). The disease-prone genotype is distributed in a majority of the Asian population, especially in the Japanese ethnicity. This indicates that there would be a clear ethnic difference in dosing when a drug is developed to target this gene.

12.7.5 Key Determinants for Successful MRCTs in CVM Field

In consideration of the accumulated scientific evidence and the fact that successful results have been obtained in the increasing opportunities for Japanese subjects to join MRCTs in CVM areas, the key determinants for successful global simultaneous approvals are to examine the potential similarities of PK and PD of Japanese subjects with those of Caucasians in the early steps of clinical trials. This can be achieved through phase I or proof-of-concept studies and will enable appropriate assessment of the feasibility of introducing new drugs to Japan at the optimum timing using MRCTs.

12.8 Issues in MRCTs

As described already, inclusion of Japanese patients in MRCTs has been increasing, and it is now obvious that MRCTs are becoming the standard approach in most therapeutic areas to obtain regulatory approvals Japan. This situation is considered to be due to the significant improvement in the environment surrounding clinical trials through the tremendous efforts of parties involved in drug development in Japan. On the other hand, it is well recognized that many issues remain as obstacles to be overcome for pharmaceutical companies to conduct MRCTs more seamlessly in Japan.

12.8.1 Ethnic Factors

As was discussed in the oncology and CVM sections, advanced considerations of intrinsic ethnic factors relating to racial genetic background are critical for meaningful MRCTs from scientific and regulatory points of view. Extrinsic factors such as the differences in lifestyle and medical practices between Japan and Western countries are identified as equally major issues from a strategic point of view. One important example is that regional differences in approved doses and indications of comparator and concomitant drugs will be used in the protocols, as described in the oncology and CVM sections.

Different situations among regions often exist in the way marketed drugs are used in medical practice, and these differences, often associated with specific dieting habits, are difficult to change in a short period, or even impossible to change. These differences usually require significant amendments to the protocols to enable Japanese patients to be enrolled, or in the worst scenario, it may turn out to be impossible for Japan to join an MRCT. To avoid the risk for Japan to be isolated from MRCTs, close communication involving early input from the Japanese side in the process of writing protocols is imperative.

12.8.2 Regulatory Requirements

Various regulatory requirements specific for Japan are identified as significant issues influencing a wide range of areas. These include the need of Japanese subanalysis to examine whether Japanese data is sufficiently similar or extrapolatable to the whole results, and the determination of acceptable sample sizes of Japanese patients for the regulatory approval. These issues have been discussed publicly in many regulatory science-related forums, and further experience with MRCTs seems to be necessary to reach general consensus. Close communication between regulatory agencies, especially the PMDA in Japan, and companies is critical to identify the critical regulatory issues for approvals and to reduce the gap in the timing of regulatory approvals among regions.

12.8.3 Operational Issues

In both the JPMA and EFPIA Japan surveys described previously, many operational issues were recognized regarding MRCTs in Japan, in addition to those already presented.

One example is the lack of commonality in various document forms. Efforts have been made to use common forms of documents necessary for the administrative tasks at all trial sites. Roughly half of the sites require their own forms. Another example is the delivery of trial drugs to the sites. Many hospitals in Japan require delivery by company personnel rather than direct delivery through couriers. Monitoring productivity, expressed as the number of sites monitored by one clinical research associate, is currently 3.5, and this number does not seem to have increased significantly from 3.1 in 2007 (EPFIA, 2010), and this may be due to operational issues such as the aforementioned.

12.9 Future Prospects

The goal for those involved in drug development, including pharmaceutical companies in Japan and the Japanese government, is to provide access to innovative drugs developed anywhere in the world to the Japanese population without delay. As discussed already, the global simultaneous development strategy for new drugs using MRCTs has been an effective approach to achieve this goal.

According to a report from the PMDA, the drug lag compared with the United States has indeed been reduced recently, from 3.4 years in 2007, to 2.2 in 2008, and to 2.0 in 2009 (Tominaga, 2011). Based on improvements in many aspects of clinical trials in Japan as described in this article, it is highly likely that a further reduction in the lag will be achieved in the next few years. However, a question has been raised recently in the public, asking whether the current trend to reduce drug lag is satisfactory for Japan.

Recently, new aspects of drug development in Japan have been discussed in symposiums and forums relating to drug development. Japan is one of the major countries where innovative drugs have been discovered and developed. Further, Japan has been playing an important role as an ICH member along with the United States and the European Union for the last few years, impacting on the advances in the global regulatory aspects. Current drug development in Japan is, however, mostly dependent on data generated in the United States or the European Union, and therefore it is highly likely that drug development in Japan will stay behind these regions, and

Japan could eventually be criticized from an ethical point of view that the Japanese people's medical benefits are gained at the sacrifice of people in other countries. Considering the situation described already, Japan seems to be at a turning point to consider in which direction the Japanese pharmaceutical industry should move to go forward.

Indeed, a strong desire exists in Japan that Japan should change its role from one of just participating in global MRCTs to one of playing a leading role in global drug development and that it should take the initiative to lead global development in particular for seed compounds discovered there.

Recently, discussions have been taking place regarding how best to utilize the strengths of Japanese capability and to contribute to the global development of innovative drugs. Topics include the promotion of early stage clinical trials in Japan, such as "First Time in Human" trials, proof-of-concept trials, or even dose-ranging trials investigating the lower doses particularly in oncology drug development, which will benefit from the high quality of Japanese clinical trials.

These ideas make some sense for the promotion of the Japanese pharmaceutical industry and academic activities for innovation. However, advantages and disadvantages for Japanese society, and most importantly for Japanese patients, must be considered from many points of view in making selection of any strategy, because in the end the drug development is for the patients, and our goal is to provide access to innovative drugs available in the world to Japanese patients.

Finally, a true partnership forged among the scientific and technological stakeholders, together with government agencies and experienced industry experts, seems to have boosted the rate of change in Japan and will hopefully revitalize Japan as a true global leading player in drug development for patients.

References

Basic principles on Global Clinical Trials. (2007). Available at: http://www.pmda.go.jp/english/service/pdf/notifications/0928010-e.pdf.

Chang, A., Parikh, P., Thongprasert, S., Tan, E. H., Perng, R. P., Ganzon, D. et al. (2006). Gefitinib (IRESSA) in patients of Asian origin with refractory advanced non-small cell lung cancer: subset analysis from the ISEL study. *Journal of Thoracic Oncology*, 1: 847–855.

European Federation of Pharmaceutical Industries and Associations. (EFPIA). (2010). Investigation of the current environment for conducting clinical studies in Japan (in Japanese). Available at: http://www.jmacct.med.or.jp/plan/files/p3_7-2.pdf.

Fujimoto, W., Leonetti, D., Kinyoun, J., Schuman, P., Stolov, W., and Wahl, P. (1987). Prevalence of diabetes mellitus and impaired glucose tolerance among second-generation Japanese–American men. *Diabetes*, 36: 721–729.

Gutierrez, M. E., Kummar, S., and Giaccone, G. (2009). Next generation oncology drug development: Opportunities and challenges. *Nature Reviews Clinical Oncology*, 6, 259–265 (May). Available at: http://www.nature.com/nrclinonc/journal/v6/n5/full/nrclinonc.2009.38.html.

Hashimoto, J., Ueda, E., and Narukawa, M. (2009). The current situation of oncology drug lag in Japan and strategic approaches for pharmaceutical companies. *Drug Information Journal*, 43: 757–765. Available at: http://www.diahome.org/product-files/8357/diaj_32437.pdf.

Hayashi, K. (2011). Current situation and issues on "companion diagnostic drug." OPIR Views and Actions (in Japanese), 34: 27–31. Available at: http://www.jpma.or.jp/opir/news/news-34.pdf.

Ichimaru, K., Toyoshima, S., and Uyama, Y. (2009). Effective global drug development strategy for obtaining regulatory approval in Japan in the context of ethnicity-related drug response factors. *Clinical Pharmacology Therapeutics*, 87(3): 362–366.

Iguchi, T. (2011). The current situation of global studies in Japan (in Japanese). Available at: http://atdd-frm.umin.jp/slide/10/iguchi.pdf.

Iwasaki, M., Hinotsu, S., and Katsura, J. (2010). Clinical trials and approval of anticancer agents. *Japanese Journal of Clinical Oncology*, 40(suppl. 1): i65–i69. Available at: http://jjco.oxfordjournals.org/content/40/suppl_1/i65.full.

Kim, K. and Johnston, S. (2011). Global variation in the relative burden of stroke and ischemic heart disease. *Circulation*, 124: 314–323.

Malinowski, H., Westelinck, A., Sato, J., and Ong, T. (2008). Same drug, different dosing: Differences in dosing for drugs approved in the United States, Europe, and Japan, *Journal of Clinical Pharmacology*, 48: 900–908.

Matsuo, H., Takada, T., Ichida, K., Nakamura, T., Nakayama, A., Ikebuchi, Y. et al. (2009). Common defects of ABCG2, a high-capacity urate exporter, cause gout: A function-based genetic analysis in a Japanese population. *Science Translational Medicine*, 1(5): 5ra11.

Matsuzawa, Y. (2006). The metabolic syndrome and adipocytokines. *FEBS Lett.* 580: 2917–2921.

Ministry of Health, Labour and Welfare of Japan. (2007). Basic principles on global clinical trials. September 28th. Available at: http://www.pmda.go.jp/english/service/pdf/notifications/0928010-e.pdf.

Ministry of Health, Labor, and Welfare Website (in Japanese). (2006). Available at: http://www.mhlw.go.jp/topics/bukyoku/isei/chiken/dl/kasseika_todokede.pdf.

Ministry of Education, Culture, Sports, Science, and Technolgoy (MEXT), Ministry of Health, Labour, and Welfare (MHLW), and the Ministry of Economy, Trade, and Industry (METI). (2007). The new five year strategy for creating innovative pharmaceuticals and medical devices (in Japanese). April 26. Available at: http://www.mhlw.go.jp/bunya/iryou/shinkou/dl/03.pdf.

Mitsudomi, T. and Yatabe, Y. (2007). Mutations of the epidermal growth factor receptor gene and related genes as determinants of epidermal growth factor receptor tyrosine kinase inhibitors sensitivity in lung cancer. *Cancer Science*, 98: 1817–1824.

Miyata, T. (2011). Recent trend in clinical development of drugs and clinical research. Paper presented at Regional Meeting for Clinical Trial Promotion, March 5th, Fukuoka. Available at: http://www.jmacct.med.or.jp/jma/act_mcnf2010.html.

Mok, T., Wu, Y., Thongprasert, S., Yang, C., Chu, D., Saijo, N. et al. (2008). Phase III, randomized, open-label, first-line study of gefitinib vs. carboplatin/paclitaxel in clinically selected patients with advanced non-small cell lung cancer (IPASS). Paper presented at the 33rd European Society for Medical Oncology Meeting, September, Stockholm, abstr LBA2. Available at: http://www.esmo.org/fileadmin/media/presentations/977/2061/Mok%20IPASS%20ESMO%20presentation%209%209%2008%20for%20uploading.ppt.pdf.

Moriyama, Y. (2011). Clinical trial notifications and scientific consultation system in Japan. Paper presented at the 2nd China–Japan Symposium on Drug Development Focusing on IND, Pre-Consultation, GMP and DMF system, April 12th, Beijing. Available at: http://www.pmda.go.jp/english/past/2011beijing_sympo/20110412-3.pdf.

Nishida, C. (2011). Current status in the drug development strategy, its issues and future prospects from the view point of pharmaceutical companies. Paper presented at the first annual Meeting of Society for Regulatory Science of Medical Products. Abstract in Japanese (S-1-2) available at: http://www.srsm.or.jp/pdf/gm2011pg.pdf.

Ohmura, C., Tanaka, Y., Mitsuhashi, N., Atsum, Y., Matsuoka, K., Onuma, T. et al. (1998). Efficacy of low-dose metformin in Japanese patients with type 2 diabetes mellitus. *Current Therapy Research,* 59(12): 889–895.

Paez, J. G., Janne, P. A., Lee, J. C., Tracy, S., Greulich, H., Gabriel, S. et al. (2004). EGFR mutations in lung cancer: correlation with clinic response to gefitinib therapy. *Science,* 304: 1497–1500.

Seino, Y., Nakajima, H., Miyahara, H., Kurita, T., Bus, M. A., Yang, F. et al. (2009). Safety, tolerability, pharmacokinetics and pharmacodynamics of albiglutide, a long-acting GLP-1-receptor agonist, in Japanese subjects with type 2 diabetes mellitus. *Current Medical Research Opinions,* 25: 3049–3057.

Takahashi, K. (2007). Drug development in Japan. *International Journal of Pharmaceutical Medicine,* 21(5): 331–338.

Thatcher, N., Chang, A., Parikh, P., Rodrigues Pereira, S., Ciuleanu, T., von Pawel, J. et al. (2005). Gefitinib plus best supportive care in previously treated patients with refractory advanced non-small-cell lung cancer: Results from a randomised, placebo-controlled, multi-centre study (IRESSA Survival Evaluation in Lung Cancer). *Lancet,* 366: 1527–1537.

Wood, A. J. and Zhou, H. H. (1991). Ethnic differences in drug disposition and responsiveness. *Clinical Pharmacokinetics,* 20(5): 350–373.

The 1st Annual Meeting of Regulatory Science of Medical Product. http://www.srsm.or.jp/gm001_pg.html.

The 11th Kitasato-Harvard symposium. http://www.pharm.kitasato-u.ac.jp/biostatis/khsympo201109/eng/index-2.html.

The 8th DIA Japan Annual. http://www.diahome.org/DIAHome/Education/FindEducationalOffering.aspx?productID=25848&eventType=Meeting&utm_source=DIAHomePageGlobal&utm_medium=Button&utm_campaign=11303.

The 2011 APEC Multi-Regional Clinical Trials TOKYO Workshop. http://www.pmda.go.jp/english/past/2011apec_workshop_e.html.

Tominaga, T. (2011). PMDA's effort for Japan–China cooperative relationship. Paper presented at the 2nd China–Japan Symposium on Drug Development Focusing on IND, Pre-Consultation, GMP and DMF System, April 12, Beijing. Available at: http://www.pmda.go.jp/english/past/2011beijing_sympo/20110412-2.pdf.

Uyama, Y. (2011). East Asian contributions to global drug developments for providing a better drug to patients. Paper presented at the 2011 APEC Multi-Regional Clinical Trials TOKYO Workshop, November 1st, Tokyo. Available at: http://www.pmda.go.jp/english/past/2011apec workshop e.html.

13

Feasibility and Implementation of Bridging Studies in Taiwan[*]

Mey Wang, Yeong-Liang Lin, and Herng-Der Chern
Center for Drug Evaluation

13.1 Overview

In the recent years, with the decoding of human genome and the advance of pharmacogenomics, issues on ethnic and population differences have become the focus in the new drug approval process, especially in Asia. Since most of the new medicines were developed in Western countries, the efficacy and safety were generally established based on Caucasian majority. It would be a major concern in the drug regulation process whether the foreign clinical data could be naively extrapolated to the population of Asian region. In 1998, a consensus had been reached as summarized in the ICH E5. The guidelines addressed both the intrinsic and extrinsic factors that are associated with characteristics, culture, and environment of a drug. They also provided a framework for investigating the impact of ethnic factors upon the medicines' effect. The principal objective of E5 is to expedite the global development and availability of new medicines to patients without sacrificing the quality, safety, and efficacy.

In general, Taiwan accepts all Asian data. A study by Lin et al. (2001) determined that the Taiwanese, accounting for 91% of the total population in Taiwan, comprised Minnan and Hakka people who are closely related to the southern Han and are clustered with other southern Asian populations, such as Thai and Malaysian in terms of HLA typing. Those who are the descendants of northern Han are separated from the southern Asian cluster and form a cluster with the other northern Asian populations, such as Korean and Japanese. The Taiwanese regulatory authority therefore accepts data from trials conducted in Taiwan as well as in other Asian countries, if those trials meet Taiwanese regulatory standards and were conducted in compliance with good clinical practice (GCP) requirements.

[*] We thank Dr. Chi-Shin Chen for his invaluable advice on the preparation of this manuscript.

From Taiwan's regulatory point of view, ethnic factor should not be defined completely by citizenship or race. In the evaluation of ethnic differences, drug characteristics and target population should be the two major elements to be considered. For example, some medicines are metabolized by the enzymes with genetic polymorphism. If there are higher percentages of poor metabolizers in the Taiwanese patient population for a particular drug, the different assessment models in the risk–benefit ratio and risk management may become necessary. Usually, hepato-toxicity and tuberculosis (TB) are two major safety concerns in the bridging assessment in Taiwan. Owing to the high incidence rate of TB (62.0 per 100,000, 2008) and high prevalence rate of HBsAg carriers (18%–20%) in Taiwan, the need for additional information with the usage of agents in reactivating TB and inducing liver toxicity may lead to the necessity of an additional bridging study (BS). Difference in the disease epidemiology and disease manifestation is another important issue. As in the case of Steven-Johnson syndrome (SJS) induced by carbamazapine, the incidence was higher in Taiwanese compared with Caucasians. It was found that the risk of SJS after administering carbamazapine was associated with the presence of HLA-B*1502 (Chung et al., 2004), and the prevalence of HLA-B*1502 carrier in Taiwan (8.6%) was much higher than that in the United States (0%), Japan (0.2%), and Korea (0.4%) (Lim, Kwan, and Tan, 2008). Therefore, Taiwan regulatory authority required adding a warning in carbamazapine labeling and advised HLA-B*1502 screening in an official announcement in 2007 after the diagnostic kit for detection of HLA-B*1502 was available. Another example is the case with female postmenopausal syndrome. Caucasian women usually present more vasomotor symptoms in contrast to the Taiwanese women, in whom the vasomotor symptoms are not predominant. Therefore, new agents whose efficacy was demonstrated by improved Kupperman Index score (which put more weight on the vasomotor-symptom domain) may not be accepted completely. Further investigations on Taiwanese postmenopausal women, using an index scale more suitable for this population (i.e., Greene Climateric Scale), may be needed. Furthermore, medical practice among the regions usually reflects one of the greatest variations and is the most difficult to harmonize. The GCP compliance, differences in diagnostic criteria for some diseases, potential of drug abuse, and possible drug–drug interactions are all essential considerations in the evaluation for BS.

13.2 Regulatory History of Bridging Strategy

Taiwan implements the bridging strategy in a stepwise manner. In 1993, the Department of Health (DOH) of Taiwan issued an announcement (the

Double-Seven Announcement) for the requirement of including data from local (Taiwan) clinical trials in the NDA dossier for every new medicine seeking marketing approval in Taiwan. The clinical trial should provide data on at least 40 evaluable study subjects and preferably should be randomized, double-blinded, and controlled. Subsequently, the DOH issued guidelines on GCP in 1996 and initiated on-site clinical trial GCP inspection in 1999. The standard and quality of local clinical trials improved significantly over time.

Considering the requirement of tremendous financial and human resources in carrying out clinical trials, special or unmet medical needs, practical difficulty with trials in certain diseases, and the desire to minimize duplication of similar or unnecessary trials, the DOH issued five successive announcements of clinical trial waiver between 1998 and 2000. Local clinical trials of drugs in the following nine categories may be waived with no requirement to verify ethnic insensitivity. These include (1) drugs for treatment of AIDS, (2) drugs for organ transplantation, (3) topical agents, (4) nutrition supplements, (5) cathartics used prior to surgery, (6) radio-labeled diagnostic pharmaceuticals, (7) the only choice of treatment for a given serious disease, (8) drugs with demonstrated breakthrough efficacy for life-threatening disease, and (9) drugs for the treatment of rare diseases, where it is difficult to enroll enough subjects for the trial. However, for drugs in other categories including (1) anticancer drugs, (2) vaccines, (3) drugs for psychiatric disorders or chronic diseases (e.g., rheumatoid arthritis, SLE), for which there is difficulty to conduct local trial, (4) drugs of single use, (5) fixed-dose combination, (6) drugs of the same compound but different salt and the same route of administration as the approved products, and (7) drugs with the same mechanism and similar pharmacological profiles as the approved products, the trials may also be waived if the sponsor can provide adequate and proper evidence that the compound is not sensitive to ethnic factors.

On December 12, 2000, the DOH issued an announcement (the Double-Twelve Announcement) for the requirement of including the BS report or the protocol in NDA dossier and recommended that the sponsors, before submitting the complete clinical data package (CCDP) to the DOH, apply for a bridging study evaluation (BSE) to assess the necessity for carrying out a BS in Taiwan. The DOH, with help of its Center for Drug Evaluation (CDE), also developed and published a sponsor self-evaluation checklist for BSE to help the sponsors organize pertinent documents for this review. During the transitional period between January 2001 and December 2003, a sponsor could choose to follow the Double-Seven Announcement and perform a clinical trial or follow the Double-Twelve Announcement and carry out a BSE, then perform a meaningful, well-designed BS, if required. By January 1, 2004, BSE was thoroughly implemented.

13.3 Assessment Experiences Based on ICH E5

In Taiwan, assessment of ethnic sensitivity proceeds entirely according to the principles described in the ICH E5 document. After the CDE receives an application, the whole clinical data package, including foreign clinical efficacy and safety data to be extrapolated to the Taiwan region, is assessed. The application is examined to see whether it meets Taiwan's regulatory requirements. If it does, regulators seek answers to key questions regarding the product's pharmarcokinetic/pharmacodynamic (PK/PD) and clinical properties to determine whether the product is ethnically sensitive or ethnically acceptable. According to concepts in the ICH E5 guideline, there are two steps in the assessment of foreign data for extrapolation. The first step is to assess the product's sensitivity to ethnic factors by obtaining knowledge of the PK/PD characteristics that have the potential to be influenced by ethnic factors. If there are concerns that the product may be sensitive to ethnic factors based on these PK/PD properties and other related questions, such as its use in a setting of multiple comedications and the possible inappropriate use of this product in the new region, then a second assessment step follows. This step consists of conducting bridging trials focusing on the concerns raised. Data generated from these trials are then compared with those derived from foreign trials.

Eight PK/PD properties are selected as major intrinsic factors for the assessment, and two clinical properties are used to assess sensitivity to extrinsic factors (Table 13.1). To reflect the special concerns in Taiwan, Lin, Chern, and Chu (2003) suggested adding five more properties to the checklist to evaluate the acceptability of the extrapolation of foreign clinical data for registration purpose more thoroughly: (1) whether notable hepatobiliary side effects exist, (2) whether clinically alarming drug resistance exists in the new region, (3) likelihood of higher incidence of an adverse event due to a different standard of care, (4) likelihood of poor tolerability because of major side effects, and (5) administration by titration or fixed dose.

Although the checklist displayed in Table 13.1 is helpful, it has a drawback of the lack of a clear-cut criterion for decision making. Being aware of this insufficiency, Wang, Ou, Chern, and Lin (2003) conducted a simulation study to address several pharmacological factors that, in conjunction with the checklist, should be useful in determining the necessity of BS for a potential ethnic-sensitive compound. The simulation results suggested that when the therapeutic index (C_{max}/C_{min} ,where C_{min} is the minimal effective concentration and C_{max} is the maximal effective concentration without adverse effect) of a new drug is sufficiently wide, such as four to eight, no BS is required in a new region if interethnic variation (μ_2/μ_1) and intraethnic variation (σ/μ) are within a reasonable limit, i.e., $\mu_2/\mu_1 < 2.5$, $\sigma/\mu < 0.8$, respectively. Fixing the interethnic variation, the clinical impact of narrow therapeutic index becomes less significant with the increment of intraethnic variation. On the

TABLE 13.1

PK/PD Properties and Clinical Properties for Assessing Ethnic Sensitivity

PK/PD Properties
1. Linearity of PK properties
2. Steep or flat concentration-effect curve for efficacy and safety
3. Narrow or wide therapeutic dose range
4. Whether the product is metabolized through one major pathway
5. Whether the product is metabolized by enzyme demonstrating genetic polymorphism
6. Whether the product is administered as a prodrug with potential for variable enzymatic conversion
7. High or low bioavailability
8. High or low intersubject variation in bioavailability
Clinical Properties
1. Likelihood of use in a setting of multiple comedications
2. Likelihood of off-level use

other hand, at a given value of intraethnic variation, the significance of therapeutic index becomes more substantial when interethnic variation increases.

From 2001 to 2007, a total of 320 applications of BSE was received and evaluated by the DOH. Among the 280 applications with completed assessment, the percentage of clinical trial waiving was 59.3%. Inadequate or insufficient data on pharmacokinetics (42%), efficacy (31%), and safety (29%) were the most common reasons for which the local clinical trials in Taiwan could not be waived. A total of 81% of the cases that failed to obtain a waiver of a BS were new chemical entities, especially drugs with new mechanisms but with little Asian data available. Follow-up analyses indicated that for those cases in which a BS in Taiwan was required, approximately 20% conducted a local trial as requested, and, in approximately 24% of the cases, the sponsor chose to resubmit a more detailed BS package for reevaluation instead of conducting a trial. Among these cases, more than half failed again to obtain the waiver. For those failure cases, 44% had no follow-up actions.

The following two cases are good examples that well document the key considerations in determining the labeling dose of a new drug through a bridging evaluation in Taiwan.

13.3.1 Case 1

Drug X, by suppression of gastric acid secretion, is one of the commonly used proton pump inhibitors for treatment of gastroesophageal reflux disease. This drug has a low oral bioavailability of 30–40% and demonstrates nonlinear pharmacokinetic behavior with doses greater than 40 mg. The oral bioavailability appears to be age-dependent and increases upon repeated administration and in disease states such as chronic hepatic disease. It is highly bound to plasma protein (95–96%) and is extensively metabolized in the liver primarily by the cytochrome P450 isoform CYP2C19, an enzyme well known for its genetic polymorphism. The proportion of CYP2C19 poor metabolizer is 15–20% in Asians compared with 2–5% in Caucasians. Since the AUC of the poor metabolizers may be 10 times higher than that of the extensive metabolizers at the same dosage, it is not surprising to observe an AUC in Asians two to four times higher than that in Caucasians.

Although the aforementioned pharmacokinetic characteristics strongly suggest this drug as an ethnically sensitive compound, this pharmacokinetics-related ethnic sensitivity may be buffered by a rather flat pharmacodynamic curve from antisecretory studies. After administration with 20 and 40 mg, the peak acid output two to six hours postdose decreases by 79% and 88%, respectively. In other studies, the decreases in 24-hour intragastric acidity were comparable for the 20 mg dose (80–97%) and 40 mg dose (92–94%).

The pharmacodynamic findings were further sustained by the clinical outcomes. In trials of gastric ulcer disease, eight-week healing rates were 74.8% and 82.7% for 20 and 40 mg doses, and they were 74% and 75% in an erosive esophagitis study, respectively. For such cases, the dose-response curves were rather flat, and patients may not benefit from the increment of the dosage. These observations indicate that the ethnic difference in PK or PD parameters is not so clinically relevant as that in clinical outcome.

For a promising new compound with PK and PD profiles similar to this drug, a dose-ranging bridging study may be requested in the Asian region if only PK and PD results are concerned. However, an argument may arise when clinical therapeutic effects are taken into account with PK and PD. More information is needed before making a more appropriate decision.

13.3.2 Case 2

Drug Y is a small molecule to increase platelet production through activation of the thrombopoietin receptor. The drug is indicated for the treatment of chronic idiopathic thrombocytopenic purpura (ITP). Different PK profiles were observed in the phase I studies in different patient population. The plasma AUC in Asian (Japanese, Chinese, Taiwanese, and Korean) ITP patients was more than 80% higher than that of Caucasian patients. The absolute PD response was also higher in Asians. Therefore, different dosing regimens were used in phase II/III studies.

In the Caucasian phase II study, patients were randomized to placebo and three doses of Drug Y (20 mg, 40 mg, or 60 mg QD). The results showed the responder (defined as platelet count ≧ 50,000/μL) rates at day 43 were 25%, 68%, and 82% for 20 mg, 40 mg, and 60 mg QD, respectively. The two higher doses were significantly superior to placebo (both $p < 0.001$). In the phase III study, Caucasian subjects were randomized to a placebo and flexible dose (40–60 mg QD). The responder rate at day 43 were 62% for Drug Y and 15%

for placebo, and the difference was also statistically significant ($p < 0.001$). The recommended dose for Caucasians is thus 40 mg–60 mg QD.

Considering the greater PK/PD response, the active treatment in the Asian phase II/III placebo-controlled study was a lower flexible dose of 10–40 mg QD. The responder rates of this study were 55% for Drug Y and 5% for placebo, and the difference was highly significant ($p < 0.001$). Based on the results, the approved dosage in Taiwan was 20–40 mg QD.

13.4 Bayesian Statistical Approach to Bridging Studies

13.4.1 Evaluating Regional Treatment Effect in a Multiregional Trial

In the ICH E5 guideline, a *bridging study* is defined as a supplemental study performed in a new region to provide pharmacodynamic or clinical data on efficacy, safety, dosage, and dose regimen that allow extrapolation of foreign clinical data to new region. The goal of such bridging, naturally facilitated by a multiregional trial, is to make valuable drugs available to patients globally without a time lag (11th Q&A of ICH E5 guideline).

For a multiregional trial, although the overall average of regional drug effect may reflect the global performance of the medication, it may not always serve as a meaningful proxy for the drug effect in a local region. This is especially the case when the interregional variability is substantial or when the sample size in the region considered is small relative to the overall sample size in the trial. Considering the statistical problem regarding how to bridge data among different regions in a multiregional trial to get a refined analysis of treatment effect for a local region, Chen, Wu, and Wang (2009) proposed a Bayesian approach to combine local and global evidence when evaluating treatment effect in a given region. Chen et al. (2009) assume that the true treatment effect θ across global regions follows a normal distribution $N(\mu, \omega^2)$, where μ and ω^2 represent, respectively, the overall (global) mean treatment effect and the interregional variance of the treatment effect. In the terminology of Bayesian statistics, the $N(\mu, \omega^2)$ distribution corresponds to the "prior" distribution for the local treatment effect θ. Applying standard results in a Bayesian statistical analysis using $N(\mu, \omega^2)$ as the "prior distribution," the posterior distribution for the local treatment effect θ, conditional on the treatment effect $\bar{x}$ observed in this region, is explicitly given by

$$N\left(\frac{\omega^2\bar{x} + \sigma^2\mu}{\omega^2 + \sigma^2}, \frac{\omega^2\sigma^2}{\omega^2 + \sigma^2}\right) \tag{13.1}$$

To avoid inconsistency between local and global inference, Equation 13.1 was refined by using an alternative "prior variance" $\tilde{\omega}^2$ instead of the crude inter-regional variance ω^2, and consider

$$\tilde{\omega}^2 = \frac{t\sigma^2\omega^2}{\mu^2} + \frac{\sigma^2\lambda^2}{\sigma^2 - \lambda^2} \tag{13.2}$$

where λ^2 and σ^2 represent, respectively, the overall (global) and local variance, the "offset" $b \equiv \sigma^2\lambda^2 / (\sigma^2 - \lambda^2)$ protects the resulting posterior variance $\tilde{\omega}^2\sigma^2 / (\tilde{\omega}^2 + \sigma^2)$ from going to 0 under the homogeneous setting ($\omega^2 \approx 0$), and the "slope" $a \equiv \sigma^2 / \mu^2 > 0$ keeps the alternative prior variance $\tilde{\omega}^2$ being proportionally varied with the crude interregional variation ω^2 so that the automatic bridging property in Equation 13.1 can still be preserved; that is, smaller interregional variation permits a larger degree of bridging of information. Parameter t is introduced as a multiplication factor for the interregional variance ω^2 that determines the degree of bridging global information to local drug evaluation. An appropriate value (or range of values) for the parameter t can be determined a priori according to past experiences, prior knowledge, features of hypothesis to be tested, and consensus between sponsor and local regulatory. The power curves in Figure 13.1 reveal that t at a range of 0.5 to 1.0 can fulfill a moderate, but not extreme, level of internal bridging in a multiregional trial such that substantial power gains are ensured for a region not too small (e.g., with a sample size allocation proportion $\geq 15\%$).

Assuming negative value of θ represents effectiveness of the treatment, we assess the efficacy of the treatment in a given region by computing the posterior probability

$$P(\theta > 0 \mid \bar{x}) = \Phi\left(\frac{\tilde{\omega}^2\bar{x} + \sigma^2\mu}{v(\tilde{\omega}^2 + \sigma^2)}\right) \tag{13.3}$$

where $v^2 = \tilde{\omega}^2\sigma^2/(\tilde{\omega}^2 + \sigma^2)$ with $\tilde{\omega}^2$ given in Equation 13.2, and Φ is the standard normal distribution function; a small value (e.g., 2.5%) of this probability would suggest effectiveness of the treatment in the local region under study.

The approach proposed by Chen, Wu, and Wang (2009) has the following distinct features: (1) it performs internal bridging in a multiregional trial, with the degree of bridging automatically determined by the interregional variability of the treatment effect across different region; (2) it usually ensures the consistency between the conclusions from local and global inference when the treatment effect is virtually homogeneous across regions and is found nonsignificant globally; and (3) it generally protects against overbridging of the global information of evaluating the treatment effect in a

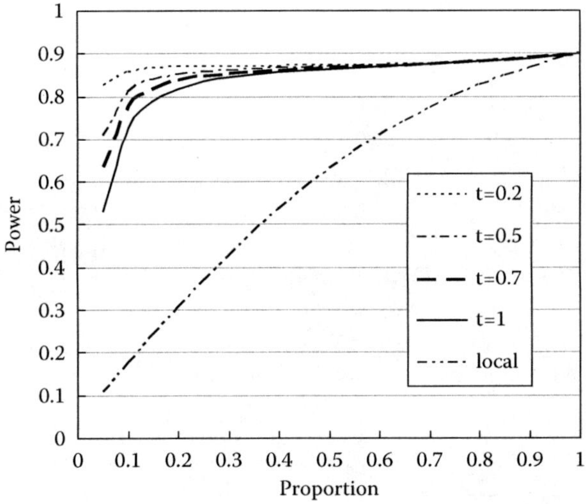

FIGURE 13.1
Power curves based on Equation 13.4 under various values of t when $\theta_1 = \mu$. The x-axis represents the proportion of the full sample size allocated to the region under consideration.

very small region. As well, this approach can be readily extended to binary and survival time response by using respectively the sample log odds-ratio and the sample log hazard-ratio as the treatment effect estimate.

13.4.2 Regional Power and Sample Size Allocation in a Multiregional Trial

Let N be the total (per group) sample size in the multiregional trial, and p the proportion of the sample size allocated to a specific region; hence the (per group) sample size for this region is Np. Chen et al. (2009) further derived the regional power (probability that $P(\theta < 0 \mid \bar{x}) > 97.5\%$), which is given as

$$\Phi\left(\frac{-1.96\, C^{1/2}\kappa - F}{W^{1/2}}\right) \tag{13.4}$$

where $\kappa = \sigma/\omega$, $C = A_1 + A_2$, $\sigma^2 = \tau^2/(Np)$ with τ^2 denoting the variance of the response difference between the treatment and the control groups (assuming constant across regions), $F = A_1 r_1 + A_2 r_2$, $W = A_1^2\kappa^2 + A_2^2\kappa^2 p/(1-p)$, $A_1 = 1 + r^2p(1-p)/[r^2p + tL(1-p)]$, $A_2 = r^2(1-p)^2/[r^2p + tL(1-p)]$, $L = p\kappa^2 + p(1-p)(r_1 - r_2)^2$, $r_i = \theta_i/\omega$, $i = 1,2$; here θ_1 is the presumed treatment effect for region 1 and $\theta_2 = (\mu - p\theta_1)/(1-p)$.

Suppose that the total sample size N for each group (treatment/control) of the multiregional trial is determined by the usual sample size formula

$$\sqrt{\frac{N}{\tau^2}}\mu = -K \tag{13.5}$$

where $K = Z_{1-\alpha/2} + Z_{1-\beta}$ and $1-\beta$ is the desired power. Then by substituting τ^2/N with μ^2/K^2 in Equation 13.4, at the study-planning stage one can determine the required sample size allocation proportion p for a region to ensure a desired power (e.g., 80%) for showing the treatment effect in this region. The power curves obtained by Equation 13.4 and Equation 13.5 are depicted in Figure 13.1, where $\theta_1 \equiv \mu$. Also shown in this figure is the power for showing the treatment effect in the local region with traditional subgroup analysis based only on the local data (without bridging).

13.5 Designing an External (Supplemental) Bridging Study

The acceptance of foreign clinical data will depend completely on its ability to extrapolate to Taiwanese population. When this is in doubt, supplemental bridging data may be requested by the regulatory authority. In general, a bridging study could be widely applicable to trials of any phase, including pharmacokinetic and pharmacodynamic studies and phase III controlled clinical trials. However, a phase III controlled clinical trial is preferred because it is the most favorable study when there are uncertainties about dose, when there is limited experience with the drug class, or when there are safety concerns. Ideally, a bridging phase III trial should have a study design identical to the foreign pivotal study. However, a full phase III clinical trial may not be practical considering the small individual market in the local region. To remedy this and to accelerate the approval of a good medicine to be marketed in Taiwan, several compromising strategies are proposed. For example, we may allow the widely accepted surrogate endpoints to serve as primary efficacy endpoints, that is, bone density in place of bone fracture in osteoporosis trials and objective tumor response rate in place of patient survival in cancer trials. Under some circumstances, the study period may be shortened if clinically justifiable. Though a sample size computed to powerfully address similar efficacy and safety to those of pivotal studies is scientifically sounder, the calculated sample size is often too large to be practical. Alternatively, a positive drug effect in Asian population (d_N) is thought to be sufficient in sample size justification given that the effect of the original pivotal studies (d_O) has been shown positive, and d_N is within an acceptable range of d_O.

When efficacy data are already available from the approval package in foreign countries, Lan, Soo, Siu, and Wang (2005) introduced weighted Z-tests and applied them to the design of bridging studies. The weighted Z-test, with constant weight $0 \leq w \leq 1$ determined by prior knowledge and clinical judgment regarding the impact of extrinsic and intrinsic factors on the inter-regional variability, is expressed as

$$Z_w = \sqrt{w}Z_{Foreigh} + \sqrt{1-w}Z_{Bridging} \quad (13.6)$$

For $Z_w > Z\alpha$, conditional on the observed value of the foreign study, $Z_{Foreign}$, the significance level of bridging study in the new region is determined by

$$\alpha_{Bridging} = 1 - \Phi((z_\alpha - \sqrt{w}z_{Foreign})/\sqrt{1-w}) \quad (13.7)$$

Thus, by incorporating prior information from the foreign study, the bridging study may be conducted with a smaller sample size and tested at a higher significance level compared with those required by a full-scale study. However, the bridging α-level should be acceptable to the local regulatory agency that, for example, may require a maximum α-level of 0.1.

13.6 Concluding Remarks

Concepts and procedures described in the ICH E5 guideline have proved feasible in the assessment of the ethnic sensitivity of a product that is to be introduced to a region for registration purposes. The PK/PD and clinical properties mentioned in the guideline are good screening tools to assess ethnic sensitivity. However, considering the insufficiency of the existing clinical properties, also reflecting special safety concerns in Taiwan, we suggest adding five more clinical properties to improve the assessment's efficacy.

The clinical relevance of ethnic factors depends on the pharmacological characteristics and clinical indication of a drug. The simulation study by Wang et al. (2003) verifies several heuristic thinking arising from a series of bridging study evaluation. First, the ethnic difference in clinical outcome is more decisive than that in PK and PD parameters. Second, the clinical impact of ethnic difference is more significant if the extent of interethnic variation increases, the extent of intraethnic variation decreases, the therapeutic index of the drug becomes narrower, and the slope of dose–response curve is steeper.

A multiregional trial serves as an important step toward global simultaneous drug development. A fundamental concept inspired by this goal is to bridge regional and global clinical data for evaluating regional treatment effect in a multiregional trial. A novel Bayesian statistical approach has been proposed for explicitly and naturally implementing such an "internal bridging" concept, where the degree of "bridging" is automatically determined by the interregional variation of the treatment effect. With a sensible proposal for the prior variance of the treatment effect, the approach is expected to ensure consistency of the local and global inference when the treatment effect is virtually homogeneous across regions and is globally nonsignificant and to protect against the over modification of the local inference by the global information when the sample size of the local study is too small. Simple formulas for predicting the regional power were also developed. To have a reasonable power of showing an effect in a local region, a sufficient number of subjects should be recruited in a multiregional study, as suggested in the ICH E5 guideline. We suggest the multiregional trial be designed to have the total sample size sufficient to achieve a 90% power (under a 5% significance level) with a traditional test for the overall treatment effect. The power analysis shows that the total sample size so determined can guarantee reasonable power (e.g., > 80%) of showing an effect in the local region comprising at least 20% of the total sample, when the effect in this region is in fact as good as the global effect. The proposed method focuses on the inference of the treatment effect in a given region. When the goal is the simultaneous inference on treatment effect for some or all of the regions in a multiregional trial, to compensate the reduction in overall power of the trial one may have to increase the sample size of the trial or allow a larger degree of bridging information.

The weighted Z-test is a practical way to design a local supplemental bridging study. The amount of bridging information required corresponding to the sample size of local bridging trial depends on the established evidence from foreign trial, the given weight, w, as well as the degree of certainty on the variability of treatment effects among regions. Since the constant weight, w, determines the degree of increased type I error, the choice of this value should reflect a consensus with the local regulatory agency on the expected amount of variability in treatment effects among regions concerned.

The requirement of a bridging study evaluation has ushered in a new paradigm for regulatory approval in Taiwan. Previous administrative regulation, such as the requirement to carry out a small-scale local registration trial for all new drugs and free-sale certification, was gradually phased out. With the implementation of ICH E5, accompanied by the establishment of sound IND consultation processes and practice of good regulatory sciences, Taiwan has become a preferred site to participate in the global research and development.

References

Chen, Y. H., Wu, Y. H., and Wang, M. (2009). A Bayesian approach to evaluating regional treatment effect in a multiregional trial. *Journal of Biopharmaceutical Statistics*, 19: 900–915.

Chung W. H., Hung S. I., Hong, H. S. et al. (2004). A marker for Stevens-Johnson syndrome. *Nature,* 428.

International Conference on Harmonisation. (ICH). (1998).*Tripartite guidance E5 ethnic factors in the acceptability of foreign data.* Available at: http://www.ich.org/LOB/media/MEDIA481.pdf.

International Conference on Harmonisation. (ICH). (2006). *Q&A for the ICH Guideline E5 on ethnic factors in the acceptability of foreign clinical data.* Available at: http://www.ich.org/LOB/media/MEDIA1194.pdf.

Lan, K. K., Soo, Y., Siu, C., and Wang, M. (2005). The use of weighted Z-tests in medical research. *Journal of Biopharmaceutical Statistics,* 15(4): 625–639.

Lim, K. S., Kwan, P., and Tan, C. T. (2008). Association of HLA-B*1502 allele and carbamazepine-induced severe adverse cutaneous drug reaction among Asians, a review. *Neurology Asia,* 13: 15–21.

Lin, M., Chu, C. C., Chang, S. L., Lee, H. L., Loo, J. H., Akaza, T. et al. (2001). The origin of Minnan and Hakka, the so-called "Taiwanese", inferred by HLA study. *Tissue Antigen,* 57: 192–199.

Lin, Y. L., Chern, H. D., and Chu, M. L. (2003). Taiwan's experience with the assessment of the acceptability of the extrapolation of foreign clinical data for registration purposes. *Drug Information Journal,* 37: 143–145.

Wang, M., Ou, S. T., Chern, H. D., and Lin, M. S. (2003). A clinical relevance of ethnic factors: A simulation study. *Drug Information Journal,* 37(4): 117s–122s.

Index

G

H

I

S

T

Z